Perioperative Pain Management for General and Plastic Surgery

PERIOPERATIVE PAIN MANAGEMENT FOR GENERAL AND PLASTIC SURGERY

Edited by

Deepak Narayan, MD
Professor of Surgery, Yale University School of Medicine, New Haven, CT

Alan D. Kaye, MD, PhD
Professor, Program Director, and Chairman, Department of Anesthesiology,
Louisiana State University Health Sciences Center, Hospital Anesthesia
Director, Louisiana State University Medical Center, New Orleans, LA

and

Nalini Vadivelu, MD
Professor, Department of Anesthesiology, Yale University School of
Medicine, New Haven, CT

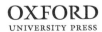

OXFORD
UNIVERSITY PRESS

Oxford University Press is a department of the University of Oxford. It furthers
the University's objective of excellence in research, scholarship, and education
by publishing worldwide. Oxford is a registered trade mark of Oxford University
Press in the UK and certain other countries.

Published in the United States of America by Oxford University Press
198 Madison Avenue, New York, NY 10016, United States of America.

© Oxford University Press 2019

Library of Congress Cataloging-in-Publication Data
Names: Narayan, Deepak, editor. | Kaye, Alan David, editor. | Vadivelu, Nalini, editor.
Title: Perioperative pain management for general and plastic surgery /
edited by Deepak Narayan, Alan D. Kaye, Nalini Vadivelu.
Description: New York, NY : Oxford University Press, [2019]
Identifiers: LCCN 2018025979 | ISBN 9780190457006 (paperback : alk. paper) |
ISBN 9780190464745
Subjects: | MESH: Pain Management—methods | Perioperative Care |
Surgical Procedures, Operative | Reconstructive Surgical Procedures
Classification: LCC RD49 | NLM WL 704.6 | DDC 617.9/192—dc23
LC record available at https://lccn.loc.gov/2018025979

9 8 7 6 5 4 3 2 1
Printed by WebCom, Inc., Canada

Contents

Preface

Our intention for writing this concise, up-to-date, evidence-based handbook, organized by anatomic location, is to equip general surgeons and plastic surgeons with the necessary knowledge to effectively and safely manage patients with pain. All surgical specialties are faced with the challenge of treating pain. The surgical and allied specialties include neurosurgeons, neuropathologists, orofacial surgeons, ear, nose, and throat surgeons, cardiothoracic surgeons, pulmonologists, radiologists, interventional radiologists, gastroenterologists, urologists, nephrologists, colorectal surgeons, obstetrics and gynecologic surgeons, vascular surgeons, plastic surgeons, orthopedic surgeons, and podiatrists, among others.

Almost all physicians are involved in the management of pain at some level. Of the various specialties and health care professions, surgeons and plastic surgeons are at the frontline delivering perioperative pain care. Perioperative pain control presents a serious challenge for the practicing surgeons and plastic surgeons who need to be able to diagnose pain and be cognizant of both common and rare painful conditions that present perioperatively so that they can manage them effectively. It is vital then for these surgeons of these many specialties to accomplish the following:

1. Understand the basics of pain management of commonly encountered conditions.
2. Have an awareness of current standards of care guidelines in pain medicine.
3. Grasp the tenets of comprehensive perioperative pain management necessary for overall patient safety.
4. Be cognizant of the latest evolving techniques and appropriate utilization of modern equipment and technology to provide care safely to these patients.

At the time of publication of this book, there was no book on the market that met the need for a comprehensive reference on pain management for general surgeons and plastic surgeons. Plastic surgeons and general surgeons often own and operate their own surgical centers and ideally need a short, accessible book with a concentrated focus on pain education that fits their specific needs. We have included practical drawings, diagrams, and illustrations to achieve this goal. Although some material may overlap among the different chapters, there is clear distinction in much of the material that is unique to general surgery or plastic surgery.

We believe this book is an invaluable resource for surgeons and plastic surgeons who wish to understand the basics of pain, current guidelines, and standard of care.

This book is an asset to surgeons, residents, medical students, and nurses involved in surgical care in both academic and private practices in the United States and abroad.

We are grateful to all of the experts who contributed to the book. We would like to extend our sincere thanks to the editorial staff of Oxford University Press, especially our editors, Andrea Knobloch and Tiffany Lu. We would also like to thank our colleagues and our families for their constant encouragement.

We hope you find *Perioperative Pain Management for General and Plastic Surgery* a practical tool for your clinical practice.

Deepak Narayan
Alan D. Kaye
Nalini Vadivelu

Contributors

Magdalena Anitescu, MD
Associate Professor
Department of Anesthesia and
Critical Care
University of Chicago Medical Center
Chicago, IL

William G. Austen Jr., MD, FACS
Chief, Division of Plastic and
Reconstructive Surgery
Massachusetts General Hospital
Associate Professor
Harvard Medical School
Boston, MA

Jarrod T. Bogue, MD
Division of Plastic and Reconstructive
Surgery
Columbia University
Medical Center
New York-Presbyterian Hospital
New York, NY

Cody Brechtel, MD
Resident
Department of Anesthesiology
Louisiana State University Health
Shreveport
Shreveport, LA

Kenneth D. Candido, MD
Chairman
Department of Anesthesiology
Advocate Illinois Masonic
Medical Center

Clinical Professor of Anesthesiology
Department of Anesthesiology
University of Illinois Chicago
Clinical Professor of Surgery
Department of Surgery
University of Illinois Chicago
Chicago, IL

Jessica Carter, MD
Assistant Professor
Department of Anesthesiology
Duke University School of Medicine
Durham, NC

Michael Casimir, MD
CA-3 Resident
Department of Anesthesiology
Yale New Haven Hospital
New, Haven, CT

Mia Castro, MD
Yale New Haven Hospital
Department of Anesthesiology
New Haven, CT

Toby C. Chai, MD
Professor
Department of Urology
Yale University School of Medicine
New Haven, CT

Daniel Chang, MD
Department of Anesthesiology
Yale New Haven Hospital
New Haven, CT

Q. Cece Chen, MD
Instructor
Department of Anesthesiology,
Perioperative Care, and Pain Medicine
New York University Langone Health
New York, NY

Grace Chen, MD
Assistant Professor
Department of Anesthesiology and
Perioperative Medicine
Oregon Health and Science University
Portland, OR

Paul K. Cheng, MD
Resident in Anesthesiology
Department of Anesthesia and
Critical Care
University of Chicago Medical Center
Chicago, IL

George C. Chang Chien, DO
Director of Pain Management
Ventura County Medical Center
Ventura, CA
Director of Center Regenerative
Medicine
Southern California University of
Health Sciences
Whittier, CA

Jacob Cole, MD, LT, MC, USN
Department of Anesthesiology
Naval Medical Center
Portsmouth, VA

Elyse M. Cornett, PhD
Assistant Professor and Director of
Research
Department of Anesthesiology
Assistant Professor
Department of Pharmacology,
Toxicology, and Neuroscience
Louisiana State University New Orleans
School of Medicine
New Orleans, LA

Sophia Delpe, MD
Chief Resident
Department of Urology
Yale University School of
Medicine
New Haven, CT

Jessica Feinleib, MD, PhD
Staff Anesthesiologist
Veterans Affairs Medical Center
West Haven, CT
Assistant Professor
Yale University School of
Medicine
New Haven, CT

Alexander J. Feng, MD
Chief Resident
Department of Physical Medicine and
Rehabilitation
Temple University Hospital
Moss Rehab
Philadelphia, PA

Charles J. Fox III, MD
Chair, Department of
Anesthesiology
Louisiana State University Health
Shreveport, LA

Timothy Furnish, MD
Associate Clinical Professor of
Anesthesiology
Center for Pain Medicine
Pain Fellowship Program Director
University of California, San Diego
Medical Center
San Diego, CA

Cyril S. Gary, BA
Section of Plastic and Reconstructive
Surgery
Department of Surgery
Yale University School of
Medicine
New Haven, CT

Evan Goodman, MD
Assistant Professor, Anesthesiology
Case Western Reserve University
School of Medicine
Cleveland, OH

Thomas Hickey, MS, MD
Assistant Professor
Yale University School of
Medicine
New Haven, CT

John Hulsen, MD
Clinical Fellow
Division of Plastic and Reconstructive
Surgery
Massachusetts General Hospital
Boston, MA

Zahid Huq
Division of Pain Management
Department of Anesthesiology
University of Miami
Miami, FL

Samuel Kim, MD
Section of Plastic and Reconstructive
Surgery
Department of Surgery
Yale University School of Medicine
New Haven, CT

Daniel Krashin, MD
Psychiatrist and Pain Specialist
University of Washington Medicine
Seattle, WA

Teresa M. Kusper, DO, MBS
Resident Physician
Department of Anesthesiology
Advocate Illinois Masonic
Medical Center
Chicago, IL

Tariq M. Malik, MD
Assistant Professor
University of Chicago
Medical Center
Department of Anesthesia and
Critical Care
Chicago, IL

Natalia Murinova, MD
Director
University of Washington Medicine
Headache Center
Seattle, WA

Amanda Norwich, MD
Research Fellow
Department of Surgery
Yale University School of Medicine
New Haven, CT

Jodi-Ann Oliver, MD
Assistant Professor of Pediatric
Anesthesiology
Director of Pediatric Regional
Anesthesiology
Yale New Haven Children
Hospital
New Haven, CT

Lori-Ann Oliver, MD
Assistant Professor of
Anesthesiology
Associate Director of Pediatric Regional
Anesthesiology
Director of Education
for Pediatric Regional
Anesthesiology
Yale New Haven Hospital
New Haven, CT

Chane Price, MD
Division of Pain Management
Department of Anesthesiology
University of Miami
Miami, FL

Srinivas Pyati, MBBS, MD, FCARCSI
Department of Anesthesiology
Duke University School of Medicine
Durham, NC

Vineetha S. Ratnamma, MBBS, MD, FRCA
Hospital-Charing Cross Hospital
Imperial School of Anaesthesia
London, United Kingdom

Victor Rivera, MD, LCDR, MC, USN
Department of Anesthesiology
Naval Medical Center
Portsmouth, VA

Christine H. Rohde, MD, MPH
Division of Plastic and Reconstructive
Surgery
Columbia University
Medical Center
New York-Presbyterian Hospital
New York, NY

Dionne Rudison, MD
Yale New Haven Hospital
Department of Anaesthesia
New Haven, CT

Ean Saberski, MD
Resident
Department of Surgery
Yale University School of Medicine
New Haven, CT

Lloyd Saberski, MD
Founder, Fellowship in Pain
Management
Yale University School of Medicine
New Haven, CT

Engy Said, MD
Department of Anesthesiology
University of California, San
Diego Health
San Diego, CA

Constantine Sarantopoulos, MD, PhD
Division of Pain Management
Department of Anesthesiology
University of Miami
Miami, FL

Harish Siddaiah, MD
Co-Director of Critical Care
Rotation
Louisiana State University Health
Shreveport, LA

Eellan Sivanesan, MD
Division of Pain Management
Department of Anesthesiology
University of Miami
Miami, FL

Katherine Stammen, MD
Residency Assistant Program
Director
Assistant Professor
Director of PACU Rotation
Louisiana State University
Health
Shreveport, LA

Anand C. Thakur, MD
Anesthesiologist
ANA Pain Management, PC
Clinton Township, MI

J. Grant Thomson, MD, FRCS, FACS
Section of Plastic and Reconstructive
Surgery
Department of Surgery
Yale University School of
Medicine
New Haven, CT

David M. Tsai, MD
Section of Plastic and Reconstructive
Surgery
Department of Surgery
Yale University School of
Medicine
New Haven, CT

Anthony Tucker, MD, CDR, MC, USN
Naval Medical Center
Department of Anesthesiology
Portsmouth, VA

Ashley Valentine, MD, PhD
Resident Physician
Oregon Health and Science University
Department of Anesthesiology and
Perioperative Medicine
Portland, OR

Alessandra Verzelloni, MD
Department of Anaesthesia
University of Modena and Reggio Emilia
Emilia-Romagna, Italy

Caroline Walker, MD
CA-2 Resident
Department of Anesthesiology
Yale New Haven Hospital
New Haven, CT

Marc E. Walker, MD, MBA
Section of Plastic and Reconstructive
Surgery
Department of Surgery
Yale University School of Medicine
New Haven, CT

Shengping Zou, MD
Clinical Associate Professor
Department of Anesthesiology,
Perioperative Care, and Pain
Medicine
Medical Director, Center for the Study
Treatment of Pain
Director, Pain Medicine Fellowship
Program
New York University Langone Health
New York, NY

Perioperative Pain Management for General and Plastic Surgery

1 Pain Pathways and Pain Physiology

Chane Price, Zahid Huq, Eellan Sivanesan, and Constantine Sarantopoulos

INTRODUCTION

The perception and experience of pain result from complex and interactive mechanisms in the nervous system. The International Association for the Study of Pain defines "pain" as a subjective unpleasant sensory and emotional experience associated with actual or potential tissue damage, or described in terms of such damage.[1] The definition highlights the notion that pain is not a strictly biological or biological problem: the experience of pain includes complex emotional, behavioral, and psychosocial dimensions as well.

Anatomically, the processing of pain involves numerous pathways that extend all the way from the peripheral tissues to the brain and the other way around (conveying signals from the peripheral sites of the pain to the brain and from the brain down to spinal sites of pain processing). Yet the conscious experience and manifestations of pain are also determined by multiple interacting environmental, social, emotional, cognitive, and behavioral factors, which highlights the need for patient-centered, comprehensive, and multimodal therapies.

Pain manifests in different forms.[1-4] These forms are characterized by different pathogenesis and by distinct pathophysiological mechanisms, and they need different therapeutic approaches. *Acute pain* is usually generated by injury, either intentional (surgery, other diagnostic or therapeutic procedures) or unintentional (trauma, fracture, environmental exposure, disease) and is expected to resolve as the underlying cause heals but in certain conditions may be recurrent (sickle cell disease, migraines). In contrast, *chronic pain* lasts much longer, by convention extends beyond the expected healing phase (usually three to six months), and besides its distinct pathophysiology is confounded by a complexity of emotional, behavioral, and psychosocial manifestations. For most patients, complete cure from chronic pain is unlikely, and several aspects of their lives are impacted negatively (self-care and well-being, work, socialization, pleasure, relationships). Both of these types of pain may initially originate from noxious (tissue-damaging) chemical, mechanical, or thermal stimuli, produced by inflammation or tissue injury, acting onto specific receptors on nociceptive peripheral sensory fibers (*nociceptive pain*). Or painful sensations may originate from the nerves themselves, after injury, disease, or other alterations (*neuropathic pain*). In either type of pain, the pain may be amplified by overresponsive peripheral or central nerves (after "peripheral" or "central sensitization," respectively).[2-4]

PAIN PATHWAYS

The pathways that convey the signals of pain from the periphery to the brain follow a chain of three afferent neurons.[4-5] The first order (or *primary afferent*) neurons respond to noxious stimuli in peripheral tissues and generate signals that are relayed to second order neurons in the dorsal horns (DHs) of the spinal cord. The second-order neurons send axons, which cross over and ascend via the spinothalamic tracts in the contralateral side of the spinal cord to the thalamus. At the thalamus, they synapse to the third-order neurons, which project to a variety of subcortical and cortical centers, wherein the sensation of pain is perceived (Figure 1.1).[4-5]

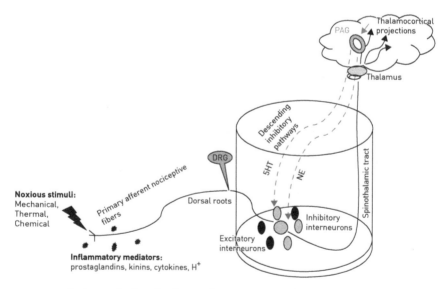

FIGURE 1.1. Basic organization of pathways of pain transmission from the periphery to the brain. Primary afferent nociceptive fibers have somata localized in the dorsal root ganglia, peripheral axons that innervate tissues and respond to noxious stimuli, and central axons that convey signals to the second-order neurons in the dorsal horns of the spinal cord. Peripheral fibers may be also sensitized by inflammatory mediators after inflammation. Second-order sensory neurons projecting from dorsal horns to higher CNS structures. An extensive network of excitatory and inhibitory interneurons in the dorsal horns of the spinal cord modulate their responses, as well as descending inhibitory pathways from supraspinal centers, such as the periaqueductal grey (PAG) that mediate analgesia. Spinothalamic tracts project to the contralateral thalamic nuclei, while other ascending tracts project to other supraspinal sites, mediating different functions. Third-order neurons project from the thalamus to brain sites involved in pain perception and pertinent responses. Descending systems, including cortical, modulate the transmission of pain.

The first-order neurons are pseudounipolar (*T-shaped*) cells, with somata in the dorsal root ganglia (DRG), peripheral axons which innervate peripheral tissues, and central axons which project to the DH of the spinal cord, wherein they synapse with second-order neurons, as well as with multiple intermediate neurons (Figure 1.1). Primary afferents, including those that convey pain, are contained in the spinal nerves and enter into the DHs of the spinal cord through the posterior (dorsal) spinal roots while the anterior (ventral roots) contain motor and autonomic efferent fibers. Each spinal nerve divides into an anterior ramus that contributes to the various plexuses and peripheral nerves of the body and into a posterior ramus that innervates the dorsal spinal and somatic muscular and cutaneous structures.[4-5]

Peripheral sensory nerves convey various sensory modalities, but pain is mediated by a subpopulation of nerves that belong to the category of small sensory fibers. The neuroanatomical and functional classification of sensory nerve fibers is based on their myelination, diameter, and conduction velocity. The Aβ are large and myelinated and conduct rapidly. They convey touch, pressure, vibration, and proprioception. The Aγ innervate muscle spindles. The Aδ fibers convey signals of touch, heat, and pain, much faster than the C fibers, which also convey similar modalities yet more slowly, as they are much smaller and nonmyelinated. Aδ and C fibers are referred as *small fibers*, while the Aβ are *large fibers*. The large fibers not only do not conduct pain but, once activated (by touch, massage, transcutaneous electrical stimulation), may suppress the input of pain from the small fibers (a property useful in analgesia).[2-5]

Pain from the viscera is also conveyed by small fibers, but these follow the course of the autonomic nerves. Nociceptive signals from the abdominal and thoracic viscera via these fibers traverse through the prevertebral ganglia (celiac or hypogastric plexus), then via the splachnic nerves enter the paravertebral sympathetic chain, and then via the rami communicans reach the spinal nerves and enter into the DH through the dorsal roots (T1 to L2). At the DH they converge onto the same second-order neurons as the somatic nerves.

Pain fibers from the sigmoid colon, rectum, bladder, prostate, and cervix of the uterus accompany the parasympathetic efferents entering the cord in the dorsal roots of S2 to S4.

Vagal afferents, with somata in the nodose ganglion, transmit signals of bloating, distention, and nausea-like sensation but not pain, except perhaps from the hypopharynx and the upper respiratory tract. Finally, pain fibers that innervate the face and head have somata in the Gasserian ganglion and, through the sensory trigeminal root, project to the spinal trigeminal nucleus in the medulla.

Pain Pathways in the Spinal Cord

As the primary afferents enter into the DH through the dorsal roots, the small (Aδ and C) fibers are distributed laterally, while the large fibers (Aβ) enter more medially. Then afferents may send a branch directly to the DH at the segment of entry, or they may send collateral branches rostrally and caudally, up to several segments beyond the segment of entry (the small fibers in the *Lissauer's tract* and the large fibers in the *dorsal columns*). The primary afferent endings are finally distributed and synapse in the DHs of the spinal cord, but this distribution is determined by the fiber type (small or large). The small fibers end in the more superficial laminae of the DHs (*substantia gelatinosa*), while the large fibers end deeper (*nucleus proprius*). The central pathways that further process nociceptive information begin at the level of the DH. They contain second-order neurons that project the signal to the thalamus or pass it on to other spinal neurons, including flexor motoneurons, and numerous intermediate neuronal networks that modulate the information. Some of the intermediate neurons in the DH sensitize the projection neurons and facilitate nociceptive transmission. Others inhibit the synaptic transmission and the projection neurons, thus contributing to analgesia.[2,4,5]

From the spinal cord, rostral transmission of nociceptive signals is via axons that ascent to supraspinal centers (Figure 1.1). Second-order neurons that relay pain project to the contralateral thalamus, periaqueductal gray (PAG), parabrachial region, and bulbar reticular formation, as well as to the limbic and other sites. Depending on the site of projection, they are classified as *spinothalamic, spinomesencephalic, spinoreticular*, and so forth. The most important relay of nociceptive information is via second-order neurons, the axons of which cross the midline and project to the thalamus via contralateral ascending spinothalamic tracts (Figure 1.1).[4,5]

Pain Pathways in the Brain

Although the primary somatosensory cortex processes the conscious perception of pain, this may not be considered as the specific pain center in the brain. The perception of pain has been thought more to be the result of interaction between various subcortical and cortical centers, therefore it is not possible to abolish the perception of pain by ablation of any specific brain centers. The thalamus receives signals from the ascending afferents and relays to the cortex (Figure 1.1), contributing to the awareness of the pain. The *neothalamus* (lateral thalamus) is projected to the sensory cortex for localization and discrimination of pain. The *paleothalamus* (medial thalamus) projects diffusely to the cortex, driving motivational-affective behavior. Affective-motivational responses to pain are also mediated by the limbic system, including the hypothalamus that regulates autonomic and neuroendocrine responses to pain. Cortical areas highly involved in pain perception include the somatosensory SI and SII regions, the anterior insula, and the anterior cingulate cortex.[4,5]

Descending Pathways that Modulate Pain

Ascending signals, in addition to resulting in pain, may alter their afferent input and its sensory perception. Incoming pain signals to higher centers, including the PAG, activate descending pathways that inhibit the input of pain via serotoninergic or noradrenergic fibers (Figure 1.1). The PAG contains a dense concentration of opioid peptides and receptors serving as a mediator for opioid analgesia. Both serotonin and norepinephrine, as well as encephalins (endorphins), are released in the DH via this negative feedback loop activated by pain, and spinal transection inhibits this effect. In addition, higher structures, including the cerebral cortex, and limbic structures contribute to analgesia, and this can be a learned response. In the DH nociceptive stimuli drive inhibitory interneurons to release encephalin, GABA, or glycine. The analgesic action from systemically administered opioids seems to be from their ability to activate an interconnected opioidergic network that spans the whole neuraxis, from the forebrain to the spinal cord, even to peripheral nerves.[2-5]

PAIN PHYSIOLOGY

The pathways of pain are not hardwired conduits of signals but capable of signal modulation. The *plasticity* of these pathways may alter dynamically the relation between the painful stimulus and the responses to it, all the way from the periphery, through the spinal cord, and to the higher centers of the brain.[2-4]

The interplay between incoming signals, numerous excitatory, and inhibitory systems will determine the intensity of perception of the signal of pain and the responses to it. Depending on particular circumstances, the response to the incoming messages may be attenuated or amplified. Amplification or even spontaneous pain can result from *peripheral* or *central sensitization* of sensory neurons, while altered perception of the localization of pain pertains to the phenomenon of *referred pain.*[4]

Referred Pain and Visceral Pain Sensations

Typically pain from visceral organs, like the heart or the abdominal viscera, is felt onto an overlying, onto an adjacent, or onto a remote somatic area and may be accompanied by deep or superficial tenderness (*hyperalgesia*), by reflexive muscle spasm, and by intense viscero-visceral, vascular, and neuroendocrine responses.[4] These, together with the muscular spasm, produce new sources of nociception that may outlast the original.

Acute and Chronic Pain States

In normal states, noxious stimuli generate pain and various responses that are proportional to the stimulus, although genetic or other factors may result in qualitative and quantitative variability. These responses, in the case of acute pain, are physiologically adaptive, transient, and self-limited, secondary to homeostatic restoration. Yet, not infrequently acute pain leads to chronicity. Transition to chronicity may manifest with the development of persistent pain, disproportional to stimulus, or spontaneous pain which is pathological and nonadaptive. Likewise, genetic and multiple internal and external factors may determine the transition from acute to chronic pain.[2-4]

Typically, prolonged or intense nociception, or loss of normal sensation, alters the properties of the somatosensory pathways to such an extent that incoming pain is amplified or spontaneous pain may be generated. This, in addition to chronic pain after injury, is particularly the case after injury or disease affecting the nerves, leading to neuropathic pain.

The Physiology of Transient, Acute Pain

Under normal conditions, no spontaneous activity is observed in the peripheral nociceptive fibers. Yet, after injury or inflammation, chemical, mechanical, or thermal noxious stimuli activate specific receptors onto their terminals. These receptors are coupled to cation channels, the opening of which generates electrical signals in the form of action potentials that will successively propagate proximally. Several receptors that respond to specific noxious stimuli have been identified onto C and Aδ nociceptive fibers. The transient receptor potential vanilloid 1, for example, responds to noxious thermal, acidic, and irritating chemical stimuli by generating nociceptive signals that are perceived as painful sensations.[4-6] Other receptors transduce noxious heat, cold, mechanical, or chemical stimuli[2,4,7] and initiate the signals that will enable the nervous system to distinguish these stimuli as painful.

The action potentials in response to noxious stimulation will then be conveyed to the DH via Aδ fibers and C fibers and elicit release of synaptic neurotransmission. The main neurotransmitters involved in the synaptic transmission of pain at the DH include excitatory amino acids, such as glutamate or aspartate, or neuropeptides, such as the tachykinin substance P. These transmit the signal of pain by acting onto cognate postsynaptic receptors. Glutamate acts by binding to receptors that mediate signaling responses by activating cation channels (ionotropic receptors such as the *a-amino-3-hydroxy-5-methyl-4-isoxazolepropionic acid [AMPA] receptor, or the N-Methyl-D-aspartate [NMDA] receptor*), or by inducing second messenger cytosolic signaling (metabotropic receptors). Substance P binds to neurokinin receptor 1 (NK_1) that also induces downstream second messengers, which in turn regulate various mediators of cellular excitability and function.[2,4,7]

The information that signals brief acute pain is generally mediated via synaptic release of excitatory amino acids (glutamate) acting at the AMPA receptors, and only to a minimal degree by substance P acting at the NK_1 receptor (Figure 1.2). Postsynaptic

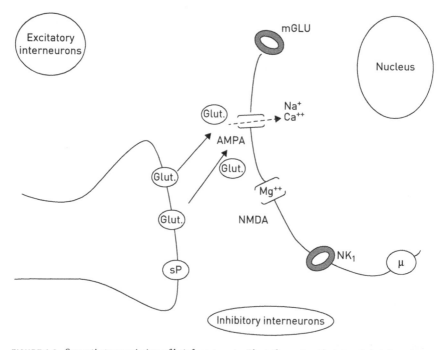

FIGURE 1.2. Synaptic transmission of brief, acute pain. The information that signals brief acute pain is generally mediated via synaptic release of excitatory amino acids (glutamate, aspartate) acting mainly at the AMPA receptors, but only to a minimal degree by substance P acting at the NK_1 receptor. The other ionotropic glutamate receptor, NMDA, is usually inactive in these states, partly as a result of magnesium (Mg^{++})-dependent blockade. Synaptic transmission of brief acute nociceptive signaling typically results in postsynaptic responses that tend to match the stimulus in terms of intensity and temporal characteristics.

responses lead to brief discharge of action potentials and subsequent activation of discriminative-sensory ascending pathways. Acute pain is considered as physiologically adaptive, transient, and self-limited.[2,4,7]

The Pathophysiology of Persistent and Chronic Pain

In contrast, tissue injury or persisting inflammation that is more spatially or temporally extensive induces plasticity to neural pathways, leading to chronic pain. Mechanical or thermal trauma or inflammation injures tissues and attracts a variety of immune, inflammatory cells, leading to a release of numerous inflammatory mediators, such as prostaglandins, protons and potassium ions, bradykinin, cytokines, growth factors, purines, and amines that constitute an *inflammatory soup*.[2,4,7,8] For example, some mediators, such as the nitric oxide (NO) and pronociceptive cytokines (interleukins, tumor necrosis factor) induce the inducible enzyme COX2 synthase, which then contributes with prostaglandins and so forth. Prostaglandins are also contributed by the constitutive COX1 enzyme as well. These further sensitize the nociceptive neurons and amplify their responses to noxious stimulation, a process that can targeted by nonsteroidal anti-inflammatory analgesics.

Some of these mediators may activate nociceptors directly and evoke pain, while others sensitize them by facilitating their easier activation (by lowering the threshold), or their increased responsiveness (by enhancing membrane excitability), thus contributing to phenomena such as spontaneous pain and pain evoked by nonpainful stimuli (allodynia) or amplified (hyperalgesia). Some of these mechanisms are rapid, subsequent to posttranslational modification (phosphorylation) of signal effectors such as membrane ion channels, while other changes are more delayed because they depend on altered gene translation, transcription, and transport of new protein to distal or proximal terminals.[2,4,9] Yet, the overall effect is the transition of the primary afferent nociceptive system to a more excitable, hyperresponsive state, driving much more heightened nociceptive input to the DH.

Downstream, this heightened traffic of signals to the central nociceptive pathways will in turn significantly enhance their responsiveness too, by inducing a series of neuroplastic alterations. *Central sensitization*, a mechanism of neuroplasticity, is the phenomenon in which prolonged, intense input of signals of pain into the DH of the spinal cord, into the spinal trigeminal nucleus in the medulla, or into higher centers, alter their neuronal phenotype which results in an amplified, exaggerated synaptic transmission of pain signaling.[2,4,9,10] The sensitized state contributes to generation of spontaneous pain signals and/or to enhanced responsiveness to painful stimuli with sensory gain amplification that clinically manifests as *allodynia* (pain evoked by a stimulus which does not normally produce pain) and *hyperalgesia* (increased pain to a stimulus which is normally painful but much less; Figure 1.3). Ultimately, a pathologic state of chronic pain may develop that involves more or less permanent changes in the central nervous system (CNS; DH neurons, interneurons, ventral horn neurons, thalamus, cortex, and other brain areas) persisting long after the original injury has healed. Adequate neural blockade prior to initiation of the noxious stimulation and throughout the perioperative period, or appropriate suppression of nociceptive signaling by multimodal analgesia, may, at least theoretically, prevent some of

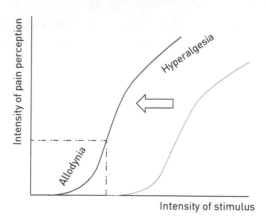

Intensity of pain perception

Hyperalgesia

Allodynia

Intensity of stimulus

FIGURE 1.3. Increased responsiveness with allodynia and hyperalgesia in chronic pain states. In chronic pain states, the response to pain is augmented as a result of the sensitization of the peripheral and central nociceptive pathway. Inflammation contributes to sensitization of the peripheral nerves so that they become hyperexcitable. Then, prolonged, intense nociception from peripheral nerves, or painful nerve injury with ectopic action potentials, drive an excessive traffic of pain signals into the spinal cord and higher center. Spontaneous pain may emerge, as well as amplified painful sensations evoked from stimulation of the injured area and from stimulation of the undamaged surrounding area. In sensitized states, the curve which describes the relation between the perceived intensity of the pain and that of the stimulus shows a leftward shift (arrow). Because of the shift of the neuronal networks to a more hyperresponsive state, stimuli that normally do not produce pain will be now perceived as painful (allodynia), and stimuli that normally are painful will be now perceived as much more painful than they normally are.

these changes, reduce postoperative pain or analgesic requirements, and transition to chronic pain.[10,11]

In contrast to acute pain wherein synaptic transmission is mainly mediated by Aδ fiber-released glutamate, acting mainly on AMPA receptors, in conditions of persisting inflammation, peripherally sensitized C fibers, in addition to Aδ, provide a more sustained input to DH. In addition to glutamate, activated C fibers release tachykinins which lead to prolonged excitatory postsynaptic responses, cumulative postsynaptic depolarization, and firing. In this case a synergistic activation of both the AMPA and the NK$_1$ receptor, if of sufficient magnitude and duration, can subsequently excite the NMDA receptor (Figure 1.4). NMDA receptors are linked to channels, permeable to Ca^{++}, and their activation results in pronounced, sustained deployment of cytosolic Ca^{++} dependent mechanisms. These include increased activity of multiple second messenger cascades, such as activation of phospholipase A2, mediators, such as NO, inositol triphosphate and diacylglycerol, activation of protein kinase C (PKC), with phosphorylation of various targets, "burst" firing of DH neurons, hyperexcitability, and amplified rostral transmission of nociceptive information.[2–4, 9–11]

Chronic opioids also mimic NMDA-mediated central events, including activation of PKC. This leads to chronic development of reduced sensitivity to opioids, further sensitization, and even to hyperalgesia induced by these drugs (opioid-induced hyperalgesia).[3]

Other mechanisms contribute too. Glial and immune cells in the periphery and within the CNS get activated by tissue injury, by inflammation, and by nerve lesions and release cytokines and other pronociceptive mediators.[12] The activation of glial by

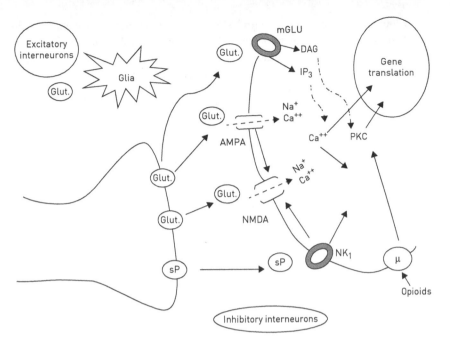

FIGURE 1.4. Complexity of synaptic transmission in chronic pain states. In contrast to acute pain wherein synaptic transmission is mainly mediated by Aδ fiber-released glutamate (acting on AMPA receptors), in conditions of persisting inflammation, peripherally sensitized small fibers provide a more sustained input to the DH. In addition to glutamate, release of substance P (sP) leads to prolonged excitatory postsynaptic responses, cumulative postsynaptic depolarization, and firing. In this case a synergistic activation of both the AMPA and the NK_1 receptor can excite the NMDA receptor. NMDA receptors are linked to channels, permeable to Ca^{++}, and their activation results in pronounced, sustained deployment of cytosolic Ca^{++}-dependent mechanisms. These include increased activity of multiple second messenger cascades, including inositol triphosphate (IP_3) and diacylglycerol (DAG), activation of protein kinase C (PKC), with phosphorylation of various targets, including altered gene translation, with hyperexcitability and amplified postsynaptic responses. Chronic opioids may mimic NMDA-mediated central events, including activation of PKC. Diminished inhibitory processes and increased excitatory influences from excitatory interneurons and activated glial cells may further exacerbate the process of central sensitization.

inflammation or drugs (opioids) may drive central sensitized responses to the point that chronic pain has been viewed also as a *gliopathy*.[13] Diminished tonic GABAergic and glycinergic inhibitory interneuronal activity can mimic and further accentuate processes of DH sensitization, contributing to the allodynia and hyperalgesia. Loss of inhibitory interneurons has been attributed to glutamate-NMDA-receptor dependent excitotoxic mechanisms (Figure 1.3).[4,9]

The Pathophysiology of Neuropathic Pain

Neuropathic pain develops after disease or injury to peripheral nerves or to the CNS itself. In pure neuropathic pain states there is no association between pain and any tissue damage; however, neuropathic pain clinically may coexist with nociceptive pain by concomitant tissue injury or inflammation.

Various neurological diseases with lesions to peripheral nerves or damage to the somatosensory system within the CNS (multiple sclerosis, strokes), infections (herpes zoster, HIV), trauma (nerve transection, nerve damage, brachial plexus injuries), and metabolic disorders (diabetes) or intoxications (alcohol) can cause neuropathic pain. Neuropathic pain can be spontaneous, or evoked, triggered by innocuous stimuli or associated with exaggerated responses to minor noxious stimuli, and accompanied by loss of motor or sensory function.

Pathogenetically, the mechanisms that generate neuropathic pain are cause specific and unique to the etiology, but a predominant abnormality that typically drives neuropathic pain is the aberrant electrical hyperexcitability and generation of ectopic firing discharge of sensory neurons after injury.[14-16] This takes place at injured neurons, at the DRG, and at the DH. Various alterations in the genetic translation and posttranslational modification of neuronal sodium channel subtypes[17,18] and other channels have been implicated,[14-16] and drugs that block sodium channels or modulate other channels may have a role as analgesics. Suppressing of the afferent initial barrage by local anesthetics may also attenuate the development of subsequent hyperalgesic manifestations. The ectopic firing and hyperexcitability that develops in injured peripheral nerves may be reciprocally related to sensitivity to humoral (cytokines, prostaglandins, catecholamines) and mechanical effects (pressure, touch) (e.g., Tinel's sign in carpal tunnel syndrome).

Abnormal firing generates signals that propagate centrally and may elicit spontaneous pain, or drive the development of central sensitization in DH and higher centers, so that central changes may also contribute to abnormal pain perception and phenomena such as allodynia and hyperalgesia.[14-16] Both peripheral and central changes are implicated with a varying contribution in each type of neuropathic pain; for example peripheral spontaneous firing and neuronal hyperexcitability in neuromas may be a dominant mechanism in neuropathic pain in the stump of amputees, while central (including cortical) mechanisms may predominate in phantom pain states.

Deficient supraspinal or descending mechanisms may also be significant, so that excitatory input predominates, and various subtypes of sensory fibers alter their phenotype; for example large Aβ fibers may develop a phenotype more consistent with nociceptors. Some types of neuropathic pain, such as the complex regional pain syndromes, may result from both peripheral and central sensitization mechanisms, with significant contribution in some cases of hyperexcitability driven by dysregulation of efferent sympathetic activity.[14-16]

REFERENCES

1. International Association for the Study of Pain. Part III: Pain terms, a current list with definitions and notes on usage. In *Classification of chronic pain*, 2nd ed., edited by H. Merskey and N. Bogduk. Seattle, WA: IASP Press, 1994:209–214.
2. Scholz J, Woolf CJ. Can we conquer pain? *Nat Neurosci.* 2002;5(Suppl):1062–1067.
3. Stucky CL, Gold MS, Zhang X. Mechanisms of pain. *Proc Natl Acad Sci U S A.* 2001;98:11845–11846.
4. Basbaum AI, Bautista DM, Scherrer G, Julius D. Cellular and molecular mechanisms of pain. *Cell.* 2009;139:267–284.
5. Willis WD, Westlund KN. Neuroanatomy of the pain system and of the pathways that modulate pain. *J Clin Neurophysiol.* 1997;14:2–31.

6. Stucky CL, Dubin AE, Jeske NA, Malin SA, McKemy DD, Story GM. Roles of transient receptor potential channels in pain. *Brain Res Rev.* 2009;60:2–23.

7. Dubin AE, Patapoutian A. Nociceptors: the sensors of the pain pathway. *J Clin Invest.* 2010;120:3760–3772.

8. Bodeke EW. Involvement of chemokines in pain. *Eur J Pharmacol.* 2001;429:115–119.

9. Latremoliere A, Woolf CJ. Central sensitization: a generator of pain hypersensitivity by central neural plasticity. *J Pain.* 2009;10:895–926.

10. Woolf CJ. Central sensitization: Implications for the diagnosis and treatment of pain. *Pain.* 2011;152(3 Suppl):S2–S15.

11. Dahl JB, Kehlet H. Preventive analgesia. *Curr Opin Anaesthesiol.* 2011;24:331–338.

12. Watkins LR, Milligan ED, Maier SF. Glial activation: a driving force for pathological pain. *Trends Neurosci.* 2001;24:450–455.

13. Ji RR, Berta T, Nedergaard M. Glia and pain: is chronic pain a gliopathy? *Pain.* 2013;154(Suppl 1):S10–S28.

14. Woolf CJ, Mannion RJ. Neuropathic pain: aetiology, symptoms, mechanisms, and management. *Lancet.* 1999;353:1959–1964.

15. Bridges D, Thompson SWN, Rice ASC. Mechanisms of neuropathic pain. *Br J Anaesth.* 2001;87:12–26.

16. Baron R. Neuropathic pain: a clinical perspective. *Handb Exp Pharmacol.* 2009;194:3–30.

17. Devor M. Sodium channels and mechanisms of neuropathic pain. *J Pain.* 2006;7:S3–S12.

18. Dib-Hajj SD, Cummins TR, Black JA, Waxman SG. Sodium channels in normal and pathological pain. *Annu Rev Neurosci.* 2010;33:325–347.

2 NMDA Receptor Antagonists, Gabapentinoids, Alpha-2 Agonists, and Dexamethasone

Alexander J. Feng, George C. Chang Chien, and Alan D. Kaye

INTRODUCTION

Effective pain management in surgical patients is of the upmost importance. Poorly controlled acute pain can lead to increased cardiorespiratory work, immunosuppression,[1] and coagulation disturbances.[2,3] In addition, undertreatment of postoperative pain can delay patient recovery, postpone discharge from the hospital, or cause unexpected hospital admissions after outpatient surgery. Furthermore, higher levels of postoperative pain are associated with an increased risk of chronic pain.[4] Despite this recognition, up to 70% of patients still complain of moderate to severe pain postoperatively.[5] It is therefore important to aggressively treat and prevent postoperative pain to optimize recovery.

Opioids and nonsteroidal anti-inflammatory drugs (NSAIDs) are the mainstay therapy for alleviating moderate to severe pain. Opioids are often limited by their side effects including decreased gastrointestinal mobility leading to nausea and vomiting, sedation, pruritus, and urinary retention with incidences reported to be 25%, 20%, 3%, 15%, and 23% respectively.[6] NSAIDs are also associated with their own complications including gastrointestinal mucosa damage, bleeding, renal toxicity, allergic reactions, and heart failure.[7] In addition, cyclooxygensase-2 selective NSAIDs may have prothrombotic properties thus increasing the risk of myocardial ischemia and cerebral vascular events.[7,8] Improved understanding of the peripheral and central mechanisms involved in nociceptive transmission provides clinicians with newer options and adjuvants to manage pain more effectively. An adjuvant medication is one that acts to decrease pain in patients and allows for a reduction in the doses of individual drugs and thus a lower incidence of adverse effects, particularly opioids. The goals of the adjuvants in pain management are to relieve suffering, achieve early mobilization, reduce the length of hospital stay, and ultimately improve patient satisfaction.

As such, studies have shown a lower incidence of adverse effects and improved analgesia with adjuvant analgesia techniques, which likely lead to improved recovery and function.[9–11]

The idea of adjuvant analgesia is not a new concept. It has been used for more than a decade to improve analgesia. The idea is that by using multiple medications of different classes of analgesics, one would be able to achieve better analgesia due to additive or synergistic effects.[12] In addition, blocking the neuronal pathway during surgery with local anesthetics does not decrease the humeral biochemical responses that occur during surgery, which have to be inhibited by administering systemic pharmacological therapy.[13] Furthermore, in the surgical patient, generation of pain is multifactorial, and clinicians must take into account the patient's pre-existing medical, psychological, and physical condition; age; surgical procedure performed; personal preferences; and response to agents given. The basis of using nonopioid analgesic adjuvants is to reduce opioid consumption, administer individual agents in optimal dosages that maximize efficacy, and attempt to minimize the side effects of one analgesic (mainly opioids).

The use of adjuvant therapy, including alpha-2 (A-2) agonists, gabapentinoids, n-methyl-D-aspartate (NMDA) receptor antagonists, and dexamethasone, is evaluated in this chapter. We review the evidence on the opioid-sparing effects of these adjuvant medications in perioperative pain management. Most available data support the use of these adjuvants in routine analgesic techniques to reduce the need for postoperative opioids and improve the quality of pain control. Current practice guidelines for acute pain management in the perioperative setting in the updated report by the American Society of Anesthesiologists Task Force on Acute Pain Management supports the use of adjuvant therapy to optimize pain control and decrease opioid use.[14]

ALPHA-2 AGONISTS

In 1908, epinephrine was applied to a cat spinal cord and showed pain modulation effects.[15] It is well known that norepinephrine is involved in the control of modulating pain-related responses through various pathways. A-2 adrenergic agonists have an analgesic profile and act as an adjunct to anesthetics and analgesics in perioperative settings. The development of subtype-selective A-2 adrenoceptor agonists produces effective and selective pain treatment with minimal side effects.

Activation of A-2 adrenergic receptor inhibits the release of noradrenaline. Initial studies hinted that the A-2 adrenergic receptor agonists exert sedative effects by suppressing noradrenaline release from the locus ceruleus;[16] however, more recent studies have found that A-2 agonists produce antinociceptive effects without affecting noradrenaline release.[17] It has been demonstrated that astrocytes and microglias in the central nervous system can be activated by noxious stimuli, such as nerve injuries and inflammation, and play an important role in the maintenance of chronic pain.[18–21] Early stages of pain appear to activate microglias with activated astrocytes emerging later and lasting longer.[22,23] Specifically following nerve injury, the activated glial cells release inflammatory factors which amplify pain signals or sensitize neighboring neurons. Membranes of glial cells express A-2 agonist receptors. Therefore, A-2 agonists inhibit activation of these microglia cells, signal regulated kinase in the spinal dorsal horn, and reduce hyperalgesia.[24] Two commonly used A-2 agonists are clonidine and dexmedetomidine.

Clonidine

Clonidine is a partial agonist with an A-2 to alpha-1 (A-1) receptor selectivity ratio of 39.[15] It can be given in various routes of administration including oral, transdermal, bolus, and continuous infusion. Its role in neuraxial blockade has been described by a number of studies. Comparing clonidine/morphine spinal plus remifentanil infusion to a sufentanil infusion for analgesia in 83 patients undergoing open heart surgery,[25] Lena et al. showed that the clonidine treatment group enabled more rapid extubation, less patient-controlled analgesia (PCA) morphine use, improved patient comfort, and decreased pain scores. Blaudszun et al. analyzed 1,792 patients in a meta-analysis and found postoperative morphine usage sparing at 24 hours with 2 to 5 ug/kg clonidine with a weighted mean difference (WMD) of −4.1 mg.[26] It is also noted that these medications did not prolong the time to postoperative recovery and extubation. There has also been a noted decreased risk of myocardial infarct, cardiac mortality, and all-cause mortality with the use of either clonidine or dexmedetomidine.[27] However, due to differences in timing and route of administration, there is no consensus for a dose-dependent effect.[28]

The A-2 agonist is a well-known antihypertensive and as such is the biggest risk factor in its use. Clonidine has an increased risk of hypotension both intraoperatively and postoperatively with the number needed to harm of 9 and 20, respectively. Therefore, these medications should be avoided in patients with simultaneous B-blockade.[26]

Dexmedetomidine

Dexmedetomidine was first approved for use in December 1999 and is a highly selective A-2 adrenoceptor agonist with a shorter terminal half-life.[29] It has an A-2 to A-1 receptor ratio of approximately 1600:1, which favors the sedative/anxiolytic actions rather than the hemodynamic actions seen in clonidine.[30] An infusion of dexmedetomidine prior to induction through wound closure (0.2–0.8 mcg/kg/h) in 80 patients undergoing laparoscopic bariatric surgery[31] led to decreased postanesthesia care unit (PACU) opioid use, reduced nausea and vomiting, and shorter PACU stay. A meta-analysis of 1,420 patients with intraoperative dexmedetomidine found lower postoperative opioid use, lower pain scores, and reduced opioid-related adverse events with optimal dosing with bolus of 1 ug/kg followed by continuous infusion of 0.5 to 1 ug/kg/h.[29] It showed a mean difference of −17 mg at 24 hours and −39 mg at 48 hours in reduced morphine consumption. The author also notes that the types of surgery might influence the degree of analgesia, with greater pain reduction during more painful surgery such as lumbar discectomy.[29] Dexmedetomidine has also been analyzed in intravenous (IV) regional anesthesia and shown to have the ability to prolong analgesia and extend the duration of motor and sensory blockade.

Dexmedetomidine has a similar side effect profile to clonidine. In one study it had an increased risk of postoperative bradycardia with a number needed to harm of 3.[15,26] A higher dose of intraoperative dexmedetomidine may require more doses of phenylephrine, but otherwise there were no differences in side effects compared to placebo.[12]

Summary

It remains unclear whether there are any significant consequences on morbidity or mortality regarding the hemodynamic effects of clonidine and dexmedetomidine. As mentioned previously, in patients with B-blockade these medications should be avoided. There is evidence that clonidine at 2 to 5 ug/kg IV and dexmedetomidine at 0.5 ug/kg bolus followed by infusion of 0.5 to 1 ug/kg/h have an effect on improving analgesia and opioid sparing.

GABAPENTANOIDS

Gabapentinoids include gabapentin and its successor, pregabalin. Gabapentin was first introduced in 1993 as an antiepileptic drug. Now it is extensively used to treat various neuropathies including diabetic polyneuropathy, postherpetic neuralgia, complex regional pain syndromes, multiple sclerosis, and neuropathic pain in general.[32] Gabapentin has now been introduced as an adjunct to managing acute postoperative pain.

Gabapentinoids are structurally derived from the alkylated analogue of gamma-aminobutyric acid (GABA). Gabapentinoids do not exert their clinical effects by interacting with GABA receptors but rather by binding to the $\alpha 2\delta 21$ subunits of the presynaptic L-type voltage-sensitive calcium channels of cortical and dorsal horn neurons, attenuating the release of the neuropeptides glutamate, norepinephrine, and substance P from the primary afferent nerve fibers in the pain pathway leading to antinociception.[7,33,34] Gabapentin also has antiallodynic and antihyperalgesic properties with only a minor effect on normal nociception.[35] It activates descending inhibitory noradrenergic pathways that regulate the neurotransmission of pain signals in the dorsal horn, reducing the hyperexcitability of dorsal horn neurons induced by tissue injury.[33,36-38]

Gabapentin

Gabapentin is available as an oral preparation. Gabapentin is not metabolized by humans. It does not bind to plasma proteins and once absorbed is eliminated unchanged in urine, with an elimination half-life of five to nine hours.[33,39] It is absorbed in a limited part of the duodenum. When the transporters are saturated, increasing dosage does not result in any increased blood concentration.[40] Bioavailability of gabapentin varies inversely with dose. The bioavailability of a 300 mg dose is 60%, whereas that of a dose of 1600 mg decreases to 35%.[41,42] The peak plasma concentration is achieved three hours after injection of a single 300 mg capsule.[42] The peak cerebrospinal fluid (CSF) for gabapentin is reported to be four to six hours.[43,44] Cimetidine decreases the clearance of gabapentin by 12% because cimetidine decreases glomerular filtration rate.[42] It has also been reported that antacids reduce the bioavailability of gabapentin by 20% when given up to two hours post-gabapentin administration.[45] Similarly, because both gabapentinoids are excreted through the kidney, dose adjustments are needed for both medications in patients with renal insufficiency.[33] Patients who undergo hemodialysis should also receive their maintenance dose of the medication after treatment.[46]

There is good evidence for gabapentin as a perioperative adjuvant. The first study in 2002 showed that a single dose of oral gabapentin 1200 mg or placebo, one hour before radical mastectomy, significantly reduced total morphine consumption from a median of 29 mg to 15 mg, and pain during movement was significantly reduced from 41 mm to 22 mm on a 100 mm visual analogue scale (VAS) two hours postoperatively and from 31 mm to 9 mm four hours postoperatively.[47] In a study of 36 patients undergoing total knee arthroplasty, administration of pre- and postoperative gabapentin decreased morphine consumption on postoperative days 2 through 4 and increased the amount of active knee flexion on those days without noted side effects.[48] Several meta-analysis have shown these adjuvant effects. In a 2006 meta-analysis of 16 trials, a single dose of preoperative 1200 mg gabapentin decreased postoperative VAS scores with a WMD of −16.5 mm at 6 hours and −10.87 mm at 24 hours and decreased 24-hour cumulative opioid consumption (WMD, −7.25mg).[28,49] A subsequent meta-analysis in 2007 of 22 trials showed after a single dose of gabapentin 300 to 1200 mg, administered one to two hours preoperatively, had an opioid-sparing effect ranging from 20% to 62%.[7] The combined effect of a single dose of gabapentin was a reduction of opioid consumption equivalent to 30+/−4 mg of morphine during the first 24 hours after surgery and was not significantly dependent on the gabapentin dose.[7] The authors also showed gabapentin decreased opioid-related adverse effects of nausea, vomiting, and urinary retention.[7] A meta-analysis of four unpublished studies in 2010 showed patients who received a 250 mg dose of gabapentin before surgery found that number needed to treat (NNT) to achieve a 50% decrease in pain was 11, and fewer participants needed rescue medications in six hours postoperatively (NNT 5.8). Perioperative use of gabapentin has been shown to also reduce both postoperative pain and opioid use after surgery.[50–52] For procedure-specific results, analysis of data from abdominal hysterectomy and spinal surgery shows patients given 1200 mg gabapentin demonstrated significantly reduced 24-hour opioids consumption and pain score.[53,54]

Gabapentin is overall tolerated well. The most common adverse effects include somnolence and dizziness, headaches, balance problems, peripheral edema, sweating, and dry mouth. The number needed to harm (NNH) to produce excessive dizziness or sedation were 12 and 35, respectively.[7] Pregabalin was also seen to have higher incidence of visual disturbances with NNH of 6.[55]

Pregabalin

Pregabalin is also an oral preparation and first appeared on the US market in 2005. Different from gabapentin, pregabalin is absorbed throughout the small intestines, and its bioavailability has a linear relationship with dosage.[56] The peak plasma concentration of pregabalin is one hour.[34] However, the peak CSF level is variable, from two hours for a 50mg dose[57] to eight hours for a 300 mg dose.[58] It is also excreted through the kidney with <2% metabolism and has a mean elimination half-life of 6.3 hours.[34,57] Because of the lack of hepatic metabolism and low protein binding, pregabalin also has no known clinically relevant drug interactions.[42]

Pregabalin has been shown to have similar positive effects as gabapentin. A meta-analysis of 18 studies of patients who received 50 to 750 mg/d of pregabalin either in a single dose or up to two weeks postoperatively found a 30.8% overall decrease in postoperative analgesic requirements with a lowest effective dose of 225 to 300 mg/d.[59] Higher dosages of pregabalin, >300 mg/d versus <300 mg/d, showed 24-hour reduced opioid consumption with a WMD of –13.4 versus –8.8 mg, respectively. Agarwal et al. showed in 30 patients undergoing laparoscopic cholecystectomy that the patients who received pregabalin 150 mg one hour preoperatively had lower VAS scores and less narcotic use with no significant side effects noted.[60] Pregabalin was also associated with decreased postoperative nausea and vomiting with a NNT of 18.[55] Lower doses of pregabalin seem to have less effect; as suggested by Hill et al., pain relief in a dental pain model 2 to 12 hours postoperatively was significant only with pregabalin of 300 mg but not 50 mg compared with placebo.[61]

The use of pregabalin has gained more attention than gabapentin because of more favorable pharmacokinetics, improved bioavailability, and faster achievement of therapeutic levels. One study showed postoperative analgesia and time to first request for analgesia was better with 300 mg pregabalin than 900 mg gabapentin and placebo, and both were better than placebo alone when given one to two hours prior to surgery.[62] A second study comparing gabapentin 600 mg twice a day and pregabalin 150 mg twice a day both pre-and postsurgery showed equivalent analgesic, adverse, and opioid-sparing effects and patient satisfaction.[63] In addition, perioperative administration of gabapentin and pregabalin were effective in reducing the incidence of chronic postsurgical pain two months after surgery and resulted in an improvement in postsurgical patient function.[64]

Summary

Both gabapentin and pregabalin effectively reduce postoperative opioid use and pain and increase patient satisfaction. The ideal dosing and timing of administration remains unclear as well as the length of postoperative usage. Both gabapentinoids have very few adverse effects of their own. While higher doses of gabapentin (1200 mg) and pregabalin (300 mg) seem to have better analgesia properties, these must be balanced with increased sedation.

N-METHYL-D-ASPARTATE RECEPTOR ANTAGONISTS

NMDA receptor antagonists are a class of drugs that work to antagonize or inhibit the action of the NMDA receptor. The NMDA receptor is an ionotropic receptor that allows for transfer of electrical signals between neurons in the brain and in the spinal column. Glutamate, which is released with noxious peripheral stimuli, bind to the receptors and open the channel, allowing for electrical signals to pass. The activation of the NMDA receptors has been associated with hyperalgesia, neuropathic pain, and reduced functionality of opioid receptors. Hyperalgesia and neuropathic pain come from increased spinal neuron sensitization, leading to a heightened level of pain.[65] Therefore, NMDA antagonists may have a role in modulating pain in these areas. There are several NMDA receptor antagonists including ketamine, dextromethorphan, memantine, and magnesium.

Ketamine was first synthesized in 1962 by Calvin Stevens. After promising research in animals, it was first introduced in humans in 1964. The first ketamine anesthesia was given to American soldiers during the Vietnam War in 1970.

In medical settings, ketamine is usually injected intravenously or intramuscularly. Ketamine can be started using the oral route, or people may be changed from a subcutaneous infusion once pain is controlled. Oral ketamine is broken down by bile acids, thus it has low bioavailability.[66] Often lozenges prepared by a compounding pharmacy are used to address this issue. Ketamine is a racemic mixture. The S (+) ketamine is three to four times more active than the R (−) form and is associated with fewer psychiatric adverse effects.[34] Ketamine is a noncompetitive NMDA receptor antagonist and is activated with intense pain stimuli; it has been shown to inhibit tumor necrosis factor-α and interleukin-6 gene expressions in lipopolysaccharide-activated macrophages.[67] It is likely that ketamine's antihyperalgesic effects are due to the modulation of proinflammatory cytokine production.[68,69]

Studies have shown that ketamine is effective in reducing hyperalgesia. These results are seen only in systemic administration of ketamine, indicating that neuraxial administration is not the route of choice.[70] In the study, subanesthetic doses of IV ketamine (0.5 mg/kg bolus followed by 0.25 mg/kg/h) given during anesthesia reduced wound hyperalgesia, significantly lowered PCA requirements, and resulted in less residual pain through six months of follow-up. Elia and Tramer performed a meta-analysis of 16 trials (889 patients) showing that IV ketamine started preincision with an average dose of 0.4mg/kg reduced pain intensity and morphine consumption at 24 hours with a WMD of −15.7mg.[71] Laskowski et al. looked at 4,701 patients in a meta-analysis in 2011 for ketamine groups versus placebo groups. The study showed particular benefit was observed in painful procedures, with a decrease in total opioid consumption with a standard difference in means of −0.631 mg, a decrease in pain intensity, and an increase in time to first rescue analgesic.[72] This was collaborated by a Cochrane Database review of 37 trials, where using ketamine doses of 0.15 to 1.0 mg/kg reduced rescue analgesic requirements, pain intensity, and 24-hour morphine PCA consumption with a mean difference of −15.08 mg.[73] Even in postincision administration, ketamine has been shown to have preventative effects with an observed significant reduction in pain and analgesic consumption beyond the clinical duration of ketamine in doses of 0.5 to 1 mg/kg regardless of pre- or postincision.[74] Patients with a history of chronic high-dose opioid use when given a ketamine infusion of 10 ug/kg/min intraoperatively saw reduced opioid consumption and pain intensity at one day, two days, and six weeks after surgery with a 71% lower opioid consumption compared with placebo and a decreased VAS score of 3.1 from 4.2.[75]

High doses of ketamine can lead to neuropsychiatric effects including agitation, nightmares, abnormal dreams, hallucinations, catatonia, dysphoria, and hypertonia. However, these effects are more dose-dependent, and lower doses of ketamine have a much lower incidence. Overall, it seems the use of ketamine in general anesthesia does not have significant side effects with the NNH in one study for the risk of hallucinations at 286. In a meta-analysis of 24 studies,[74] 12 showed no adverse effects, 7 found no difference in adverse effects between control and treatment groups, and 1 found an increase in psychomimetic effects related to epidural use of ketamine. This is supported further in a 37-trial study where 21 trials specifically reported no psychomimetic side

Dextromethorphan

Dextromethorphan is of the morphinan class, a D-isomer of the codeine analog levorphanol, most commonly used as an antitussive. It possesses only weak affinity to μ-opioid receptors and has no analgesic effect. It is a noncompetitive NMDA antagonist and has pain modulation abilities.[68] Dextromethorphan comes as a liquid-filled capsule, a chewable tablet, a dissolving strip, a solution, an extended-release suspension, and a lozenge to take by mouth. One study specifically looking at the effect of preoperative oral dextromethorphan after hysterectomy showed a 30% reduced use of PCA morphine from zero to four hours after operation in patients receiving dextromethorphan 150 mg one hour before surgery but no effect on hyperalgesia surrounding the surgical wound, nor did it reduced residual postoperative pain from 5 to 24 hours postoperatively.[76] In a 2006 systemic review of 28 studies,[77] patients receiving dextromethorphan seemed to report less pain in the early postoperative period with significant decreases in time to first analgesic request and supplemental opioid consumption in the majority of parenteral dextromethorphan studies and in about one-half of the oral studies. The study concluded that it was not possible to state the consistency of dextromethorphan's potential opioid-sparing and pain-reducing effects, and the authors could not recommend a dose regimen or routine clinical use guidelines regarding its use in postoperative pain, but they suggested that more consistent results can be observed when dextromethorphan is given via the parenteral route, because the oral bioavailability of the drug is low and oral administration leads to extensive first-pass metabolism. There was no statistical difference between adverse effects related to either opioids or dextromethorphan.[28] Side effects of dextromethorphan include blurred vision, confusion, difficulty in urination, drowsiness, nausea or vomiting, unsteadiness, unusual excitement, and slowed breathing.

Magnesium

Magnesium ion is also a noncompetitive NMDA antagonist. Magnesium can be given via IV, intramuscularly, and oral preparations. Studies have shown no direct analgesic effect, but magnesium ions seem to have synergistic effects. In an animal study, magnesium significantly increased morphine analgesia regardless of loading dose used (30 or 90 mg/kg).[78] It also potentiates morphine analgesia when co-administered intrathecally in an incisional pain model allodynia, suggesting intrathecal administration of magnesium sulfate may be a useful adjunct to spinal morphine analgesia and that it acts on the spinal NMDA receptors.[79] In humans, magnesium ion has a limited ability to cross the blood-brain barrier and reach the CSF, and IV infusion of magnesium does not increase CSF magnesium concentration or improve pain management.[80] This is further supported by several other studies which did not show any reduction of postoperative pain and analgesic requirement after perioperative IV magnesium sulfate (50 mg/kg bolus dose followed by continuous infusion of 15/mg/kg/h for six hours).[80–82] But although magnesium seems to only have minimal or no analgesic effect, the combination of ketamine and magnesium acts in a super-additive manner and may provide more effective analgesics than either compound alone without exceeding safe doses of each medication.[83] High doses of magnesium might cause build-up in the body, leading to stomach upset, nausea, vomiting, diarrhea, and serious side effects including irregular heartbeat, low blood pressure, confusion, slowed breathing, coma, and death. Doses less than 350 mg daily are safe for most adults.

Memantine

Memantin was first synthesized in the 1960s and is an NMDA receptor antagonist. The major site of action is the blockade of current flow through the NMDA receptor channel. Memantine is completely absorbed from the gastrointestinal tract with maximal plasma concentration occurring between three and eight hours after oral administration with a half-life of 6-=100 hours. Because it is orally administered, it could be a more useful analgesia adjunct. Schley et al. showed daily doses of memantine 30 mg decreased phantom pain temporarily by up to 80% at one month following upper extremity amputations in combination with brachial plexus block.[84] Memantine is well tolerated; instances of psychotic side effects have been reported though their incidence is low.

Summary

Ketamine has analgesia effects and reduces opioid use when given at subanesthetic doses (≤ 1 mg/kg bolus and 0.25 ug/kg/min infusion) and is much more evident in more painful surgeries. Psychiatric assessment must be carefully followed and the drug stopped if found to have any negative impact. The other NMDA receptor antagonists may need further study to clarify their positive effects.

GLUCOCORTICOIDS

Glucocorticoids, such as dexamethasone, have extensive therapeutic potential to treat many inflammatory and autoimmune conditions with an increased expression of inflammatory genes from cytokines, enzymes, receptors, and adhesion molecules, including asthma, inflammatory bowel diseases, rheumatoid arthritis, and autoimmune disease. Dexamethasone can be given in IV and oral routes. Glucocorticoids can modulate several components of the inflammatory response to surgery. Glucocorticoids inhibit expression of multiple inflammatory genes. This is most likely due to a direct inhibitory interaction between activated glucocorticoid receptors and activated transcription factors, such as nuclear factor-kappa B and activator protein-1 that regulate the inflammatory gene expression.[85] It also increases transcription of glucocorticoid-responsive genes by binding to glucocorticoid-response elements, thus increasing the transcription of gene coding for anti-inflammatory proteins from liocortin-1, interleukin-10, interleukin-1 receptor antagonist, and neutral endopeptidase.[85] Studies have also shown that it has antiemetic properties and is commonly used for the prevention of postoperative nausea and vomiting.[86–88] The onset of dexamethasone is thought to be one to two hours, allowing time to diffuse across the cell membrane and alter gene transcription.[89]

Dexamethasone

A meta-analysis of 45 studies in patients receiving 1.25 to 20 mg of intraoperative dexamethasone found that a single dose of IV perioperative dexamethasone had small but statistically significant analgesic benefits.[90] The study showed patients receiving dexamethasone had lower pain scores at two hours with a mean difference of −0.49 and at 24 hours with a mean difference of −4.8 after surgery. Dexamethasone-treated patients also used less opioids at two hours (about a 13% decrease in pooled opioid consumption) and 24 hours (a 10.3% reduction) and required less rescue analgesia, had a longer time to first dose of analgesic, and had shorter stays in the PACU. This study, however, did not find a dose response with regard to the opioid-sparing effect.[90] An earlier meta-analysis of 24 studies, however, showed the use of doses less than 0.1 mg/kg dexamethasone did not reduce pain scores or opioid consumption.[91] A meta-analysis of five studies looking at the effect of epidural dexamethasone showed a significant decrease in postoperative morphine consumption, with a mean difference of −7.89 mg, and a reduction in number of patients who required postoperative rescue analgesic boluses.[92] This study stated the optimum epidural dose of dexamethasone is unclear, although 4 to 8 mg seems to be the ideal dosing for significant opioid-sparing effects.

Glucocorticoid use is associated with many adverse effects, although most of these are in the setting of prolonged or high-dose glucocorticoid use. Some of the concerns in the use of glucocorticoid in operative patients include wound infection, gastrointestinal complications, delayed healing, avascular bone necrosis, and hyperglycemia. Multiple studies have shown no increase in infection associated with steroid administration.[87,88,93] Significant gastrointestinal complications including perforation and bleeding are seen only with dexamethasone at high doses (16–100 mg) and long-time (24 days) use.[94] Prolonged use of dexamethasone is also associated with avascular necrosis of the femoral head but has not been described with a single low-dose of dexamethasone.[28,95] A single perioperative dose of dexamethasone also does not impair wound healing and is not a concern for impaired wound healing.[96] This is supported by two additional retrospective studies showing no evidence of significant delayed wound healing in patients undergoing orbital wall factures or mandibular factures repairs.[97,98] There is a significant increase in blood glucose even with low-dose dexamethasone, although the clinical significance of this hyperglycemia is unclear; this does warrant more cautious use in diabetes mellitus patients.[90]

Summary

There is certainly potentially important biologic modifiers of perioperative inflammatory responses to dexamethasone use, and there is evidence that high-dose dexamethasone has an analgesic effect. There is also evidence that a small single dose of dexamethasone used for nausea and vomiting (4–8mg) also has opioid-sparing and analgesic effects. Anti-inflammatory effects of dexamethasone have been demonstrated in many procedures, but administration later than one to two hours before surgery is likely too late to benefit patients. Patients with diabetes mellitus or a history of poor wound healing may have an increased risk of such complications, and clinicians may choose to avoid the use of dexamethasone in these patients.

CONCLUSION

Postoperative pain for patients is a real issue that not only affects the comfort of patients but also can lead to physiological changes that impede recovery. Traditional opioid medications for pain control can lead to their own complications and further complicate recovery. Adjuvant medications have been demonstrated to be beneficial in perioperative pain care and to reduce reliance on traditional analgesics such as opioid medications. Importantly, these adjuvant medications may result in a reduced risk for development of dependency, addiction, or toxicity. We discussed the use of NMDA receptor antagonists, gabapentinoids, A-2 agonists, and dexamethasone and their positive effects on pain. The overall idea of using adjuvant medications for pain management is to optimize comfort and recovery for patients. By using the synergistic or additive effects of these adjuvants, we can use lower dosages of certain medications and thus accomplish greater pain control with less likelihood of side effects. An astute pain medicine physician would be well advised to add them to their armamentarium.

REFERENCES

1. Page GG. The immune-suppressive effects of pain. *Adv Exp Med Biol*. 2003;521:117–125.
2. Joshi GP, Ogunnaike BO. Consequences of inadequate postoperative pain relief and chronic persistent postoperative pain. *Anesthesiol Clin N Am*. 2005;23(1):21–36.
3. Rosenfeld BA, Faraday N, Campbell D, Dise K, Bell W, Goldschmidt P. Hemostatic effects of stress hormone infusion. *Anesthesiology*. 1994;81(5):1116–1126.
4. Katz J, Jackson M, Kavanagh PB, Sandler AN. Acute pain after thoracic surgery predicts long-term post-thoracotomy pain. *Clin J Pain*. 1996;12(1):50–55.
5. Pyati S, Gan TJ. Perioperative pain management. *CNS Drugs*. 2007;21(3):185–211.
6. Dolin SJ, Cashman JN. Tolerability of acute postoperative pain management: nausea, vomiting, sedation, pruritus, and urinary retention. Evidence from published data. *Br J Anaesth*. 2005;95(5):584–591.
7. Tiippana EM, Hamunen K, Kontinen VK, Kalso E. Do surgical patients benefit from perioperative gabapentin/pregabalin? A systematic review of efficacy and safety. *Anesth Analg*. 2007;104(6):1545–1556.
8. Ghosh R, Alajbegovic A, Gomes AV. NSAIDs and cardiovascular diseases: role of reactive oxygen species. *Oxid Med Cell Longev*. 2015;2015:536962.
9. Buvanendran A, Kroin JS, Tuman KJ, et al. Effects of perioperative administration of a selective cyclooxygenase 2 inhibitor on pain management and recovery of function after knee replacement: a randomized controlled trial. *JAMA*. 2003;290(18):2411–2418.
10. Shen B, Yang J, Zhou Z-K, Pei F-X, Tang X, Li Y, Kang PD. [Effects of perioperative administration of celecoxib on pain management and recovery of function after total knee replacement]. *Zhonghua Wai Ke Za Zhi*. 2009;47(2):116–119.
11. White PF, Sacan O, Tufanogullari B, Eng M, Nuangchamnong N, Ogunnaike B. Effect of short-term postoperative celecoxib administration on patient outcome after outpatient laparoscopic surgery. *Can J Anaesth*. 2007;54(5):342–348.
12. Buvanendran A, Kroin JS. Multimodal analgesia for controlling acute postoperative pain. *Curr Opin Anaesthesiol*. 2009;22(5):588–593.
13. Buvanendran A, Kroin JS, Berger RA, et al. Upregulation of prostaglandin E2 and interleukins in the central nervous system and peripheral tissue during and after surgery in humans. *Anesthesiology*. 2006;104(3):403–410.

14. Practice guidelines for acute pain management in the perioperative setting: an updated report by the American Society of Anesthesiologists Task Force on Acute Pain Management. *Anesthesiology.* 2012;116(2):248–273. practice-guidelines-for-acute-pain-management-in-the-perioperative-setting.pdf

15. Giovannoni MP, Ghelardini C, Vergelli C, Dal Piaz V. Alpha2-agonists as analgesic agents. *Med Res Rev.* 2009;29(2):339–368.

16. De Sarro GB, Ascioti C, Froio F, Libri V, Nisticò G. Evidence that locus coeruleus is the site where clonidine and drugs acting at alpha 1- and alpha 2-adrenoceptors affect sleep and arousal mechanisms. *Br J Pharmacol.* 1987;90(4):675–685.

17. Engelhard K, Kasper S, Werner C, et al. Effect of the alpha2-agonist dexmedetomidine on cerebral neurotransmitter concentrations during cerebral ischemia in rats. *Anesthesiology.* 2002;96(2):450–457.

18. Hansson E. Could chronic pain and spread of pain sensation be induced and maintained by glial activation? *Acta Physiol.* 2006;187(1–2):321–327.

19. McMahon SB, Malcangio M. Current challenges in glia-pain biology. *Neuron.* 2009;64(1):46–54.

20. Ren K, Dubner R. Neuron-glia crosstalk gets serious: role in pain hypersensitivity. *Curr Opin Anaesthesiol.* 2008;21(5):570–579.

21. Watkins LR, Milligan ED, Maier SF. Glial activation: a driving force for pathological pain. *Trends Neurosci.* 2001;24(8):450–455.

22. Mika J, Osikowicz M, Rojewska E, et al. Differential activation of spinal microglial and astroglial cells in a mouse model of peripheral neuropathic pain. *Eur J Pharmacol.* 2009;623(1–3):65–72.

23. Xu M, Bruchas MR, Ippolito DL, Gendron L, Chavkin C. Sciatic nerve ligation-induced proliferation of spinal cord astrocytes is mediated by kappa opioid activation of p38 mitogen-activated protein kinase. *J Neurosci.* 2007;27(10):2570–2581.

24. Obata H, Eisenach JC, Hussain H, Bynum T, Vincler M. Spinal glial activation contributes to postoperative mechanical hypersensitivity in the rat. *J Pain.* 2006;7(11):816–822.

25. Lena P, Balarac N, Lena D, et al. Fast-track anesthesia with remifentanil and spinal analgesia for cardiac surgery: the effect on pain control and quality of recovery. *J Cardiothorac Vasc Anesth.* 2008;22(4):536–542.

26. Blaudszun G, Lysakowski C, Elia N, Tramèr MR. Effect of perioperative systemic alpha2 agonists on postoperative morphine consumption and pain intensity: systematic review and meta-analysis of randomized controlled trials. *Anesthesiology.* 2012;116(6):1312–1322.

27. Wijeysundera DN, Bender JS, Beattie WS. Alpha-2 adrenergic agonists for the prevention of cardiac complications among patients undergoing surgery. *Cochrane Database Syst Rev.* 2009(4):CD004126.

28. Low YH, Gan TJ. NMDA receptor antagonists, gabapentinoids, alpha-2 agonists, and dexamethasone and other non-opioid adjuvants: do they have a role in plastic surgery? *Plast Reconstr Surg.* 2014;134(4 Suppl 2):69S–82S.

29. Schnabel A, Meyer-Frießem CH, Reichl SU, et al. Is intraoperative dexmedetomidine a new option for postoperative pain treatment? A meta-analysis of randomized controlled trials. *Pain.* 2013;154(7):1140–1149.

30. Ramadhyani U, Park JL, Carollo DS, et al. Dexmedetomidine: clinical application as an adjunct for intravenous regional anesthesia. *Anesthesiol Clin.* 2010;28(4):709–722.

31. Tufanogullari B, White PF, Peixoto MP, et al. Dexmedetomidine infusion during laparoscopic bariatric surgery: the effect on recovery outcome variables. *Anesth Analg.* 2008;106(6):1741–1748.

32. Dworkin RH, Backonja M, Rowbotham MC, et al. Advances in neuropathic pain: diagnosis, mechanisms, and treatment recommendations. *Arch Neurol.* 2003;60(11):1524–1534.

33. Schmidt PC, Ruchelli G, Mackey SC, et al. Perioperative gabapentinoids: choice of agent, dose, timing, and effects on chronic postsurgical pain. *Anesthesiology.* 2013;119(5):1215–1221.

34. Weinbroum AA. Non-opioid IV adjuvants in the perioperative period: pharmacological and clinical aspects of ketamine and gabapentinoids. *Pharmacol Res.* 2012;65(4):411–429.

35. Iannetti GD, Zambreanu L, Wise RG, et al. Pharmacological modulation of pain-related brain activity during normal and central sensitization states in humans. *Proc Natl Acad Sci U S A.* 2005;102(50):18195–18200.

36. Gilron I. Is gabapentin a "broad-spectrum" analgesic? *Anesthesiology.* 2002;97(3): 537–539.

37. Hayashida K, DeGoes S, Curry R, et al. Gabapentin activates spinal noradrenergic activity in rats and humans and reduces hypersensitivity after surgery. *Anesthesiology.* 2007;106(3):557–562.

38. Werner MU, Perkins FM, Holte K, et al. Effects of gabapentin in acute inflammatory pain in humans. *Reg Anesth Pain Med.* 2001;26(4):322–328.

39. Blum RA, Comstock TJ, Sica DA, et al. Pharmacokinetics of gabapentin in subjects with various degrees of renal function. *Clin Pharmacol Ther.* 1994;56(2):154–159.

40. Stewart BH, Kugler AR, Thompson PR, et al. A saturable transport mechanism in the intestinal absorption of gabapentin is the underlying cause of the lack of proportionality between increasing dose and drug levels in plasma. *Pharm Res.* 1993;10(2):276–281.

41. Richens A. Clinical pharmacokinetics of gabapentin. In: Chadwick D, ed. *New Trends in Epilepsy Management: The Role of Gabapentin.* London: Royal Society of Medicine;1993:41–46.

42. Rose MA, Kam PC. Gabapentin: pharmacology and its use in pain management. *Anaesthesia.* 2002;57(5):451–462.

43. Ben-Menachem E, Persson LI, Hedner T. Selected CSF biochemistry and gabapentin concentrations in the CSF and plasma in patients with partial seizures after a single oral dose of gabapentin. *Epilepsy Res.* 1992;11(1):45–49.

44. Ben-Menachem E, Söderfelt B, Hamberger A, et al. Seizure frequency and CSF parameters in a double-blind placebo controlled trial of gabapentin in patients with intractable complex partial seizures. *Epilepsy Res.* 1995;21(3):231–236.

45. Busch JA, Radulovic LL, Bockbrader HN, et al. Effect of Maalox TC on single-dose pharmacokinetics of gabapentin capsules in healthy subjects. *Pharm Res.* 1992;9(Suppl 2):S315.

46. Wong MO, E.M., Keane WF, et al. Disposition of gabapentin in anuric subjects on hemodialysis. *J Clin Pharmacol.* 1995;35:622–626.

47. Dirks J, Fredensborg BB, Christensen D, et al. A randomized study of the effects of single-dose gabapentin versus placebo on postoperative pain and morphine consumption after mastectomy. *Anesthesiology.* 2002;97(3):560–564.

48. Clarke H, Pereira S, Kennedy D, et al. Gabapentin decreases morphine consumption and improves functional recovery following total knee arthroplasty. *Pain Res Manag.* 2009;14(3):217–222.

49. Ho KY, Gan TJ, Habib AS. Gabapentin and postoperative pain--a systematic review of randomized controlled trials. *Pain.* 2006;126(1–3):91–101.

50. Hurley RW, Cohen SP, Williams KA, et al. The analgesic effects of perioperative gabapentin on postoperative pain: a meta-analysis. *Reg Anesth Pain Med.* 2006;31(3):237–247.

51. Peng PW, Wijeysundera DN, Li CC. Use of gabapentin for perioperative pain control—a meta-analysis. *Pain Res Manag.* 2007;12(2):85–92.

52. Seib RK, Paul JE. Preoperative gabapentin for postoperative analgesia: a meta-analysis. *Can J Anaesth.* 2006;53(5):461–469.

53. Turan A, Karamanlioğlu B, Memiş D, et al. The analgesic effects of gabapentin after total abdominal hysterectomy. *Anesth Analg.* 2004;98(5):1370–1373.

54. Mathiesen O, Moiniche S, Dahl JB. Gabapentin and postoperative pain: a qualitative and quantitative systematic review, with focus on procedure. *BMC Anesthesiol.* 2007;7:6.

55. Zhang J, Ho KY, Wang Y. Efficacy of pregabalin in acute postoperative pain: a meta-analysis. *Br J Anaesth.* 2011;106(4):454–462.

56. Piyapolrungroj N, Li C, Bockbrader H, et al. Mucosal uptake of gabapentin (Neurontin) vs. pregabalin in the small intestine. *Pharm Res.* 2001;18(8):1126–1130.

57. Randinitis EJ, Posvar EL, Alvey CW, et al. Pharmacokinetics of pregabalin in subjects with various degrees of renal function. *J Clin Pharmacol.* 2003;43(3):277–283.

58. Buvanendran A, Kroin JS, Kari M, et al. Can a single dose of 300 mg of pregabalin reach acute antihyperalgesic levels in the central nervous system? *Reg Anesth Pain Med.* 2010;35(6):535–538.

59. Engelman E, Cateloy F. Efficacy and safety of perioperative pregabalin for postoperative pain: a meta-analysis of randomized-controlled trials. *Acta Anaesthesiol Scand.* 2011;55(8):927–943.

60. Agarwal A, Gautam S, Gupta D, et al. Evaluation of a single preoperative dose of pregabalin for attenuation of postoperative pain after laparoscopic cholecystectomy. *Br J Anaesth.* 2008;101(5):700–704.

61. Hill CM, Balkenohl M, Thomas DW, et al. Pregabalin in patients with postoperative dental pain. *Eur J Pain.* 2001;5(2):119–124.

62. Ghai A, Gupta M, Hooda S, et al. A randomized controlled trial to compare pregabalin with gabapentin for postoperative pain in abdominal hysterectomy. *Saudi J Anaesth.* 2011;5(3):252–257.

63. Ozgencil E, Yalcin S, Tuna H, et al. Perioperative administration of gabapentin 1,200 mg day-1 and pregabalin 300 mg day-1 for pain following lumbar laminectomy and discectomy: a randomised, double-blinded, placebo-controlled study. *Singapore Med J.* 2011;52(12):883–889.

64. Clarke H, Bonin RP, Orser BA, et al. The prevention of chronic postsurgical pain using gabapentin and pregabalin: a combined systematic review and meta-analysis. *Anesth Analg.* 2012;115(2):428–442.

65. Bennett GJ. Update on the neurophysiology of pain transmission and modulation: focus on the NMDA-receptor. *J Pain Symptom Manage.* 2000;19(1 Suppl):S2–S6.

66. Lankenau SE, Sanders B, Bloom JJ, et al. First injection of ketamine among young injection drug users (IDUs) in three U.S. cities. *Drug Alcohol Depend.* 2007;87(2–3):183–193.

67. Wu GJ, Chen TL, Ueng YF, et al. Ketamine inhibits tumor necrosis factor-alpha and interleukin-6 gene expressions in lipopolysaccharide-stimulated macrophages through suppression of toll-like receptor 4-mediated c-Jun N-terminal kinase phosphorylation and activator protein-1 activation. *Toxicol Appl Pharmacol.* 2008;228(1):105–113.

68. De Kock MF, Lavand'homme PM. The clinical role of NMDA receptor antagonists for the treatment of postoperative pain. *Best Pract Res Clin Anaesthesiol.* 2007;21(1):85–98.

69. Kawamata T, Omote K, Sonoda H, et al. Analgesic mechanisms of ketamine in the presence and absence of peripheral inflammation. *Anesthesiology*. 2000;93(2):520–528.

70. De Kock M, Lavand'homme P, Waterloos H. "Balanced analgesia" in the perioperative period: is there a place for ketamine? *Pain*. 2001;92(3):373–380.

71. Elia N, Tramer MR. Ketamine and postoperative pain--a quantitative systematic review of randomised trials. *Pain*. 2005;113(1–2):61–70.

72. Laskowski K, Stirling A, McKay WP, et al. A systematic review of intravenous ketamine for postoperative analgesia. *Can J Anaesth*. 2011;58(10):911–923.

73. Bell RF, Dahl JB, Moore RA, et al. Perioperative ketamine for acute postoperative pain. *Cochrane Database Syst Rev*. 2006;1:CD004603.

74. McCartney CJ, Sinha A, Katz J. A qualitative systematic review of the role of N-methyl-D-aspartate receptor antagonists in preventive analgesia. *Anesth Analg*. 2004;98(5):1385–1400.

75. Loftus RW, Yeager MP, Clark JA, et al. Intraoperative ketamine reduces perioperative opiate consumption in opiate-dependent patients with chronic back pain undergoing back surgery. *Anesthesiology*. 2010;113(3):639–646.

76. Ilkjaer S, Bach LF, Nielsen PA, et al. Effect of preoperative oral dextromethorphan on immediate and late postoperative pain and hyperalgesia after total abdominal hysterectomy. *Pain*. 2000;86(1–2):19–24.

77. Duedahl TH, Rømsing J, Møiniche S, et al. A qualitative systematic review of perioperative dextromethorphan in post-operative pain. *Acta Anaesthesiol Scand*. 2006;50(1):1–13.

78. Begon S., Pickering G, Eschalier A, et al. Magnesium increases morphine analgesic effect in different experimental models of pain. *Anesthesiology*. 2002;96(3):627–632.

79. Kroin JS, McCarthy RJ, Von Roenn N, et al. Magnesium sulfate potentiates morphine antinociception at the spinal level. *Anesth Analg*. 2000;90(4):913–917.

80. Ko SH, Lim HR, Kim DC, et al. Magnesium sulfate does not reduce postoperative analgesic requirements. *Anesthesiology*. 2001;95(3):640–646.

81. Paech MJ, Magann EF, Doherty DA, et al. Does magnesium sulfate reduce the short- and long-term requirements for pain relief after caesarean delivery? A double-blind placebo-controlled trial. *Am J Obstet Gynecol*. 2006;194(6):1596–1602; discussion 1602–1603.

82. Wilder-Smith CH, Knopfli R, Wilder-Smith OH. Perioperative magnesium infusion and postoperative pain. *Acta Anaesthesiol Scand*. 1997;41(8):1023–1027.

83. Liu HT, Hollmann MW, Liu WH, et al. Modulation of NMDA receptor function by ketamine and magnesium: Part I. *Anesth Analg*. 2001;92(5):1173–1181.

84. Schley M., Topfner S, Wiech K, et al. Continuous brachial plexus blockade in combination with the NMDA receptor antagonist memantine prevents phantom pain in acute traumatic upper limb amputees. *Eur J Pain*. 2007;11(3):299–308.

85. Barnes PJ. Anti-inflammatory actions of glucocorticoids: molecular mechanisms. *Clin Sci*. 1998;94(6):557–572.

86. Gan TJ, Meyer TA, Apfel CC, et al. Society for Ambulatory Anesthesia guidelines for the management of postoperative nausea and vomiting. *Anesth Analg*. 2007;105(6):1615–1628.

87. Henzi I, Walder B, Tramer MR. Dexamethasone for the prevention of postoperative nausea and vomiting: a quantitative systematic review. *Anesth Analg*. 2000;90(1):186–194.

88. Holte K, Kehlet H. Perioperative single-dose glucocorticoid administration: pathophysiologic effects and clinical implications. *J Am Coll Surg*. 2002;195(5):694–712.

89. Sapolsky RM, Romero LM, Munck AU. How do glucocorticoids influence stress responses? Integrating permissive, suppressive, stimulatory, and preparative actions. *Endocr Rev.* 2000;21(1):55–89.

90. Waldron NH, Jones CA, Gan TJ, et al. Impact of perioperative dexamethasone on postoperative analgesia and side-effects: systematic review and meta-analysis. *Br J Anaesth.* 2013;110(2):191–200.

91. De Oliveira GS Jr, Almeida MD, Benzon HT, et al. Perioperative single dose systemic dexamethasone for postoperative pain: a meta-analysis of randomized controlled trials. *Anesthesiology.* 2011;115(3):575–588.

92. Jebaraj B, Khanna P, Baidya DK, et al. Efficacy of epidural local anesthetic and dexamethasone in providing postoperative analgesia: A meta-analysis. *Saudi J Anaesth.* 2016;10(3):322–327.

93. Sauerland S, Nagelschmidt M, Mallmann P, et al. Risks and benefits of preoperative high dose methylprednisolone in surgical patients: a systematic review. *Drug Saf.* 2000;23(5):449–461.

94. Fadul CE, Lemann W, Thaler HT, et al. Perforation of the gastrointestinal tract in patients receiving steroids for neurologic disease. *Neurology.* 1988;38(3):348–352.

95. Gogas H, Fennelly D. Avascular necrosis following extensive chemotherapy and dexamethasone treatment in a patient with advanced ovarian cancer: case report and review of the literature. *Gynecol Oncol.* 1996;63(3):379–381.

96. Ali Khan S, McDonagh DL, Gan TJ. Wound complications with dexamethasone for postoperative nausea and vomiting prophylaxis: a moot point? *Anesth Analg.* 2013;116(5):966–968.

97. Snall J, Kormi E, Lindqvist C, et al. Impairment of wound healing after operative treatment of mandibular fractures, and the influence of dexamethasone. *Br J Oral Maxillofac Surg.* 2013;51(8):808–812.

98. Thoren H., Snäll J, Kormi E, et al. Does perioperative glucocorticosteroid treatment correlate with disturbance in surgical wound healing after treatment of facial fractures? A retrospective study. *J Oral Maxillofac Surg.* 2009;67(9):1884–1888.

3 Barriers to Optimal Pain Management in the General Surgery Population

Anand C. Thakur

Albert Schweitzer once said, "We must always die. But that I can save a person from days of torture, that is what I feel is my great and ever-new privilege. Pain is a more terrible lord of mankind than even death itself."

Pain as described and defined by the International Association for the Study of Pain is "An unpleasant sensory and emotional experience associated with actual or potential tissue damage, or described in terms of such damage."

There has been a 30-year-plus assessment by multiple national health organizations and societies examining the factors which influence the treatment of pain in both the acute and chronic setting, adequate versus inadequate pain relief, and long-term and short-term pain management. Organizations such as the American Pain Society (APS), the Joint Commission on Accreditation of Healthcare Organizations (JCAHO) and the American Society of Anesthesiology (ASA) have helped the initial and on-going efforts and in this constantly changing and challenging environment.[1,2] In 2005, the APS made revisions with an expanded and updated reform of its 1999 criteria and recommendations regarding the management of acute postoperative and cancer pain.[1,2]

Revised APS standard recommendations focus on a safety driven, cost-effective, efficacious, patient-centered interdisciplinary approach with emphasis on improved assessment and cultural appropriateness and with a basis in evidence-based medicine.[1]

JCAHO has also focused on pain management with analysis of metrics that evaluate pain assessment and progress throughout the entire hospitalization stay encompassing initial evaluation, ongoing care, and discharge planning. Particular focus was also placed on education of doctors, nurses, and other team members upon the nature, subtype, and qualitative and quantitative assessment of pain.[2,4]

In 2012 the ASA presented updated criteria regarding safe and effective pain management in the perioperative time period, maintenance of the patient's function and well-being, reduction of potential adverse outcomes, and improvement of the patient's quality of life in the perioperative period.[3]

Unfortunately, despite the ongoing education reforms, attempts of standardization of care and updating of pathways, guidelines, and assessment strategies there continues to be a significant population of patients that continues to suffer from inadequate pain relief.[4,5]

There are significant barriers to the implementation of what is deemed to be adequate pain relief. We examine these significant barriers to pain management in the acute postoperative general surgery population. For the purposes of this chapter we allow general surgery to encompass both general surgical and subspecialty surgical populations. It would be quite difficult to stratify and separate each surgical subspeciality in regards to the specific surgical procedure and concomitant postoperative pain management. That would be beyond the scope of this chapter.

Suffice it to say that postsurgical pain regardless of the anatomical location and specific operation pathophysiologically travels the similar pain spinothalamic pathways and has similar treatment options medically and procedurally.

Barriers to the implementation of adequate pain control are multifactorial and extensive. A complete list of barriers to adequate pain control would involve biopsychosocial factors, the physiological factors, pharmacological concerns, and medical legal concerns that could compose a book itself.

A short list of barriers to adequate pain control can be separated into physician knowledge, expectations and perceptions, nurses' and other ancillary providers' knowledge, expectations and perceptions, patient expectations and perception, management of acute pain, management of chronic pain, discrepancies of pain perception and different population groups, and both regulatory and formulary issues.

Based on 2010 estimates, in the United States there were approximately 4,647 operations per 100,000 people.[6] Extrapolating to today's population of approximately 324 million, there are approximately 15 million operations in the United States performed yearly. We define a surgical operation as an operation that necessitates a general anesthetic, regional anesthetic, and/or a combination of both. This is a significant number of surgical patients with multiple outcomes and varying functional needs that require adequate and definitive postoperative pain management and control. Acute postoperative pain is experienced by greater than 80% of patients who undergo surgical procedures and about 70% of the population has described that pain as moderate, severe, or extremely painful. Less than 50% of patients who undergo surgery report adequate pain relief.[5] When pain is less than adequately controlled, there is a risk of transition from acute (less than 12weeks) to chronic pain (greater than 12 weeks), increased risk of postsurgical complications, decreased quality of life, and decreased functional recovery postsurgery.

Pain relief has been recognized as a basic human right according to the World Health Organization and the International Association for the Study of Pain.[7] Postoperative pain can be best addressed by a multimodal approach. A standard approach in the treatment of postoperative pain involves a complete history and physical with particular emphasis on functionality, age, and physician understanding of pain generators, as well as current opioid, non-opioid, and adjuvant medications, along with previously failed opioid and non-opioid medication.

Pain management during surgery is divided into three phases: the preoperative, intraoperative, and postoperative. Assessment of the baseline opioid usage, scope, and duration of the surgical procedure and anatomic regions of the body affected by this operation are evaluated during the preoperative phase. The next stage involves an intraoperative management by the anesthesiologist of the analgesic requirement commensurate to the operative procedure and its dynamic changes. The third stage postoperatively involves appropriate use of oral or intravenous non-opioid and/or opioid-related medication options in a scheduled versus as-needed dosing format. In some studies, intravenous acetaminophen has been shown to have an opioid dose-sparing effect of almost 20%.[8,9] Patient-controlled analgesia via intravenous fixed-dose opioid basal dosing and demand dosing is also an option. Anesthetic regional and/or neuraxial anesthetic either single-dose blockade and continuous dosing catheters are other options which allow us to minimize pain and discomfort the pain postoperatively.

The net sum result of well-managed, multimodal perioperative pain management can lead to a decrease in negative potential postoperative outcomes such as tachycardia, hypertension, myocardial infarction, decreased alveolar ventilation, and poor wound healing,[10] as well as a potential decreased hospital stay.[3,11–15]

The negative effects of undertreated pain in the postoperative patient can lead to multiple adverse outcomes. Inadequate postsurgical pain relief can lead to increases and catecholamines, heart rate, and systemic vascular resistance with an endpoint of increased risk of myocardial ischemia postoperative bleeding, stroke, and other adverse postoperative outcomes.

Also, the undertreatment of acute postoperative pain can cause pathophysiological changes in neural pathways leading to both peripheral and central neural sensitization, that ultimately have an endpoint of chronic pain. Chronic pain further devolves into psychologic, social, and familial outcomes which are maladaptive. Physiologically chronic pain can lead to immune dysfunction, sleep disturbances, limited mobility, functional impairment, codependency, and untoward secondary gain behavior. This constellation of biopsychosocial factors is a basic disease entity.

Studies have shown that physicians, nurses, and other members of the interdisciplinary health care team do not readily or accurately assess and/or recognize the patient's pain and pain complaints and behaviors.[16]

PHYSICIAN-RELATED BARRIERS

Poor understanding of the mechanisms of pain and pain management, coupled with inadequate pain assessment skills, negative perceptions and attitudes toward prescribing opioids, and fear of recrimination for the use of opioids can lead to poor outcomes and treatment of pain.[17,18]

The origin of this phenomenon starts in medical school. A significant number of physicians report inadequate teaching, training, and education in the pathophysiology of pain medicine. This lack of proper training and education of principles and practices of multidisciplinary pain management in medical school leads to anecdotal pain management practices being reinforced both in residency and fellowship, without using an evidence-based pathway.

Approximately 88% of physicians reported that their medical school education in pain management was poor. Additionally 73% of physicians reported that residency training was still fair to poor.[17,19]

A study by the Eastern Cooperative Oncology Group showed that approximately 900 physicians with direct patient care responsibilities documented their own sense of low competence with usage of opioid pain medications (76%). This is a major barrier towards effective pain management.[17,20]

The second most common barrier was physician reluctance (61%) to prescribed opioid medication. Pain medications usage by physicians was also limited due to fears of addiction, abuse, and inappropriate use by patients.[21,22] The combination of these two barriers have led to a decrease in treatment of acute and chronic nonmalignant pain.[17,20]

NURSING-RELATED BARRIERS

The patient's pain is usually assessed most frequently by nurses. Regular patient assessment, standardized pain rating scales, and consistent documentation are the main stays of nursing care that can lead to improved pain relief.[23]

There are multiple pain assessment tools such as pain thermometers, numeric rating scales, verbal descriptor scales, and facial pain scales, all of which are valid and reliable pain assessment tools.[22,24]

Nurse-related barriers as perceived by nurses were as follows: high patient to nurse ratio, low psychosocial support services, inadequate time for health teaching with patients, inadequate knowledge of pain mechanisms and pain management, and, to a much lesser degree, indifference toward the patient's pain management.[25]

In the scope of nursing care, there are multiple barriers to pain management. An observational study in Melbourne, Australia, identified six main themes: managing pain effectively, prioritizing pain experiences for pain management, missing pain cues for initiation and or maintenance of pain management, stimulating and non-stimulating factors related to pain, pain prevention, and reactive management of pain. The study emphasized the importance of communication between patients and nursing care-givers.[26]

PATIENT-RELATED BARRIERS

Each patient is a unique individual opportunity to treat pain.[1] Patients' racial, ethnic, cultural, socioeconomical, historical, and geographical perspectives influence their perception of pain and concomitantly physicians' and nurses' interpretation and treatment of their pain.[4] Patient-related factors include psychological, emotional, sensory, and communicative challenges in relating and describing their pain to caregivers.[22]

Pain is defined as a subjective and emotional experience with actual or potential tissue damage as referenced earlier. It is influenced by multiple factors including age, sex, culture, communication skills, demographics, psychological comorbidities, and fear of addiction.[22, 27–29] Patients typically regard a decrement of pain scores from 33% to 50% to be meaningingful.[1]

Communication barriers are a primary problem between patients' description and explanation of their pain (or lack thereof) to doctors and nurses and doctors' and nurses' subsequent understanding and interpretation of their reported pain.

Poor communication between patients and doctors leads to poor pain outcomes and results as well.[30] Specific barriers to opioid use come from patient attitudes toward pain and opioid medication. Fears of addiction to opioids, tolerance, and plateaus to pain relief, along with opioid-related side effects of constipation, nausea, and vomiting, were significant barriers to opioid medication use. The patient's wanting to please the physician is also a significant barrier to optimal pain relief.[31]

There are also other factors that limited a patient's reporting of pain and pain generators. Patients did not expect to obtain pain relief by taking medication. They also associated pain with worsening of the disease process and fatalism in cancer patients, which led to underreporting pain. Some patients also believe that pain is a natural and expected outcome of a disease process. Other patients also feel that their ability to tolerate pain is an admirable and/or beneficial quality. Patients' expectation of pain relief was low.[31]

MANAGEMENT OF ACUTE PAIN

Numerous consequences of acute pain have been described.[32–37] In the typical general surgery setting, management of acute pain revolves around evaluation of the acute abdomen, blunt and penetrating trauma in the emergency department, and acute postoperative pain. Abdominal pain is one of the most common reasons for emergency room visits and comprises about 5% of all visits to the emergency department each year.[35] Acute pain is a homeostatic function of the body, offering a protective function and/or barometer of a potential adverse bodily event.[38] Almost 80% of patients who come into the emergency department have a chief complaint of pain.[39] Management of acute pain is a challenge to all physicians in the emergency department. Despite the presence of emergency doctors, nurses, and other consulting physicians, the treatment of acute pain is still lacking. Some factors which contribute to this are the patient is often interviewed for a short period of time, consultation and diagnostic testing can be time consuming until a diagnosis is established, and delivery of pain medication is often delayed during this workup. This unfortunately leaves the patient at risk of the adverse sequelae of untreated pain.[4,40,41] An observational, prospective study at 20 emergency departments in the United States and Canada examining 842 patients with moderate to severe pain demonstrated that the acute pain was not well managed.[39] Pain scores examined at admission and discharge were relatively unchanged. Patients' expectations of pain relief were not met, and there was still a large time disparity between chief complaint of pain at onset and pain medication delivery.[39]

Unfortunately, physician-related barriers and nurse-related barriers as mentioned earlier are rate-limiting steps in the delivery of adequate pain relief.[4,39]

MANAGEMENT OF CHRONIC PAIN

Chronic pain occurs from 12 to 30 weeks postacute pain. It is characterized by sensitization of both the peripheral central nervous systems which leads to a maladaptive process and persistence of acute pain. Simply put, this is pain which goes past its expected time period and normal tissue healing time.[42] This evolves into a primary disease process where pain is a primary pathologic state.[43] The sequelae of chronic pain leads to anatomical, physiological, psychological, and functional changes in the patient which ultimately leads to decreased quality of life, decreased patient compliance and satisfaction, and increased morbidity, mortality, and medical costs of care.[5,43,44]

The appropriate use of both long-acting and short-acting opioids for the treatment of chronic pain is supported by both the APS and the American Academy of Pain Medicine joint consensus statement.[45] The prevalence of treatment of chronic noncancer pain with chronic opioid therapy has increased over the last 30 years.[46] The use of chronic opioid therapy for the treatment of noncancer pain is well supported.[46] Unfortunately, despite the appropriate use of opioid medication with clinical and regulatory guidelines there continues to be a challenge to the medical health system with risks of abuse, diversion, addiction, and inappropriate medication usage leading to a systemic public health problem. Careful initiation, maintenance, and titration of opioid usage is paramount in this population. Endpoints to be evaluated are adverse effects, dose escalation, analgesic tolerance, and functionality.[47,48] In 2004 a study in the *Journal of Anesthesiology* examined patients' expectations of pain relief versus adverse effects of medications. Patients placed relatively equal importance on limitation adverse effects and pain relief.[47] We are able to use a multimodal perioperative anesthetic plan including patient education and teaching and adjuvant and non-opioid medication in the perioperative phase to decrease opioid usage and increase regional anesthesia and minimally invasive surgeries to help patients reach this balance.[49]

DISCREPANCIES OF PAIN IN DIFFERENT POPULATION GROUPS

The treatment of all patients who have pain is not equal. There are fractures along the lines of racial, ethnic, and gender divisions. The groups that are at most risk for inadequate pain relief are racial and ethnic minorities.[2] In a 13-year (1993–2005) study examining pain management and opioid delivery from the National Hospital Ambulatory Medicine Care Survey, despite a steady increase in the use of opioids over 13 years from 23% in 1993 to 37% 2005, there was still higher utilization of opioids for pain treatment for whites 40% versus nonwhites 32%.[2] In decreasing order, the utilization rates of opioid for pain was 31% for whites, 28% for Asians, 24% for Hispanics, and 23% for blacks.[2] There was still a significant difference in opioid-prescribing habits for all degrees of pain (mild, moderate, severe) and subtypes of pain.[2] This shows that there is a clear imbalance in the delivery of pain medication and relief in different populations.

A patient's gender male or female can also play significant role in the patient's treatment of pain. In a cross-sectional survey of 368 physicians using clinical vignettes in the treatment of pain, more physicians chose to provide optimal pain relief for many versus when and after surgery. In the study, the clinical scenarios examined for postoperative pain were four prostatectomy, myomectomy, and cesarean section. The survey showed that approximately 56% of physicians provided optimal care for prostatectomy patients, 45% for cesarean section patients, and 42% for myomectomy patients.[50]

REGULATORY ISSUES

Since the early 1990s, there has been an increase in the amount of opioids prescribed for both acute and chronic pain syndromes. Despite this increased awareness of pain and pain treatment options, there still remains a population of physicians who are unwilling, not adequately trained, and/or afraid to prescribe opioids in appropriate doses.[2,51] A major concern for most physicians is the degree of scrutiny by regulatory authorities such as the Food and Drug Administration, Drug Enforcement Administration, and state medical boards. The Federation of State Medical boards updated 1998 policy in 2004 regarding recommendations of the use of controlled substances for the treatment of pain.[51] This policy validates the use of opioids for the treatment of acute and chronic pain.[52] A national survey of physician attitudes and knowledge for prescribing opioids in pain management was examined in 1991, 1997, and 2004 by the Wisconsin Pain and Policy Studies Group and the Federation of State Medical Boards.[53] The treatment of cancer pain with opioids was found to be acceptable by 75% of respondents in 1991, 82% of respondents 1997, and 87% of respondents in 2004. For chronic pain of noncancer origin utilization rates were 12% in 1991, 33% in 1997, and 67% in 2004.[53] On the surface, this does not appear to be significant progress, but 33% of respondents still questioned the use of opioids for the management of chronic pain of noncancer origin. There is a lot of confusion with physician understanding of the differences in addiction, dependency, and tolerance. Most physicians are unfamiliar with these guidelines and standards from the 1998 and 2004 APS recommendations regarding opioid usage. Unfortunately, there remains a population of physicians (41%) who believes that dose utilization greater than those listed in the physician's desk reference or package insert are excessive and worrisome. Twenty-eight percent of physicians questioned usage of more than one opioid for an individual patient. There was an improvement in the understanding of the differences in condition, dependency, and tolerance.[53] Despite an awareness and increased emphasis on pain treatment, guidelines, and standards, there is not uniform understanding and application of these principles by physicians.

FORMULARY ISSUES

Despite all the aforementioned regulatory concerns, formulary concerns regarding pharmaceutical company manufacture of opioid medication and the availability and accessibility of these medications continues to be a significant problem. There are many new and emerging opioids and mixed opioid formulations which can offer durable pain relief. Almost two-thirds of physicians who are prescribing opioid medications are not aware of the formulary status of the medications that they are prescribing, as described by the national ambulatory medical care survey in 2000.[54] Many new and effective medications are not on the formulary plans for patients because of high cost concerns, changing insurance platforms with higher cost for copays and third-tier status medications, and/or preauthorization requirements. This leads to a disconnect in patients receiving prescriptions for pain medication who cannot afford them or who do not have access through their insurance.[54] More awareness for both patients and physicians regarding what medications are and are not covered by insurance will hopefully help improve more adequate pain management.

A 17-year-old right-handed African American female presents in the emergency room with a chief complaint of mild periumbilical abdominal pain, right upper quadrant pain, and low back pain. She also has nausea and vomiting prior to right upper quadrant and abdominal pain.

Past Medical History: Type 2 diabetes, juvenile rheumatoid arthritis, and mild obesity

Past Surgical History: Tonsillectomy

Meds: Methotrexate, Prednisone, and Hydrocodone/APAP 5/325 1 po tid (three years)

Allergies: NKDA

Family History: Negative

Social History: Negative × 3

ROS: Generalized malaise, anorexia, abdominal pain as mentioned, otherwise negative

Physical Exam: 5 feet 5 inches, 150 pounds. Vital signs are stable. Her exam is otherwise normal except for the abdominal exam which shows right upper quadrant tenderness and periumbilical tenderness; bowel sounds are positive, and abdomen is mildly tender and nondistended.

Initial Triage and Management: Placement of routine monitors and intravenous access. The FAST exam by the emergency room physician is initially unremarkable. Her urine HCG is negative. A general surgery consult is requested.

The patient starts to complain about diffuse joint pain in addition to her abdominal pain. Her abdominal pain is a 8/10 on a Visual Analog Scale (VAS) score. Her joint pain is a 6/10 VAS score and her usual baseline pain. She requests pain medication. You have reviewed her medical history. How would you proceed?

Discussion

The patient is opioid tolerant: Is she on sufficient opioids or does she require further opioid treatment?

The patient has abdominal pain: Do you continue her daily opioid medication?

Diagnostic testing FAST scan: The patient is stable clinically. A computed tomography (CT) scan of the abdomen, with and without contrast, is pending. How would you manage the patient's pain during the waiting time for the CT scan?

The patient has a chronic autoimmune disease: How do you manage her chronic nonmalignant pain? Does she need a rheumatology consult?

This is an acute pain on chronic pain condition: Is a pain management consult necessary?

If the patient presentation transforms into an acute abdomen, what are the perioperative measures that would decrease the patient's pain postoperatively?

This would be a good exercise to discuss with your colleagues and team to better address your ideas of undertreatment of pain in this challenging patient. There is no right answer to this scenario. The goal here is to challenge yourself and your thinking. Are you following best care guidelines and evidence-based principles, or are you practicing anecdotal medicine?

CONCLUSION

In conclusion, the barriers to the effective management of pain in the general surgery population is multifactorial and encompasses all caregivers. We have simplified these barriers into eight basic categories. It is important to have an understanding of the most up-to-date recommendations and standards regarding evidence-based pain management. This requires a multimodal approach with a team of physicians including surgeons, anesthesiologists, internists and other subspecialty physicians, nurses, and social workers. We have access to new regional anesthesia techniques including ultrasound guided regional anesthesia blockade, extended-release and immediate-release opioids with abuse deterrent technology, and minimally invasive surgical procedures, all of which help increase the ability to limit inadequate pain relief in postsurgical patients. We all have a role to play in the biopsychosocial treatment and management of pain. Hopefully taking a careful look at our own personal and professional barriers to pain relief for our patients will help advance our ability to offer more adequate and universal pain relief.

REFERENCES

1. Gordon DB, Dahl JL, Miaskowski C, et al. American Pain Society recommendations for improving the quality of acute and cancer pain management. *Arch Intern Med.* 2005;165:1574–1580.
2. Pletcher MJ, Kertesz SG, Kohn MA, Gonzales R. Trends in opioid prescribing by race/ethnicity for patients seeking care in US emergency departments. *JAMA.* 2008;299:70–78.
3. American Society of Anesthesiologists Task Force on Acute Pain Management Practice guidelines for acute pain management in the perioperative setting: an updated report by the American Society of Anesthesiologists Task Force on Acute Pain Management. *Anesthesiology.* 2012;116(2):248–273.
4. Rupp T, Delaney KA. Inadequate analgesia in emergency medicine. *Ann Emerg Med.* 2004;43:494–503. Abstract
5. Apfelbaum JL, Chen C, Mehta SS, Gan TJ. Postoperative pain experience: results from a national survey suggest postoperative pain continues to be undermanaged. *Anesth Analg.* 2003;97:534–540. Abstract
6. John Rose, MD, Thomas G Weiser, MD, et.al. Estimated need for surgery worldwide based on prevalence of diseases: a modelling strategy for the WHO Global Health Estimate *Lancet.* 2015 Apr 27;3:S13–S20.
7. Brennan F, Carr DB, Cousins M. Pain management: a fundamental human right. *Anesth Analg.* 2007;105(1):205–221.
8. American Society of Anesthesiologists Task Force on Acute Pain Management. Practice guidelines for acute pain management in the perioperative setting: an updated report by the American Society of Anesthesiologists Task Force on Acute Pain Management. *Anesthesiology.* 2012;116:248–273.
9. Gonzales, AM, Romero RJ, Ojeda-Vaz MM, Rabaza JR. Intravenous acetaminophen in bariatric surgery: effects on opioid requirements. *J Surg Res.* 2015;195(1):99–104.

10. Vadivelu N, Mitra N, Narayan D. Recent advances in postoperative pain management. *Yale J Biol Med*. 2010 Mar; 83(1):11–25.

11. Momeni M, Crucitti M, De Kock M. Patient-controlled analgesia in the management of postoperative pain. *Drugs*. 2006; 66:2321–2337.

12. Block BM, Liu SS, Rowlingson AJ. Efficacy of postoperative epidural analgesia: a meta-analysis. *JAMA*. 2003;290:2445–2463.

13. Hudcova j, Mcnicol E, Quah C, Lau J, Carr DB. Patient-controlled opioid analgesia versus conventional opioid analgesia for postoperative pain. *Cochrane Database Syst Rev* 2006;18(4):CD003348.

14. Gan TJ, Habib AS, Miller TE, White W, Apfelbaum JL. Incidence of patient satisfaction, and perceptions of her surgical pain: results from the last national survey. *Current Med Res Opin*. 2014;30:149–160.

15. Kehlet H, Jensen T, Woolf C. Persistent postsurgical pain: risk factors and prevention. *Lancet*. 2006;367:1618–1625.

16. Guru V, Dubinsky I. The patient vs caregiver perception of acute pain in the emergency department. *J Emerg Med*. 2000;18:7–12.

17. Von Roenn JH, Cleeland CS, Gonin R, Hatfield AK, Pandya KJ. Physician attitudes and crackles in cancer pain management: a survey from the Easton and Cooperative Oncology Group. *Ann Intern Med*. 1993;119:121–126.

18. Cleeland CS. Strategies for improving cancer pain management. *J Pain Symptom Manage*. 1993;8.361–364.

19. Von Gumten, Von Roenn JH, Barriers to pain control: ethics and knowledge. *J Pallait Care*. 1994;10:52–54.

20. Portenoy PK. Opioid therapy for chronic nonmalignant pain: a review of the critical issues: *J Pain Symptom Manage*. 1996:11(4):203–217.

21. Marcus, NJ. *Loss of Productivity Due to Pain*. New York: New York Pain Treatment Program, Lenox Hill Hospital; 1996.

22. Turk DC, Okifuji A. directions in prescriptive chronic pain management based on diagnostic characteristics of the patient. *Bull Am Pain Soc*. 1998;8:5–11.

23. Horgas AL. Pain management in elderly adults. *J Infusion Nurs*. 2003;26:161–165.

24. American Geriatric Society Panel on Chronic Pain in Older Persons. The management of persistent pain in older persons: AGS panel on persistent pain in older persons. *J Am Geriatr Soc*. 2002;6(50 Suppl):205–224.

25. Elcigil A, Maltepe H, Esrefgil G, Mutafoglu K. Nurses proceed to barriers to assessment and management of pain in the university hospital. *J Pediatr Hematol Oncol*. 2011 Apr;33(Suppl 1):S33–S38..

26. Manias E, Bucknall T, Botti M. Nurses' strategies for managing pain in the postoperative setting. *Pain Manag Nurs*. 2005 Mar;6(1):18–29.

27. McCarberg BH. Pharmacologic Management of Pain Expert Column. What are we afraid of? Barriers to providing adequate pain relief. *Medscape Neurol*. 2008:

28. IASP Task Force on Taxonomy. Part III: Pain terms, a current list with definitions and notes on usage. In: Merskey H, Bogduk N, eds. *Classification of Chronic Pain*, 2nd ed. Seattle: IASP Press; 1994:209–214.

29. Turk, DC. System is in treatment for chronic pain patients: who, what and why? *Clin J Pain* 1990;6(2):55–70.

30. Glajchen M, Fitzmartin RD, Blum D, Swanton R. Psychosocial barriers to cancer pain relief. *Cancer Pract*. 1995;3:76–82.

31. Ward SE, Goldberg N, Miller–McCauley V, et al. The patient-related barriers to management of cancer pain. *Pain*. 1993;52:319–324.

32. Carr DB, Jacox AK, Chapman, C.R., Ferrell, B., Field, H.L., Heidrich, G. Acute pain management operative or medical procedures and trauma. Clinical Practice Guidelines. AH CRP., Pub Number 92–0 032. Rockville, MD: Agency for Health Care Policy and Research, Public Health Service, US Department of Health and Human Services; 1992.

33. McIntyre P, on behalf of the Working Party of the Australia and New Zealand College Anesthetists. *Acute Pain Management: Scientific Evidence*, 2nd ed. Melbourne: Australia and New Zealand College of Anesthetists; 2005. http://www.nhmrc.gov.au.publications/synopses/cp104syn.htm

34. European Federation of IASP Chapters. EFIC's declaration on chronic pain as a major healthcare problem: the disease in its own right. Presented at the European Parliament, Brussels, Belgium, October 9, 2001. http://www.painreliefhumanright.com/pdf/06declaration.pdf

35. Siddall PJ, Cousins MJ. Persistent pain as a disease entity: implications for clinical management. *Anesth Analg*. 2004:99;510–520.

36. Resnik DB, Rehm M, Minard RB. The undertreatment of pain: scientific, clinical, cultural, and philosophical factors. *Med Health Care Philos*. 2001;4:277–288.

37. Kamin RA, Nowicki TA, Courtney DS, Powers RD. Pearls and pitfalls in the emergency department evaluation of abdominal pain. *Emerg Med Clin North Am*. 2003;21(1):61–72.

38. Malnar G. Neural mechanisms of pain. *Int J Fertil Womens Med*. 2004;49:155–158.

39. Todd KH, Ducharme J, Choinicre M, et al. Pain in the emergency department: results of the Pain and Emergency Medicine Initiative (PEMI) multicenter study. *J Pain*. 2007;8:460–466.

40. Fosnocht DE, Swanson ER, Barton ED. Changing attitudes about pain and pain control in emergency medicine. *Emerg Med Clin North Am*. 2005;23:297–306.

41. Pain management in the emergency department. *Ann Emerg Med*. 2004;44:198.

42. International Association for the Study of Pain, Subcommittee on Taxonomy. Classification of chronic pain: description of chronic pain syndromes and definition of pain terms. *Pain Suppl*. 1986;3:S1–S226.

43. Gilson AM, Maurer MA, Joranson DE. State medical board members' beliefs about pain, addiction, and diversion and abuse: a changing regulatory environment. *J Pain*. 2007;8:682–691.

44. Green CR, Wheeler JRC. Physician variability in the management of acute postoperative and cancer pain: a quantitative analysis of the Michigan experience. *Pain Med*. 2003;4:8–20.

45. Chou R, Fanciullo GJ, Fine PG, et al. Opioid treatment guidelines: clinical guidelines for the use of chronic opioid therapy in chronic noncancer pain. *J Pain*. 2009;10(2):113–130.

46. American Academy of Pain Medicine, American Pain Society. The use of opioids for the treatment of chronic pain: a consensus statement from the American Academy of Pain Medicine and the American Pain Society. *Clin J Pain*. 1997;13:6–8.

47. Joranson DE, Gilson AM, Dahl JL, Haddox JD. Pain management, controlled substances, and state medical board policy: a decade of change. *J Pain Symptom Manage*. 2002;23:138–147.

48. Portenoy RK, Farrar JT, Backonja M-M, et al. Long-term use of controlled-release oxycodone for noncancer pain: results of a 3-year registry study. *Clin J Pain*. 2007;23:287–299.

49. Gan TJ, Lubarsky, DA, Flood EM, et al. Patient preferences for acute pain treatment. *Br J Anaesth*. 2004;92:681–688.

50. Green CR, Wheeler JRC. Physician variability in the management of acute postoperative and cancer pain: a quantitative analysis of the Michigan experience. *Pain Med.* 2003;4:8–20.

51. Joranson DE, Gilson AM, Dahl JL, Haddox JD. Pain management, controlled substances, and state medical board policy: a decade of change. *J Pain Symptom Manage.* 2002;23:138–147.

52. Fishman SM. *Responsible Opioids Prescribing: A Physician's Guide.* Dallas, TX: Federation of State Medical Boards; 2007.

53. Gilson AM, Maurer MA, Joranson DE. State medical board members' beliefs about pain, addiction, and diversion and abuse: a changing regulatory environment. *J Pain.* 2007;8:682–691.

54. Shih YT, Sleath BL. Health care provider knowledge of drug formulary status in ambulatory care settings. *Am J Health Syst Pharm.* 2004;61:2657–2663.

4 Preemptive, Preventive, and Multimodal Analgesia

Daniel Chang, Mia Castro, Vineetha S. Ratnamma, Alessandra Verzelloni, Dionne Rudison, and Nalini Vadivelu

INTRODUCTION

It has been long known that there is a possible relationship between intraoperative tissue damage and an intensification of acute pain and long-term postoperative pain, now referred to as central sensitization. Nociceptor activation is mediated by chemicals that are released in response to cellular or tissue damage. Preemptive analgesia is an important concept in understanding treatment strategies for postoperative analgesia. Preemptive analgesia focuses on postoperative pain control and the prevention of central sensitization and chronic neuropathic pain by providing analgesia administered preoperatively. Preventive analgesia reduces postoperative pain and consumption of analgesics, and this appears to be the most effective means of decreasing postoperative pain. Preventive analgesia, which includes multimodal preoperative and postoperative analgesic therapies, results in decreased postoperative pain and less postoperative consumption of analgesics.

The concept of preemptive analgesia is based on advances and research in the basic science of pain and evidence-based clinical research. It is now thought that surgical incision alone is not the trigger for central sensitization.[1] But that there are other factors, such as preoperative pain and additional painful noxious intraoperative inputs such as retraction, as well as postoperative inflammatory processes, related peripheral and central neuromodulators, and ectopic neural activity that can all cause an intensification of acute pain and long-term postoperative pain as a result of central sensitization.[2] At present, there are several multimodal strategies covering the perioperative period that can help to decrease postoperative pain and minimize consumption of analgesics.

Left untreated, acute pain can result in emotional and psychological distress; even worse, it can develop into a chronic pain state, which becomes significantly more difficult to manage.[3] With the growing concern of undertreating pain, patients and their providers must be able to properly assess the character and severity of surgery-related pain along with the different treatment modalities available for analgesia. Several advances have been made in our understanding of pain signaling pathways, which have since enabled caregivers to treat pain using a multimodal (or "balanced") approach to provide adequate pain relief while minimizing side effects. This allows for a reduction in the doses of individual drugs and thus a lower incidence of adverse effects from any particular medication used for analgesia.

Current evidence suggests that improvements in patient outcome related to pain control can best be accomplished by using a combination of both centrally and peripherally acting analgesics to achieve additive or even synergistic effects. Frequently used analgesics that have reported efficacy in the management of perioperative pain include opioids, acetaminophen, nonsteroidal anti-inflammatory drugs (NSAIDs), selective cyclooxygenase (COX)-2 inhibitors, gabapentinoids, N-methyl-D-aspartate (NMDA) receptor antagonists, alpha (α)-2 adrenergic agonists, glucocorticoids, and local anesthetics.[4] Other approaches to minimizing pain include use of novel methods for drug delivery and favoring the use of minimally invasive surgical techniques that result in less postoperative pain. Still, pain management in the perioperative setting remains a challenge. However, with the increasing implementation of standardized pain evaluations, development of novel analgesic drugs, and more routine use of multimodal analgesia, adequate pain management can be achieved more readily and with fewer side effects.

OPIOIDS

Opioids remain the primary treatment option for patients who require analgesia for moderate to severe pain in the postoperative period. To review, opioids bind to several receptors in the central nervous system as well as other tissues. There are four major receptors that have been identified: mu, kappa, delta, and sigma. When an agonist binds to these G-protein coupled receptors, they cause membrane hyperpolarization through the inhibition of adenylyl cyclase and voltage-gated calcium channels and activation of phospholipase C along with inwardly rectifying potassium channels. The overall result is the inability of presynaptic release and postsynaptic response to excitatory neurotransmission from nociceptive neurons.[5] Opioids exert their greatest analgesic effects within the central nervous. However, because opioids are capable of binding to receptors located in the somatic and sympathetic peripheral nerves, they are frequently associated with many undesirable effects throughout the body. Opioids are most commonly reported to cause gastrointestinal side effects, including constipation as a result of slow gut motility, and nausea and vomiting. Urinary retention is another frequently reported adverse effect. From a neurological perspective, opioids may cause somnolence, which can decrease ventilation and even cause periods of apnea. All of these reactions resulting from opioid administration may contribute to longer hospital stays, delayed recovery and function, and increased health care costs. However, because opioids still possess potent analgesic properties, they will likely remain the primary treatment option for patients who require rescue analgesic therapy.

NSAIDS/SELECTIVE COX-2 INHIBITORS

Non-opioid analgesics are increasingly being used as adjuncts before, during, and after surgery to facilitate the recovery process after ambulatory surgery because of their anesthetic and analgesic sparing effects and ability to reduce postoperative pain with movement, opioid analgesic requirement, and side effects, thereby shortening hospital stay.

There are two main types of COX enzymes—COX-1 and COX-2. COX-1 is widely distributed throughout the body, including platelets and the gut, while COX-2 is produced in response to inflammation. Traditional NSAIDs, such as aspirin and ibu-profen, exert their effects through the nonselective inhibition of COX, which is in-volved in the synthesis of prostaglandin H1 from arachidonic acid. Prostaglandins reduce the pain threshold at the sight of injury which results in central sensitization and a lower pain threshold in surrounding uninjured tissue. Thus, as NSAIDS inhibit the synthesis of prostaglandins in both spinal cord and periphery, the hyperalgesic and inflammatory state after surgical trauma becomes diminished. Use of selective COX-2 inhibitors, which include celecoxib and etoricoxib, can avoid some of the gas-trointestinal upset and bleeding risks associated with traditional NSAIDs. However, the overall safety profile of COX-2 inhibitors has been questioned as several studies have shown that certain medications have been associated with adverse cardiovas-cular events.[5]

ACETAMINOPHEN

The use of Tylenol in conjunction with other non-opioids has also facilitated the re-covery of patients. Acetaminophen is frequently used for its antipyretic and analgesic qualities. Unlike NSAIDS, it does not have anti-inflammatory effects. The mechanism of action of acetaminophen is unknown, although there is evidence to suggest that it acts centrally. Several sites of action have been postulated including COX-1 to -3 inhibition. It is also theorized to modulate the endocannabinoid, opioid, and seroto-nergic systems.[6] There is a quick onset of action with the use of acetaminophen, espe-cially if given intravenously, which has resulted in higher patient satisfaction scores postoperatively.[7,8]

PREEMPTIVE ANALGESIA

Anytime an incision is made, central sensitization can occur, eventually resulting in inflammation and increased nociception. Preemptive analgesia has been defined as treatment that (a) starts before surgery; (b) prevents the establishment of central sen-sitization caused by incisional injury, which covers only the period of surgery; and (c) prevents establishment of central sensitization caused by inflammatory injuries, which covers the period extending into the initial postoperative phase.[9]

In the 1980s it was demonstrated that peripheral tissue injury was linked to motor and sensory changes associated with peripheral activation of afferent C-type noci-ceptive nerve fibers.[10] Activation of nociceptors is mediated by chemicals that are released in response to cellular or tissue damage. For example, injured cells release leukotrienes and potassium, platelets release serotonin, and vascular injury causes a release of bradykinin from plasma.[11] Central sensitization can then occur from these nociceptive signals releasing neurotransmitters and substances that serve to amplify the response from dorsal horn neurons. These substances include substance P, calcitonin gene-related peptide, and the excitatory amino acids, glutamate and aspartate.[12–14] This concept of central sensitization ultimately results in increased pain sensitivity described as hyperalgesia and tactile allodynia, where there is pain to light touch and persistent chronic pain. In addition to increased excitability, there is a concurrent reduction in the release of inhibitory neurotransmitters from inhibitory interneurons.[15] Thus, given the importance of central sensitization, it would be prudent that analgesic treatment modalities involve modulating central sensitization, as it would be beneficial to the patient not only in the immediate postoperative period but long term as well.

Several preemptive analgesic regimens have been tried in humans. These include intravenous doses of opioids, peripheral nerve blocks (PNBs), local infiltration of the surgical site, epidural administration of opioids and local anesthetics, and multimodal combinations.[16–24] Treatment with NSAIDs given systemically and NMDA receptor antagonists has also been tried preemptively. In humans, these trials, along with meta-analytic studies, demonstrate the need for perioperative and not just preoperative analgesic interventions.[25]

PREVENTIVE ANALGESIA

Preventive analgesia that is started preoperatively utilizing a multimodal method was found to be more effective in terms of decreasing postoperative pain and reducing analgesic consumption in the postoperative period. This approach has been found to reduce unwanted side effects, thus allowing for more rapid recovery and earlier discharge from the hospital.[26–28]

GABAPENTOIDS

The gabapentinoids, specifically gabapentin and pregabalin, were initially developed as anticonvulsant medications but were subsequently found to be useful for the treatment of pain.[26] Gabapentinoids modulate pain via blockade of the neuronal voltage-gated calcium channels by binding to the $\alpha 2\delta$ subunit.[6] Some evidence suggests that gabapentinoids may also affect the NMDA receptors and inflammatory cytokines. Gabapentin is administered orally and has low bioavailability, which may increase the time it takes to have an effect. On the other hand, pregabalin has higher bioavailability, more rapid absorption rate, and is more potent than gabapentin.[26,29] However, high cost has limited its use and study in comparison to gabapentin. The most common side effects of gabapentinoids are gastrointestinal upset and sedation.[30]

Gabapentin is often used in multimodal pain regimens. Several studies have shown its efficacy for treatment and prevention of neuropathic pain, most notably diabetic neuropathy, trigeminal neuralgia, postherpetic neuralgia, and burn-related neuropathy.[6,26,29] The administration of gabapentin or pregabalin preoperatively and postoperatively has been shown to result in decreased opioid use.[29,30] Optimal gabapentinoid dosing and timing are under current study.[30]

NMDA RECEPTOR ANTAGONISTS

Ketamine

Ketamine is a noncompetitive antagonist that binds the open channel configuration of the NMDA receptor. It is also a weak opioid receptor agonist. It is most often administered intravenously or intramuscularly but can be given orally, nasally, or subcutaneously.[5] Ketamine produces a dissociative state and can cause psychotic symptoms if not administered concomitantly with a benzodiazepine.

Ketamine is used in multimodal regimens for treatment of both perioperative and chronic pain.[26] Although ketamine has inherent analgesic properties, it is rarely used as a sole agent for pain treatment due to high dose requirements and consequent side effects. Typically, it is used in low doses as an adjunct to opioid regimens.[26] Some studies have found that when given as a bolus at the beginning of surgery followed by intraoperative low dose infusion, ketamine produces an opioid sparing effect and reduced pain scores.[29] Ketamine has also been studied for management of phantom limb pain and was found to provide short-term phantom limb pain relief and improved pain scores.[31] Low-dose ketamine has also been effective as an adjunct treatment for chronic regional pain syndrome.[32] There is also growing evidence that ketamine is beneficial in the management in refractory cancer pain.

Memantine

Similar to ketamine, memantine is noncompetitive NMDA antagonist that blocks the open calcium channel. Memantine is Food and Drug Administration–approved for the treatment of Alzheimer's disease but has also been studied for the treatment of pain. Memantine is administered orally and has a greater than 80% bioavailability. In general, it is well tolerated without many significant side effects, unlike ketamine which is frequently associated with amnesia and psychosis. The role of memantine in pain treatment is still under review. It was discovered that administration of memantine decreased opioid withdrawal symptoms, suggesting that it may have a role in prevention and treatment of opioid dependence. Other studies suggest that when combined with brachial plexus block, memantine reduced the incidence of phantom limb pain after upper extremity amputations.

Magnesium

Occasionally utilized in perioperative pain treatment, magnesium is also capable of NMDA receptor antagonism both centrally and peripherally. Studies suggest that intravenous magnesium aids in the reduction of intra- and postoperative opioid requirements.[29,33,34] Comparatively, low-dose intrathecal magnesium has been shown to be an effective adjunct to intrathecal fentanyl infusion. Optimal dosing and timing are currently under study.

A-2 RECEPTOR ANTAGONISTS

Drugs such as clonidine and dexmedetomidine are included in the group of α-2 adrenoreceptor agonists that are useful adjuvants in acute pain management. α-2 agonists reduce perioperative analgesic and anesthetic requirements.

Clonidine and dexmedetomidine are both imidazole ring compounds. The relative selectivity of these two drugs for α-2 receptors compared to α-1 receptors differs. Both clonidine and dexmedetomidine are selective agonists of α-2 adrenergic receptors with an α-2 to α-1 ratio of 200:1 and 1,620:1 respectively.[35] Clonidine can be administered orally, intravenously, neuraxially or perineurally in combination with local anesthetics. Dexmedetomidine is mainly administered intravenously.

Central and peripheral stimulation of the α-2 receptors is believed to be the basic mechanism behind analgesia. The α-2 adrenergic receptor has high density in the substantia gelatinosa of the dorsal horn in humans. That is believed to be the primary site of action by which α-2 adrenergic agonists can reduce pain.[26] In the spinal cord, clonidine acts at α-2 adrenergic receptors to stimulate acetylcholine release, which acts at both muscarinic and nicotinic receptor subtypes with analgesic effects.[36] The analgesic effects of dexmedetomidine are exerted through stimulation of α2-adrenoceptors in the dorsal horn of the spinal cord, which inhibits substance P release.[37] Systemic administration of dexmedetomidine or clonidine can cause hypotension, bradycardia, and sedation.

On the basis of evidence from clinical trials and recent reviews, the use of clonidine and dexmedetomidine in the perioperative period lowers pain scores postoperatively, reduces intraoperative and postoperative opioid requirements, and improves patient satisfaction.[29] Studies also showed that both reduce postoperative nausea and vomiting, potentially related to the decreased administration of narcotics, as well as intrinsic properties of these medications themselves.

Clonidine improves the analgesic efficacy of local anesthetics and morphine, in addition to providing postoperative analgesia. The evidence supporting the postoperative analgesic effect of clonidine is strongest when it is used regionally, particularly as adjunct to PNB and also when via the intrathecal and epidural route. Multiple randomized controlled trials and several meta-analyses have demonstrated that the duration of nerve block was significantly prolonged when clonidine was added to local anesthetics for epidural or perineural analgesia.[29,36] Similarly, dexmedetomidine was first used as additive in regional anesthesia.[26] There are trials showing prolongation of analgesia and duration of motor and sensory blockade when dexmedetomidine is added to regional solutions. There are multiple randomized controlled trials and meta-analysis examining the effectiveness of dexmedetomidine as a PNB additive. A recent study found that the duration of sensory and motor block when dexmedetomidine was added to bupivacaine supraclavicular blocks was almost twice as compared to the addition of clonidine.[38]

GLUCOCORTICOIDS

Synthetic corticosteroids have anti-inflammatory, analgesic, and antiemetic properties that are useful in perioperative pain management. Corticosteroids can provide pain relief in many cancer pain syndromes, including bone pain associated with metastasis, neuropathic pain from either spinal cord compression or nerve infiltration by direct tumor infiltration, pain from lymphedema or due to bowel obstruction, headache due to increased intracranial pressure, and arthralgia.[35] Dexamethasone is a synthetic glucocorticoid with high potency and a long duration of action (half-life: two days) and low mineralocorticoid activity.

Glucocorticoids block the enzyme phospholipase, thus blocking the arachidonic acid cascade and ultimately inflammation. Analgesic action is mediated by the decrease in edema around pain-sensitive structures and a potential decrease in the ephaptic neural discharges.[35]

Glucocorticoids are mainly used in acute pain management is in the perioperative period, particularly in dental surgery, laparoscopic cholecystectomy, and to a lesser extent in orthopedic, ambulatory, and pediatric ear, nose, and throat (ENT) surgery.

Dexamethasone is usually effective in a low-dose regimen (at a dose of 2–12 mg daily) for achieving analgesia. It reduces pain and postoperative nausea and vomiting. Dexamethasone when used in dental surgery reduces severe postoperative swelling. When used as an adjuvant, dexamethasone decreases oxycodone consumption and helps to reduce postoperative pain.[30]

Various studies, retrospective reviews, and meta-analyses of randomized placebo-controlled trials demonstrated that dexamethasone prolonged a variety of upper and lower extremity PNBs when used with local anesthetics.[39] Particular attention should be given to the risk of side effects like gastrointestinal bleeding, severe dyspepsia, wound infection, and candidiasis. A single dose of dexamethasone causes no or mild adverse effects, whereas chronic usage may create major problems.

LOCAL ANESTHETICS/NERVE BLOCKS

Neuraxial Blocks

There is increasing evidence that epidural anesthesia has the potential to improve patient outcome after major surgical procedures by reducing postoperative morbidity and duration of recovery. Probable benefits include the attenuation of cardiac complications, earlier return of gastrointestinal function associated with an increase in overall patient comfort, decreased incidence of pulmonary dysfunctions, beneficial effects on the coagulation system, and, of course, a reduction in the inflammatory response. Since local anesthetics, reabsorbed from the epidural space, seem to contribute to these effects, it is not easy to differentiate between the systemic effects of local anesthetics and the effects of neuraxial blockade by epidural anesthesia. The beneficial effects of the epidural administration of local anesthetics have been attributed to the changes in physiology induced by neuraxial anesthesia and better pain management. Perioperative pain control using regional anesthesia techniques may be a powerful tool for reducing perioperative stress. Serum markers that may reflect the humoral stress response (i.e., catecholamines, corticotropin, thromboxane A2, and antidiuretic hormone) are decreased by epidural blockade but not by general anesthesia. Epidural anesthesia is not suitable for all types of surgical procedures and/or under all conditions (e.g., in anticoagulated patients); most of the alternative effects, obtained when epidural anesthesia with local anesthetics is used, do also occur when local anesthetics are administered differently, suggesting that these beneficial effects are not dependent on pure blockade of spinal nerves but instead on systemic levels of local anesthetics.[40]

Peripheral Nerve Blocks

PNBs are increasingly used as a component of multimodal analgesia and may be administered as a single injection (sPNB) or continuous infusion via a perineural catheter (cPNB).[41] PNBs have been associated with improvement in postoperative pain control and reduction in the use of opioids in a variety of surgical procedures; other benefits include reduction in hospital length of stay, prevention of hospital readmissions, reduction in postoperative nausea and vomiting, earlier participation in physical therapy, and improved patient satisfaction.

PNBs are now a common component of analgesia for both upper extremity (i.e., brachial plexus block using interscalene, supra- or infraclavicular, and axillary nerve approaches) and lower extremity (i.e., lumbar plexus, femoral, sciatic, and popliteal sciatic blocks, among others) procedures. The ideal PNB technique would have a duration of action sufficient to provide pain relief for the most intense period of postoperative pain but not result in a dense motor block that could be unpleasant to the patient or lead to safety issues such as falls. Moreover, the risk of infection, neurologic complications, bleeding, and local anesthetic systemic toxicity should be minimized to the extent possible. The technique should be easy to perform and thus independent of the technical skills of the anesthesiologist and with minimal chance of failed procedures. Finally, the ideal PNB technique should be convenient for patients and easy to manage in the postoperative period. sPNB is simple to perform, avoids the concerns associated with indwelling cPNB catheters, and does not require the patient to be responsible for medication administration at home, but the duration of block is often insufficient to manage pain beyond the first postoperative day. cPNB has the advantages of a prolonged duration of analgesia while administering more dilute local anesthetic solutions (and thus minimizing risk of toxicity). However, catheter dislodgement rates may be unacceptable, not all patients are willing to accept the responsibility of home cPNB, and extensive education and follow-up are required for successful use.[41]

The efficacy of sPNB in improving short-term pain control has been shown in a number of upper and lower extremity surgical procedures. A meta-analysis of randomized trials comparing sPNB to intravenous patient-controlled analgesia opioids showed a significant reduction in pain at rest and on movement for up to 24 and 48 hours, respectively, with significantly less opioid consumption for up to 48 hours.[42] Administration of local anesthetics via continuous infusion allows for a duration of analgesia significantly longer than that of a single injection.

CONCLUSION

The most effective strategy to significantly decrease pain is a combination of a preemptive analgesia and the use of multimodal analgesic medications. Multimodal therapy allows for lower dosages of any one medication to be used in combination, which reduces the risk of a significant side effects arising from administration of a single analgesic drug. Preventive analgesia effectively includes preemptive analgesia aimed at reducing central sensitization caused by pain. Effective multimodal analgesia is an important component of preventive analgesia, resulting in an increased duration of analgesia along with decreased long-term pain sensitivity at the peripheral and central levels. Preventive analgesia is not time-constrained in the same manner as preemptive analgesia but instead focuses on the use of various analgesic interventions in the entire perioperative setting.

REFERENCES

1. Katz J. Pre-emptive analgesia: evidence, current status and future directions. *Eur J Anaesthesiol Suppl.* 1995;10:8–13.
2. Katz J, Seltzer Z. Transition from acute to chronic postsurgical pain: risk factors and protective factors. *Expert Rev Neurother.* 2009;9(5):723–744.
3. Cohen SP, Raja SN. Prevention of chronic postsurgical pain: the ongoing search for the holy grail of anesthesiology. *Anesthesiology.* 2013;118(2):241–243.
4. American Society of Anesthesiologists Task Force on Acute Pain Management. Practice guidelines for acute pain management in the perioperative setting: an updated report by the American Society of Anesthesiologists Task Force on Acute Pain Management. *Anesthesiology.* 2012;116(2):248–273.
5. Mackey DC, Butterworth JF, Mikhail MS, Morgan GE, Wasnick JD. *Morgan and Mikhail's Clinical Anesthesiology,* 5th ed. New York: McGraw-Hill Education; 2013.
6. Barash P, Cullen, B, Stoelting, R, Calahan, M, Stock, C, Ortega, R. *Clinical Anesthesia,* 7th ed. New York: Lippincott Williams & Wilkins; 2013.
7. Wininger SJ, Miller H, Minkowitz HS, et al. A randomized, double-blind, placebo-controlled, multicenter, repeat-dose study of two intravenous acetaminophen dosing regimens for the treatment of pain after abdominal laparoscopic surgery. *Clin Ther.* 2010;32(14):2348–2369.
8. Gorocs TS, Lambert M, Rinne T, Krekler M, Modell S. Efficacy and tolerability of ready-to-use intravenous paracetamol solution as monotherapy or as an adjunct analgesic therapy for postoperative pain in patients undergoing elective ambulatory surgery: open, prospective study. *Int J Clin Pract.* 2009;63(1):112–120.
9. Kissin I. Preemptive analgesia. *Anesthesiology.* 2000;93(4):1138–1143.
10. Woolf CJ, Wall PD. Relative effectiveness of C primary afferent fibers of different origins in evoking a prolonged facilitation of the flexor reflex in the rat. *J Neurosci.* 1986;6(5):1433–1442.
11. Woolf CJ. Evidence for a central component of post-injury pain hypersensitivity. *Nature.* 1983;306(5944):686–688.
12. Costigan M, Woolf CJ. Pain: molecular mechanisms. *J Pain.* 2000;1(3 Suppl):35–44.
13. Julius D, Basbaum AI. Molecular mechanisms of nociception. *Nature.* 2001;413(6852):203–210.
14. Woolf CJ, Salter MW. Neuronal plasticity: increasing the gain in pain. *Science.* 2000;288(5472):1765–1769.
15. Simonnet G. Preemptive antihyperalgesia to improve preemptive analgesia. *Anesthesiology.* 2008;108(3):352–354.
16. Bugedo GJ, Carcamo CR, Mertens RA, Dagnino JA, Munoz HR. Preoperative percutaneous ilioinguinal and iliohypogastric nerve block with 0.5% bupivacaine for post-herniorrhaphy pain management in adults. *Reg Anesth.* 1990;15(3):130–133.
17. Ejlersen E, Andersen HB, Eliasen K, Mogensen T. A comparison between preincisional and postincisional lidocaine infiltration and postoperative pain. *Anesth Analg.* 1992;74(4):495–498.
18. Fu ES, Miguel R, Scharf JE. Preemptive ketamine decreases postoperative narcotic requirements in patients undergoing abdominal surgery. *Anesth Analg.* 1997;84(5):1086–1090.
19. Gottschalk A, Smith DS, Jobes DR, et al. Preemptive epidural analgesia and recovery from radical prostatectomy: a randomized controlled trial. *JAMA.* 1998;279(14):1076–1082.

20. Jahangiri M, Jayatunga AP, Bradley JW, Dark CH. Prevention of phantom pain after major lower limb amputation by epidural infusion of diamorphine, clonidine and bupivacaine. *Ann R Coll Surg Engl.* 1994;76(5):324–326.

21. Kehlet H, Dahl JB. The value of "multimodal" or "balanced analgesia" in postoperative pain treatment. *Anesth Analg.* 1993;77(5):1048–1056.

22. Kundra P, Gurnani A, Bhattacharya A. Preemptive epidural morphine for postoperative pain relief after lumbar laminectomy. *Anesth Analg.* 1997;85(1):135–138.

23. Richmond CE, Bromley LM, Woolf CJ. Preoperative morphine pre-empts postoperative pain. *Lancet.* 1993;342(8863):73–75.

24. Tverskoy M, Cozacov C, Ayache M, Bradley EL Jr, Kissin I. Postoperative pain after inguinal herniorrhaphy with different types of anesthesia. *Anesth Analg.* 1990;70(1):29–35.

25. Ong CK, Lirk P, Seymour RA, Jenkins BJ. The efficacy of preemptive analgesia for acute postoperative pain management: a meta-analysis. *Anesth Analg.* 2005;100(3):757–773.

26. Buvanendran A, Kroin JS. Multimodal analgesia for controlling acute postoperative pain. *Curr Opin Anaesthesiol.* 2009;22(5):588–593.

27. Wall PD. The prevention of postoperative pain. *Pain.* 1988;33(3):289–290.

28. Woolf CJ, Chong MS. Preemptive analgesia—treating postoperative pain by preventing the establishment of central sensitization. *Anesth Analg.* 1993;77(2):362–379.

29. Young A, Buvanendran A. Recent advances in multimodal analgesia. *Anesthesiol Clin.* 2012;30(1):91–100.

30. Elvir-Lazo OL, White PF. The role of multimodal analgesia in pain management after ambulatory surgery. *Curr Opin Anaesthesiol.* 2010;23(6):697–703.

31. Van Zundert J, Hartrick C, Patijn J, Huygen F, Mekhail N, van Kleef M. Evidence-based interventional pain medicine according to clinical diagnoses. *Pain Pract.* 2011;11(5):423–429.

32. Schwartzman RJ, Alexander GM, Grothusen JR, Paylor T, Reichenberger E, Perreault M. Outpatient intravenous ketamine for the treatment of complex regional pain syndrome: a double-blind placebo controlled study. *Pain.* 2009;147(1–3):107–115.

33. Shariat Moharari R, Motalebi M, Najafi A, et al. Magnesium can decrease postoperative physiological ileus and postoperative pain in major nonlaparoscopic gastrointestinal surgeries: a randomized controlled trial. *Anesth Pain Med.* 2014;4(1):e12750.

34. Koinig H, Wallner T, Marhofer P, Andel H, Horauf K, Mayer N. Magnesium sulfate reduces intra- and postoperative analgesic requirements. *Anesth Analg.* 1998;87(1):206–210.

35. Gupta K, Rastogi B, Gupta PK, Singh I, Singh VP, Jain M. Dexmedetomidine infusion as an anesthetic adjuvant to general anesthesia for appropriate surgical field visibility during modified radical mastectomy with I-Gel(R): a randomized control study. *Korean J Anesthesiol.* 2016;69(6):573–578.

36. Svirskii DA, Antipin EE, Uvarov DN, Nedashkovskii EV. [Abdominal cross section space blockade as a component of the multimodal postoperative analgesia in patients after cesarean section: blockade efficiency analysis]. *Anesteziol Reanimatol.* 2012(6):33–35.

37. Roberts MS, Grant. Dexmedetomidine in Paediatric Anaesthesia and Intensive Care. 2013. https://www.aagbi.org/sites/default/files/293 Dexmedetomidine in Paediatric Anaesthesia and Intensive Care.pdf

38. Waldron NH, Jones CA, Gan TJ, Allen TK, Habib AS. Impact of perioperative dexamethasone on postoperative analgesia and side-effects: systematic review and meta-analysis. *Br J Anaesth.* 2013;110(2):191–200.

39. Kirksey MA, Haskins SC, Cheng J, Liu SS. local anesthetic peripheral nerve block adjuvants for prolongation of analgesia: a systematic qualitative review. *PLoS One.* 2015;10(9):e0137312.

40. Hahnenkamp K, Herroeder S, Hollmann MW. Regional anaesthesia, local anaesthetics and the surgical stress response. *Best Pract Res Clin Anaesthesiol.* 2004;18(3):509–527.

41. Joshi G, Gandhi K, Shah N, Gadsden J, Corman SL. Peripheral nerve blocks in the management of postoperative pain: challenges and opportunities. *J Clin Anesth.* 2016;35:524–529.

42. Chan EY, Fransen M, Parker DA, Assam PN, Chua N. Femoral nerve blocks for acute postoperative pain after knee replacement surgery. *Cochrane Database Syst Rev.* 2014(5):CD009941.

5   Tumescent Anesthesia in General Surgery

Jacob Cole, Victor Rivera,
and Anthony Tucker

HISTORY

The tumescent technique of anesthesia was first reported in 1987 by a dermatologist named Dr. Jeffrey Klein. At that time liposuction was primarily performed under general anesthesia and often complicated by major blood loss. Prior to tumescent anesthesia, standard liposuction was performed by the rapid aspiration of adipose tissue. Suctioning was only stopped when there was more blood than fat in the aspirate. Thus, major blood loss was the primary factor limiting the amount of adipose tissue that could be safely removed and blood transfusions were routine. A 1992 study reported blood transfusion in 108 of 108 cases of liposuction performed under general anesthesia.[1] A report the following year described the novel tumescent liposuction procedure in 112 patients and reported an average blood loss of less than 20mL.[2] Gradually tumescent anesthesia for liposuction came into the mainstream.

THE FIRST TUMESCENT ANESTHESIA PROCEDURES

Dr. Klein first described the tumescent technique of liposuction in 1987. He developed a tumescent fluid formulation of 1 g lidocaine and 1 mg epinephrine in 1 L of normal saline (0.1% lidocaine with 1:1,000,000 solution).[3] This solution was infiltrated via a syringe attached to a cannula until volumes occasionally in excess of 1000 mL of infiltrate were injected and the skin was firm and blanched. Dr. Klein described the skin as "tumescent." This initial publication reported infiltrating an average lidocaine dose of 18.4 mg/kg into the subcutaneous fat. Despite this apparently high dose of lidocaine, mean serum lidocaine levels were less than 0.36 μg/mL one hour after infiltration. The highest peak serum concentration measured was 0.614 μg/mL. Mean change in hematocrit 48 to 72 hours after the procedure was insignificant, confirming the blood sparing nature of this procedure.

This initial study was controversial due to the large dosages of lidocaine administered. While follow-on liposuction studies using tumescent local anesthesia exclusively continued to demonstrate its safety and lack of lidocaine toxicity,[4,5] the tumescent infiltration procedure was not readily adopted in other surgical procedures. This may have been secondary to the lack of procedure standardization as many physicians elected to use minimal to no lidocaine in the tumescent solution due to local anesthetic safety concerns.[6] The poor results of this technique only served to further skepticism about this new procedure and hindered its mainstream acceptance. Even in more recent years this technique has struggled to find a niche for itself outside of the liposuction and cutaneous surgeries, though its role in general surgical procedures is expanding.

TUMESCENT INFILTRATE SOLUTION

The two primary constituents of a tumescent infiltrate remain the same as when Dr. Klein first proposed the technique—a local anesthetic and a vasoconstrictor. While additional medications can be added to modify the action of the infiltrate, tumescent anesthesia is defined by the presence of these two components. Local anesthetics other than lidocaine have been used, but lidocaine remains the most thoroughly studied and vetted drug for this technique. Lidocaine is used for its obvious anesthetic effects, and epinephrine is included as a vasoconstrictor in an attempt to prevent systemic absorption of the lidocaine following infiltration of the subcutaneous tissues. Given the large doses of these substances involved in tumescent anesthesia, a brief review of their mechanisms of action is indicated.

Lidocaine

Lidocaine is an amino-amine type local anesthetic that acts primarily by blocking the fast voltage-gated sodium channels in excitable tissues. In neuronal tissue, this action essentially inhibits signal propagation at the synaptic cleft.[7] By blocking depolarization of the presynaptic membrane, no signal is transmitted to the postsynaptic neuron, blocking nociceptor activation.

Systemic Effects

Systemic effects of lidocaine and all local anesthetics follow logically from their mechanism of action and affect primarily both the central nervous and the cardiac conduction systems. In systemic circulation the threshold for mild lidocaine toxicity has an accepted value of 6 μg/mL.[8,9] The effects of lidocaine toxicity are listed in Figure 5.1. If lidocaine toxicity is suspected in a patient recently infiltrated with a tumescent solution, prompt and effective airway management is crucial to preventing hypoxia and acidosis, which are known to potentiate the toxicity.[10] Prompt treatment with benzodiazepines is indicated for any local anesthetic-induced seizures. The evidence supporting lipid emulsion therapy is not as strong as these first two recommendations; however, its administration should be considered at the first signs of toxicity, and no large doses of local anesthetic should ever be administered without ready access to lipid emulsion. Table 5.1 includes other recommendations for treatment of systemic local anesthetic toxicity.

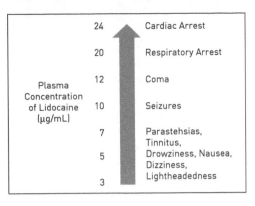

FIGURE 5.1. Side effects of lidocaine toxicity with corresponding plasma lidocaine concentration.

Table 5.1. Checklist for Treatment of Local Anesthetic Systemic Toxicity

The Pharmacologic Treatment of Local Anesthetic Systemic Toxicity (LAST) is Different from Other Cardiac Arrest Scenarios

---

❏ **Get Help**
❏ **Initial Focus**
   ❏ **Airway management**: ventilate with 100% oxygen
   ❏ **Seizure suppression**: benzodiazepines are preferred; **AVOID propofol** in patients having signs of cardiovascular instability
   ❏ **Alert** the nearest facility having **cardiopulmonary bypass** capability
❏ **Management of Cardiac Arrhythmias**
   ❏ **Basic and Advanced Cardiac Life Support (ACLS)** will require adjustment of medications and perhaps prolonged effort
   ❏ **AVOID vasopressin, calcium channel blockers, beta blockers, or local anesthetic**
   ❏ **REDUCE epinephrine dose to <1 mcg/kg**
❏ **Lipid Emulsion (20%) Therapy** (values in parenthesis are for 70kg patient)
   ❏ **Bolus 1.5 mL/kg** (lean body mass) intravenously over 1 minute (~100mL)
   ❏ **Continuous infusion 0.25 mL/kg/min** (~ 18 mL/min; adjust by roller clamp)
   ❏ Repeat bolus once or twice for persistent cardiovascular collapse
   ❏ Double the infusion rate to 0.5 mL/kg/min if blood pressure remains low
   ❏ **Continue infusion** for at least 10 minutes after attaining circulatory stability
   ❏ Recommended upper limit: Appproximately 10mL/kg lipid emulsion over the first 30 minutes
❏ **Post LAST events at** www.lipidrescue.org and report use of lipid to www.lipidregistry.org

Source: Reprinted with permission of Wolters Kluwer Health, Inc. Rubin, D, Matsumoto, M, Weinberg, G, et al. Local Anesthetic Systemic Toxicity in Total Joint Arthroplasty: Incidence and Risk Factors in the United States From the National Inpatient Sample 1998–2013. *Reg Anesth Pain Med*. 2018 Feb;43(2):131–137.

Local Effects

The local effects of lidocaine are well known. In the tumescent anesthesia literature, blockage of small cutaneous nerve fibers can be routinely obtained with a 0.05% lidocaine solution,[11] albeit for a shorter duration,[12] while other nerve blocks that utilize 1% to 2% lidocaine solution can achieve temporary large motor neuron signal suppression and a flaccid paralysis of the corresponding motor units.

When administered independently of epinephrine, lidocaine causes a marked vasodilation of peripheral vessels due primarily to the chemical sympathectomy but also from a release of nitric oxide.[13] This initial vasodilation may enhance epinephrine absorption[14] when administered together, though epinephrine rapidly overpowers this response, and the net effect is primarily a local vasoconstriction when these two medications are coadministered. While this is likely of minimal clinical relevance at typical local anesthetic doses, it becomes significant at the large doses given during tumescent anesthesia.

Pharmacodynamics

Lidocaine is 65% bound to plasma protein (primarily α-acid glycoprotein) in vivo and is metabolized by a first-pass mechanism in the liver. It undergoes N-dealkylation by the CYP3A4 isoenzyme of the cytochrome P450 complex. Following dealkylation, it is hydrolyzed to monoethylglycinexylidide and glycinxylidide. Both of these metabolites are pharmacologically active. Lidocaine has a clearance of 0.95 L/min[15] and an elimination half-life of 100 to 120 minutes.[16] Table 5.2 contains a list of potential medication interactions that might inhibit the metabolism of lidocaine, increasing the risk of toxicity. All patients should be screened for usage of these medications and supplements prior to administration of tumescent anesthesia.

Table 5.2. Potential CYP 450 3A4 Inhibitors

Protease Inhibitors
Macrolide Antibiotics
Chloramphenicol
-azole Antifungals
Aprepitant
Valerian
Grapefruit Juice
Fluoxetine
Buprenorphine
Gabapentin/Pregabalin

List of medications that may inhibit lidocaine
metabolism. This list is not comprehensive.

EPINEPHRINE

Epinephrine is a nonselective agonist of all adrenergic receptors. Table 5.3 represents signs and clinical manifestations of an epinephrine overdose.[17] Most instances of epinephrine toxicity are of a short duration and require only supportive therapy,[18] as the half-life of intravenous epinephrine is only one to three minutes and symptoms are typically self-limiting. However, in the cases of subcutaneous injection symptoms can persist for up to 120 minutes as the epinephrine depot is slowly absorbed.[19]

Epinephrine was first included in the original formulation of the tumescent infiltrate used in liposuction due to its potent vasoconstrictive action. The goal was twofold: (a) slow systemic absorption of the lidocaine thereby decreasing peak plasma concentration and systemic toxicity[20,21] and (b) provide time for the surgeon to suction out as much of the subcutaneous lidocaine as possible prior to it being absorbed. This "chemical tourniquet" effect has been well documented and is used routinely when administering local anesthetics. There is a theoretical ischemic risk of administration of a tumescent infiltrate containing epinephrine to an area of the body with no collateral blood flow such as fingers, toes, ears, nose, or penis. Previous studies have demonstrated little evidence to support this, and tissue necrosis has rarely if ever been reported.[22]

OTHER CONSTITUENTS

Sodium Bicarbonate

Sodium bicarbonate is routinely added to Dr. Klein's original formula. This addition reduces the pain of infiltration by buffering the acidity of commercial lidocaine[23] while still providing effective local anesthesia.[24] Interestingly, the weak antibacterial effects of lidocaine seem to be enhanced by co-injection with sodium bicarbonate and may provide some antiseptic properties during tumescent procedures, particularly against gram positive organisms.[25,26]

Table 5.3. Signs and Symptoms of Epinephrine Overdose

Fear
Restlessness
Tremor
Headache
Perspiration
Respiratory Difficulty
Dizziness
Pallor
Weakness
Palpitations

Bicarbonate also raises the pH of the tumescent solution, increasing the proportion of undissociated lidocaine molecules. These noncharged molecules penetrate lipid membranes more effectively, resulting in more rapid diffusion of the local anesthetic throughout the tumescent field and a denser block. Typical concentrations of sodium bicarbonate that are used in tumescent infiltration solutions range from 0.5% to 1%.[27]

Carrier Fluid

Any isotonic crystalloid fluid can be used as the carrier when preparing the tumescent solution. Both normal saline (0.9%) and lactated ringer's solution have been used effectively in past reports, though the majority of surgeons seem to prefer normal saline. Some administer the solution cooled to about 4°C and others warm it to 40°C prior to administration.[28] In the majority of cases the temperature of the infiltrate does not seem to have clinical relevance, and for practical reasons it seems reasonable to infiltrate a room-temperature solution for smaller procedures. In larger procedures, warming the solution to physiologic body temperature might reduce the pain of the infiltration as well as decrease potential risk of inducing hypothermia.[29]

Anti-Inflammatory Medications

The addition of steroids to the tumescent infiltrate is controversial at best, with limited prospective research demonstrating benefit to a steroid infiltration when compared to systemic steroid administration.[30,31] Steroids were initially included due to their anti-inflammatory effects in an effort to minimize pain once the local anesthetic had worn off; however, they also provide a slight psychological euphoric effect during long procedures that may minimize the need for benzodiazepines or other forms of sedation. The initial formulation of tumescent infiltrate proposed by Dr. Klein did incorporate 1% triamcinolone with no evidence of systemic toxicity noted.[3]

Co-Administered Medications

Given the chronotropic effects of epinephrine, it is reasonable to consider premedicating patients with an α2-agonist such as oral clonidine prior to administration of the tumescent infiltrate. Benzodiazepines such as midazolam or lorazepam can counteract the anxiety for patients undergoing conscious procedures. Prophylactic atropine administration has also been reported in patients with a history of vasovagal syncope to prevent loss of consciousness during the procedure.

Tumescent Solution Recipes

Tumescent anesthesia is the infiltration of a dilute solution of local anesthetic to anesthetize and cause swelling or tumescence of the integument. No standard tumescent solution exists. In general, the concentration of local anesthetic necessary for adequate anesthesia is directly proportional to the surface area to be infiltrated. The American Society for Dermatologic Surgery (ASDS) has a recommended formulation found in Table 5.4.[32]

Table 5.4. American Society for Dermatologic Surgery Recommended Tumescent Infiltrate Formulation

Active Substance	Dose
Lidocaine	500 to 1000 mg (0.05% to 0.1% Solution)
Epinephrine	0.5 to 1 mg (1 to 2:2,000,000)
Sodium Bicarbonate	10 mEq
Triamcinolone Acetonide	10 mg
Sodium Chloride (0.9%)	1000 mL

Maximum Dose

It should be noted that the formulation in Table 5.4 will exceed the U.S. Food and Drug Administration (FDA) and manufacturer's maximal dosage of 7 mg/kg for infiltration of lidocaine in local anesthesia. The ASDS recommends a maximal safe tumescent lidocaine dose of 55 mg/kg.[32] Interestingly, the widely accepted 7 mg/kg maximum dosage for infiltrated lidocaine was established by the FDA in 1948 specifically for epidural anesthesia.

A recent prospective investigation to determine maximum safe doses of tumescent lidocaine involved patients receiving a series of tumescent infiltrations of the ASDS recommended recipe with serial serum lidocaine measurements following the infiltration. Lidocaine dosages in this prospective analysis ranged from 19.2 to 45 mg/kg in patients who did not undergo liposuction. Hence, all of the administered lidocaine was absorbed and none was removed by liposuctioning. In this group the mean peak serum concentration was 2.38 µg/mL, which is well below the accepted serum concentration threshold for mild lidocaine toxicity of 6 µg/mL. The time of peak concentration was 13.1 hours following tumescent infiltration, and the total dose of tumescent lidocaine ranged from 1800 to 3600 mg of lidocaine in 2 to 4 L of fluid.[33]

An older study, upon which the ASDS recommendation is primarily based, gave patients up to 76.7 mg/kg of lidocaine via the ASDS formulation with the highest peak plasma lidocaine concentration reaching 3.6 µg/mL. These massive amounts of lidocaine produced no clinical signs or symptoms, despite being an order of magnitude higher than the FDA and manufacturer's recommended maximal dose. Given these findings, tumescent anesthesia is a safe and efficacious means of delivering large quantities of local anesthetic into the subcutaneous space, aiding in both dissection and decreasing intraoperative time, as well as decreasing postoperative analgesic requirements.

PROCEDURES INCORPORATING TUMESCENT ANESTHESIA

Surgical procedures that utilize tumescent anesthesia take advantage both of the analgesia from the local anesthetic as well as the hydrodissection that occurs when achieving tumescence. This hydrodissection can allow for faster and easier blunt/sharp dissection, while maintaining the same level of safety as traditional techniques.[34] These benefits allow for faster throughput of traditional cases, decreased need for postoperative pain medications, and faster discharge times for ambulatory procedures.[35] The implementation of tumescent anesthesia into surgical procedures normally performed under general anesthetic has also begun to increase the accessibility of these procedures to patients who may not be able to tolerate a general anesthetic by allowing those procedures to be performed on an awake patient.

LYMPH NODE BIOPSY

Sentinel Lymph Node Biopsy

Sentinel lymph node excision performed under tumescent local anesthesia technique has been shown to be noninferior to a sentinel node biopsy performed under general anesthesia in patients with malignant melanoma and breast cancer.[36-38] In those patients who received tumescent anesthesia, a 0.1% lidocaine solution was generally used with 1:1,000,000 concentration of epinephrine. No sodium bicarbonate was used, and dosages of lidocaine never exceeded 35 mg/kg. Complication rates between the general and tumescent anesthesia groups were not significantly different, and no cases of lidocaine or epinephrine toxicity were reported. Another author postulated that hydrodissection might be responsible for the faster localization of the sentinel node in patients undergoing tumescent local anesthesia.[36]

Complete Lymph Node Excision

A recent analysis by the same group who performed the aforementioned sentinel lymph node biopsy study investigated 60 patients for complete node dissection and found that tumescent anesthesia was a safe and cost-effective alternative to general anesthesia.[36] In patients who received tumescent anesthesia, the same 0.1% lidocaine solutions with epinephrine and without sodium bicarbonate were used as in the sentinel lymph node excision cases. The solution was infiltrated into the subcutaneous tissue along the surgical field until tumescence and blanching of the skin was achieved.

As previously, complication rates between general anesthesia and tumescent lidocaine anesthesia were not significantly different in this study and were restricted to occasional seromas and wound infections. No complications such as vascular injuries or nerve damage occurred, and there was no significant time difference between operating times in the general and tumescent anesthetic groups.

INGUINAL HERNIA REPAIR

Open Tension-Free Herniorrhaphy

Anesthetic choices for this procedure include general, neuraxial, or local anesthesia. Of these, awake local anesthesia has been shown to be superior to other techniques with regards to complication rate, postoperative pain, and duration of hospital stay.[39] A tumescent local anesthesia technique has emerged for this procedure that effectively negates concerns for local anesthetic toxicity and consequent conversion to general anesthesia while still providing all of the benefits of local anesthesia.[40]

This procedure was described with a tumescent solution consisting of 0.05% lidocaine and 0.125% bupivacaine in normal saline with 1 mg/L epinephrine and 10 mEq/L of sodium bicarbonate. The herniorrhaphy was performed according to Gilbert et al.[41] This anesthetic effectively blocks the ilioinguinal and iliohypogastric nerves, as well as the genital branch of the genitofemoral nerve. It also greatly facilitates blunt dissection of the preperitoneal space following the 40 mL dose that effectively hydrodissects the peritoneum from the preperitoneal space. In one study following this procedure, intraoperative sedation was required in only 1.5% of patients, and pain medication in the early postoperative period was required in only 13.6%.[45]

Laparoscopic Transabdominal Preperitoneal Herniorrhaphy

Laparoscopic inguinal hernia repair has emerged in recent years as a more effective alternative to the standard open mesh repair of inguinal hernias. In order to facilitate the laparoscopic technique and ease its technical difficulty, a new technique utilizing laparoscopic tumescent local anesthesia has been proposed.

The tumescent solution in this technique consists of 0.1% lidocaine and 0.66 mg/ L epinephrine. The laparoscopic transabdominal preperitoneal (TAPP) procedure is carried out using the standard surgical technique[42] with the exception that prior to incising the peritoneum, a laparoscopic needle is utilized to inject through the peritoneum in three different places. The hydrodissection of the peritoneum, preperitoneal space, and transverse fascia in this technique allows surgeons to more easily confirm anatomy, and sharp dissection is able to be utilized given the vasoconstrictive effect of the injected epinephrine and consequent hemostasis. Postoperative complications utilizing this tumescent TAPP technique are comparable to the traditional TAPP technique, though prospective analyses are lacking.

Mastectomy

Awake Mastectomy

Case reports of mastectomy utilizing tumescent anesthesia have been published, though there is limited prospective or controlled data comparing it to standard general anesthetic techniques.[43,44] This technique utilized the original Klein formulation and involved four primary tumescent injections: (a) along the parasternal and (b) midaxillary lines from the second to sixth intercostal spaces, (c) along the infraclavicular line, and (d) in the space between the pectoralis and the mammary gland.

Tumescent Anesthesia in Skin-Sparing Mastectomy

Skin-sparing mastectomy entails complete removal of breast tissue while preserving as much of the overlying skin as possible for immediate reconstruction.[45] The hydrodissection afforded by tumescent infiltration can help facilitate the removal of breast tissue from the posterior aspect of the skin flap in this procedure. A generic tumescent solution may be used for this procedure, and multiple different formulations have been used with success. Following the standard skin-sparing mastectomy incision around the areola, a spinal needle is introduced fully into the subcutaneous space and tumescent solution volumes ranging from 20 to 60 mL are infiltrated under the anticipated skin flap. This technique allows for easier sharp dissection as well as decreased need for electrocautery given the vasoconstrictive effects of the epinephrine.[46]

The safety of this tumescent technique was recently challenged due to concerns for increased rates of flap necrosis due to epinephrine.[43,47] Follow-on studies[48,49] have not supported these concerns.

LIPECTOMY

Lipectomy is often performed under general anesthesia when large lipomas cannot not be safely excised with traditional local anesthesia due to toxicity risks. Tumescent anesthesia has been performed excision of lipomas with a long axis measuring up to 22 cm.[50] In these cases a generic tumescent solution is infiltrated around the area of the lipoma to provide a field block.

Alternatively, tumescent local anesthesia can be used to facilitate liposuction of large lipomas in an effort to decrease their size prior to their excision through a smaller skin incision.[51] Some providers express concerns regarding the use of liposuction for removal of lipomas given the risk for retained fragments of the original mass and consequent reoccurrence. A recent cohort of 25 patients with 48 lipomas were followed for 1 to 10 years post-tumescent liposuction assisted excision of their lipomas and none reported recurrence.[52]

PHLEBECTOMY AND LONG SAPHENOUS STRIPPING

Muller phlebectomy has become the first choice of treatment for varicose veins given the low recurrence rate, high patient satisfaction, and potential long-term cost effectiveness.[53] This procedure involves the removal of veins through a 2 mm incision with a specially designed phlebectomy hook and can be performed in the ambulatory setting without sedation given liberal use of local anesthetic. Over the past decade tumescent anesthesia has become relatively standard in the execution of Muller phlebectomy.

The procedure involves a generic tumescent solution, though one study has shown that the inclusion of sodium bicarbonate is of particular use in phlebectomy in preventing injection pain.[54] Tumescent anesthesia is incorporated into Muller phlebectomy by subcutaneous infiltration of the tumescent solution over the entire span of the previously marked varicose vein with the tumescent wheal extending at least 3 inches to each side of the vein.[55] Surgeons who use this technique find that patients rarely require a supplemental femoral nerve block for pain relief postoperatively.

PILONIDAL DISEASE

Excisional and flap procedures can be performed under tumescent anesthesia in patients with sacrococcygeal pilonidal disease without the need for sedation, neuraxial, or regional anesthesia.[56] By infiltrating a generic tumescent solution consisting of lidocaine and epinephrine subcutaneously around and under the affected area until tumescence is achieved, sufficient anesthesia can be achieved to allow both excision and filling of the area with either an advancement or rotational flap. As in the skin-sparing mastectomy technique, there is a potential that the flap will be adversely affected by the epinephrine utilized in this technique; however, no prospective data to date has demonstrated an increased risk of skin necrosis following a tumescent excisional technique for pilonidal disease.

BURN SURGERY

Tumescent infiltration of lidocaine and epinephrine has been shown to greatly assist in escharotomies following deep dermal burns where the zone of coagulation extends into the reticular dermis.[57,58] The primary benefit of tumescent anesthesia in escharotomy is related to the epinephrine infiltration providing hemostasis during excision of eschar, debridement of necrotic tissue, and excision of granulation tissue. This hemostasis allows for rapid identification of necrotic eschar with minimal bleeding into the surgical field. Lidocaine is not entirely necessary in this tumescent infiltrate; however, it may provide pain relief depending on the nature of the burn.

SUMMARY

The technique of tumescent anesthesia is no longer relegated to only dermatologic practice. Today both general surgeons and surgically active generalists may benefit from the utilization of the tumescent technique. This method of local anesthesia opens up many procedures that previously required general anesthesia to the ambulatory setting and does so with a proven track record of safety and efficacy.

This chapter has presented the basic physiology of tumescent anesthesia, as well as a brief review of the common procedures indicated for this anesthetic technique. It is the hope of the authors that these lessons will be carried forward and continue the expansion of tumescent anesthesia for surgery.

ACKNOWLEDGMENTS

The authors are military service members. This work was prepared as part of official duties. Title 17 U.S.C. 105 provides that "Copyright protection under this title is not available for any work of the United States Government." Title 17 U.S.C. 101 defines a United States Government work as a work prepared by a military service member or employee of the United States Government as part of that person's official duties.

REFERENCES

1. Courtiss EH, Choucair RJ, Donelan MB. Large-volume suction lipectomy: an analysis of 108 patients. *Plast Reconstr Surg.* 1992;89:1068–1079.
2. Klein JA. Tumescent technique for local anesthesia improves safety of large-volume liposuction. *Plast Reconstr Surg.* 1993;92:1085–1098.
3. Klein JA. The tumescent technique for liposuction surgery. *Am J Cosmet Surg.* 1987;4:263–267.
4. Abramson DL. Tumescent abdominoplasty: an ambulatory office procedure. *Aesthet Plast Surg.* 1998;22:404–407.
5. Habbema L. Safety of liposuction using exclusively tumescent local anesthesia in 3,240 consecutive cases. *Dermatol Surg.* 2009;35:1728–1735.

6. Klein JA. Clinical biostatistics of safety. In: Klein JA, ed. *Tumescent Liposuction: Tumescent Anesthesia and Microcannular Liposuction*, vol. 1. St. Louis: Mosby; 2000:27–31.

7. Carterall WA. Molecular mechanisms of gating and drug block of sodium channels: sodium channels and neuronal hyperexcitability. *Novartis Found Symp*. 2001;241:206–225.

8. Gianelly R, von der Groeben JO, Spivack AP, Harrison DC. Effect of lidocaine on ventricular arrhythmias in patients with coronary heart disease. *N Engl J Med*. 1967;277:1215–1219.

9. Scott DB. Evaluation of the toxicity of local anaesthetic agents in man. *Br J Anaesth*. 1975;47:56–61.

10. Weinberg GL. Treatment of local anesthetic systemic toxicity (LAST). *Reg Anes Pain Med*. 2010;35:188–193.

11. Kucera IJ, Lambert TJ, Klein JA, Watkins RG, Hoover JM, Kayne AD. Liposuction: contemporary issues for the anesthesiologist. *J Clin Anes*. 2006;18:379–387.

12. Covino BG, Vassallo HG: *Local Anesthesics—Mechanisms of Action and Clinical Use*. New York, Grune & Stratton; 1976:63.

13. Newton DJ, McLeod GA, Khan F, Belch, JJF. Mechanisms influencing the vasoactive effects of lidocaine in the human skin. *Anesthesia*. 2007;63:146–150.

14. Flynn N, O'Toole DP, Bourke E, O'Malley K, Cunningham AJ. The effect of local anaesthetics on epinephrine absorption following rectal mucosal infiltration. *Can J Anaesth*. 1989;36:397–401.

15. Tucker GT. Local anesthetic drugs – mode of action and pharmacokinetics. In: Nimmo WS, Smith G, eds. *Anesthesia*. Oxford: Blackwell; 1989:983–1010.

16. Roden DM. Antiarrhythmic drugs. In: Hardman JG, Limbird LE, Mollinoff PB, Ruddon RW, Goodman Gillman A, eds. *Goodman's and Gillman's The Phamacological Basis of Therapeutics*. New York: McGraw-Hill; 1996:839–874.

17. Cassidy JP, Phero JC, Grau WH. Epinephrine: systemic effects and varying concentrations in local anesthesia. *Anesthesia Progress*. 1986;33(6):289–297.

18. Malamed S, ed. *Handbook of Local Anesthesia*, 1st ed. St. Louis: Mosby; 1980:27–35, 222–224.

19. Simons FER, Gu X, Simons KJ. Epinephrine absorption in adults: intramuscular vs. subcutaneous injection. *J Allergy Clin Immunol*. 2001;108(5):871–873.

20. Eisenach JC, Grice SC, Dewan DM. Epinephrine enhances analgesia produces by epidural bupivacaine during labor. *Anesth Analg*. 1987;66:447–451.

21. Rubin JP, Bierman C, Roslow CE. The tumescent technique: the effect of high tissue pressure and dilute epinephrine on absorption of lidocaine. *Plast Reconstr Surg*. 1999;103:997–1002.

22. Chowdhry S, Seidenstricker L, Cooney DS, Hazani R, Wilhelmi BJ. Do not use epinephrine in digital blocks: myth or truth? *Plast Reconst Surg*. 2001;126(6):393–397.

23. McKay W, Morris R, Mushlin P. Sodium bicarbonate attenuates pain on skin infiltration with lidocaine, with or without epinephrine. *Anesth Analg*. 1987;66: 572–574.

24. Stewart JH, Cole GW, Klein JA. Neutralized lidocaine with epinephrine for local anesthesia. *J Dermatol Surg Oncol*. 1989;15:1081–1083.

25. Lu CW, Lin TY, Sheih JS, Wang, MJ, Chiu KM. Antimicrobial effects of continuous lidocaine infusions in a Staphylococcus aureus-induces wound infection in a mouse model. *Ann Plast Surg*. 2014;73:598–601.

26. Thompson KD, Wellykyj S, Massa MC. Antibacterial activity of lidocaine in combination with a bicarbonate buffer. *J Derm Surg Oncol*. 1993;19:219–220.

27. dos Reis Gadelha A, de Miranda Leao TL. Rule of four: a simple and safe formula for tumescent anesthesia in dermatologic surgical procedures. *Surg Cosmetic Derm.* 2009;1:99–102.

28. Kaplan B, Moy RL. Comparison of room temperature and warmed local anesthesia solution for tumescent liposuction: a randomized double-blind study. *Dermatol Surg.* 1996;22:707–709.

29. Fialkor JA, McDougal EP. Warmed local anesthetic reduces pain on infiltration. *Ann Plast Surg.* 1996;36:11–13.

30. Neil-Dwyer JG, Evans RD, Jones BM, Hayward RD. Tumescent steroid infiltration to reduce postoperative swelling after craniofacial surgery. *Br J Plast Surg.* 2001;54:565–569.

31. Chiarello SE. Tumescent infiltration of corticosteroids, lidocaine, and epinephrine into dermatomes of acute herpetic pain or postherpetic neuralgia. *Arch Dermatol.* 1998;134:279–281.

32. Coldiron B, Coleman WP III, Cox SE, Jacob C, Lawrence N, Kaminer M, Narins RS. ASDS guidelines of care for tumescent liposuction. *Dermatol Surg.* 2006;32:709–716.

33. Klein JA, Jeske DR. Estimated maximal safe dosages of tumescent lidocaine. *Anesth Analg.* 2016;122:1350–1359.

34. Stoffels I, Dissemond J, Schulz A, Hillen U, Schadendorf D, Klode J. Reliability and cost-effectiveness of complete lymph nodedissection under tumescent local anaesthesia vs. general anaesthesia: a retrospective analysis in patients with malignant melanoma AJCC stage III. *J Euro Acad Derm Vener.* 2011;26:200–206.

35. Nordin P, Zetterstrom H, Carlsson P, Nilsson E. Cost-effectiveness analysis of local, regional and general anaesthesia for inguinal hernia repair using data from a randomized clinical trial. *Br J Surg.* 2007;94:500–505.

36. Stoffels I, Dissemond J, Körber A, et al. Reliability and cost-effectiveness of sentinel lymph node excision under local anaesthesia versus general anaesthesia for malignant melanoma: a retrospective analysis in 300 patients with malignant melanoma AJCC Stages I and II. *J Euro Acad Derm Vener.* 2010;25:306–310.

37. Kongdan Y, Chirappapha P, Lertsithichai P. Effectiveness and reliability of sentinel lymph node biopsy under local anesthesia for breast cancer. *Breast.* 2008;17(5):528–531.

38. Smidt ML, Janssen CMM, Barendregt WB, Wobbes T, Strobbe LJA. Sentinel lymph node biopsy performed under local anesthesia is feasible. *Am J Surg.* 2004;187(6):684–687.

39. Nordin P, Zetterstrom H, Carlsson P, et al. Cost-effectiveness analysis of local, regional and general anaesthesia for inguinal hernia repair using data from a randomized clinical trial. *Br J Surg.* 2007;94:500–505.

40. Narita M, Sakano S, Okamoto S, Uemoto S, Yamamoto M. Tumescent local anesthesia in inguinal herniorrhaphy with a PROLENE hernia system: original technique and results. *Am J Surg.* 2009;198:e27–e31.

41. Gilbert AI, Graham MF, Voigt WJ. A bilayer patch device for inguinal hernia repair. *Hernia.* 1999;3:161–166.

42. Bittner R, Leibl BJ, Jäger C, Kraft B, Ulrich M, Schwarz J. TAPP—Stuttgart technique and result of a large single center series. *J Minim Access Surg.* 2006;2:155–159.

43. Sleth JC, Servais R, Saizy C. Tumescent infiltrative anesthesia for mastectomy: about six cases. *Ann Francaises anesthes eReanim.* 2008;27:941–944.

44. Carlson GW. Total mastectomy under local anesthesia: the tumescent technique. *Breast J.* 2005;11:100–102.

45. Cunnick GH, Mokbel K. Skin-sparing mastectomy. *Am J Surg.* 2005;188:78–84.

46. Chun YS, Verma K, Rosen H, et al. Use of tumescent mastectomy technique as a risk factor for native breast skin flap necrosis following immediate breast reconstruction. *Am J Surg.* 2011;201:160–165.

47. Abbott AM, Miller MT, Tuttle TM. Outcomes after tumescence technique versus electrocautery mastectomy. *Ann Surg Onc.* 2012;19:2607–2611.

48. Vargas CR, Koolen PG, Ho OA, et al. Tumescent mastectomy technique in autologous breast reconstruction. *J Surg Res.* 2015;198:525–529.

49. Khavanin N, Fine NA, Bethke KB, et al. Tumescent technique does not increase the risk of complication following mastectomy with immediate reconstruction. *Ann Surg Oncol.* 2014;21:384–388.

50. Morioka D, Sato N, Ohkubo F. Excision of large lipomas using tumescent local anesthesia. *J Cutan Med Surg.* 2016;20:263–265.

51. Choi CW, Kim BJ, Moon SE, Youn SW, Park KC, Huh CH. Treatment of lipomas assisted with tumescent liposuction. *J Eur Acad Derm Ven.* 2007;21:243–246.

52. Copeland-Halperin LR, Pimpinella V, Copeland M. Combined liposuction and excision of lipomas: long-term evaluation of a large sample of patients. *Plast Surg Int.* 2015;Article ID 625396.

53. de Roos J, Niemand FHM, Martino Neuman HA. Ambulatory phlebectomy versus compression sclerotherapy: results of a randomized controlled trial [1076e0512]. *Dermatol Surg.* 2003;29:221–226.

54. Krasznai AG, Sigterman TA, Willems CE, et al. Prospective study of a single treatment strategy for local tumescent anesthesia in Muller phlebectomy. *Ann Vasc Surg.* 2015;29:586–593.

55. Bush RG, Hammon KA. Tumescent anesthetic technique for long saphenous stripping. *J Am Coll Surg.* 1999;189:626–628.

56. Kayaalp C, Olmez A, Aydin C, Piskin T. Tumescent local anesthesia for excision and flap procedures in treatment of pilonidal disease. *Dis Colon Rectum.* 2009;52:1780–1783.

57. Orgill DP. Excision and skin grafting of thermal burns. *N Engl J Med.* 2009;360:893–901.

58. Gumus N. Tumescent infiltration of lidocaine and adrenaline for burn surgery. *Ann Burn Fire Disast.* 2011;24:144.

6 Pain Management for General Surgery

Acetaminophen, NSAIDS, and COX-2 Selective Inhibitors Update

Katherine Stammen, Harish Siddaiah, Cody Brechtel, Elyse M. Cornett, Charles J. Fox III, and Alan D. Kaye

INTRODUCTION

Pain or lack of pain control is a major fear that patients have regarding surgical procedures. In a recent article, nearly 80% of patients experienced pain after surgery, which they stated was inadequately treated.[1] Pain is multidimensional and subjective, which makes it difficult to treat. And many negative outcomes have been associated with poor pain control and pain treatment, including the development of chronic pain. Undertreated pain can lead to serious consequences, including morbidity and mortality.[2] To better recognize and treat pain, recognition and assessment tools have been developed by organizations, such as the American Pain Society. Additionally, the Joint Commission on Accreditation of Healthcare Organizations (JCAHO) has standards for assessing, monitoring, and treating acute pain.[3] Treatment modalities such as acetaminophen, non-steroidal anti-inflammatory drugs (NSAIDS) and cyclooxygenase-2 (COX-2) inhibitors are a component of many multimodal therapeutic regimens that attempt to produce perioperative analgesia and decrease inflammation.[4] In recent years, newer treatment modalities have been under development to take advantage of the multifactorial components to pain development and treatment, including such agents as ketamine, capsaicin, gabapentin, pregabalin, long-acting opioids, peripheral nerve blockade, and patient-controlled analgesia.[2] Overall, adequate perioperative pain control is important both in an acute setting and in preventing the development of a chronic pain condition.

IMPORTANCE OF CONTROLLING PAIN

Undertreated pain can have many harmful effects. Patients with undertreated pain may have decreases in alveolar ventilation and vital capacity related to respiratory splinting, which may lead to pneumonic consolidation, predisposing them to hypoxia and possibly infections.[3] Inadequate pain relief may mediate or modulate various cardiovascular associated untoward events, including tachycardia, hypertension, myocardial infarction, insomnia, dementia, poor glucose control, and predisposition to infections and to poor wound healing.[3] Postoperative pain control is an important variable in patient discharge from ambulatory surgery, and lack of adequate pain control contributes to unplanned admissions and increases in overall health care costs. Inadequate pain control is one of the three most common reasons leading to delayed discharge from ambulatory surgery.[2]

Inadequate pain control can also lead to additional complications. Clinically, patients may become less mobile and become predisposed to deep venous thromboses, pulmonary embolism, pneumonia, or delayed wound healing; develop chronic pain syndromes; and potentially become physically dependent on opioid medications.[3] Up to 50% of patients may develop chronic postoperative pain symptoms, which may include depression, anxiety, and sleep issues, and a late return to work.[5] Inadequate postoperative pain treatment can lead to chronic pain syndromes leading to allodynia and hyperalgesia. Allodynia refers to a triggering of a pain response which does not normally produce pain similar to sunburn, for example, a burning sensation triggered by light touch to the skin. Hyperalgesia refers to an increased pain response to a stimulus that is normally painful. This occurs related to central pain sensitization, which may be a result of uncontrolled acute nociceptive pain. It is estimated that the economic burden of treating chronic pain which develops from acute pain in a 30-year-old individual over a lifetime could cost as much as $1 million.[1]

The mechanism by which pain is produced is important to understand the significance of multimodal therapies of pain management. Primary hyperalgesia is pain related to peripheral alterations of the sensory endings at the site of injury, whereas secondary hyperalgesia is the result of a change in the sensory processing by the central nervous system.[2] Peripheral sensitization involves inflammatory mediators such as bradykinins, histamine, and leukotrienes. These mediators stimulate the release of substance P, calcitonin gene-related protein, and cholecystokinin at the site of injury. Impulses travel down peripheral nociceptors via A delta and C fibers to lamina II and lamina V of the spinal cord. Neurotransmitters produce synaptic transmission by binding receptors that regulate sodium and potassium influx. These receptors then start the priming of N-methyl-D-aspartate (NMDA) receptors, which regulate the flow of sodium and calcium ions into the cell and potassium out of the cell.[3] NMDA receptors can have rapid and independent firing due to accumulation of calcium, even without stimulation, which is referred to as "wind up." This activation of the NMDA receptors at the level of the spinal cord can lead to long-term potentiation of pain. The central sensitization of pain is a reversible process if it causes LTP, but transcription- independent sensitization, which can occur by an alteration in the dorsal root ganglion and dorsal horn, can lead to irreversible modifications in the central nervous system.[3] Related to this response, the preemptive treatment of pain and multimodal approaches to the management of pain to avoid not only the acute effects but also pain-related modulation of the central nervous system is critical for short- and long-term benefits for each patient.[3] Preemptive analgesia has been typically defined as treatment that is initiated before surgical incision, prevents the establishment of central sensitization related to incisional injury, and prevents the establishment of central sensitization resulting from incisional and inflammatory injuries.

UNDERTREATMENT OF PAIN

Although pain is a predictable part of the perioperative process, severe uncontrolled pain is unfortunately common and can have serious negative implications. One of the principle fears that patients have prior to their surgery regards the pain that they will have after surgery. In the United States, more than 73 million surgeries are performed annually, and up to 75% of patients have pain after surgery.[1] There are many deleterious effects to undertreated pain, such as those highlighted in the previous section. In a recent article, a national survey was completed that showed 80% of patients reported inadequate pain control perioperatively; of those 85% had moderate or severe pain. Causes for the undertreatment of pain are multifactorial and include lack of patient education, pressure on physicians to discharge patients quickly, adverse effects of pain medications, hospital staffing shortages, and fear of opioid addiction. As previously stated, the JCAHO has noticed the importance of appropriately managing pain and set standards for pain management. Other organizations such as the American Society of Anesthesiologists have published guidelines for acute perioperative pain management. These guidelines promote multimodal analgesia, patient-controlled analgesia, epidurals, and peripheral nerve blockade. They also promote preemptive planning, including a history regarding pain and discussions regarding preoperative, intraoperative, and postoperative pain treatment. Despite these standards and guidelines, additional efforts are required to improve adequate pain control in surgical patients.

HARMFUL EFFECTS OF UNTREATED PAIN

Postoperative pain can affect many body systems including cardiovascular, gastrointestinal, endocrine, and metabolic and immune systems. The cardiovascular system is affected by pain because it activates the sympathetic nervous system, which in turn causes many adverse effects such as increased heart rate and blood pressure and thus, increased myocardial work, resulting in a mismatch of myocardial oxygen demand and supply. In the elderly and other high-risk cardiac patients, this physiological derangement can result in myocardial ischemia and death.

Pain can affect the gastrointestinal system by increasing sphincter tone due to activation of the sympathetic nervous system. It also results in delayed gastric emptying, and eventually both of these mechanisms can lead to ileus. Ileus can progress to small and large bowel obstruction in severe cases.[6] The endocrine system responds to pain by releasing various catabolic hormones, which can result in weight loss, fever, metabolic acidosis, shock, and even death.

Pain can also affect the immune system, especially cell-mediated immunity. Pain affects the natural killer cells, which play an important role in preventing tumor growth and metastasis. Hence inadequate pain control can result in tumor growth and increased risk of metastasis. It can also result in increased postsurgical infection and wound healing. Lastly, inadequately treated acute postoperative pain can progress to chronic pain, which can have long-term physical, physiological, psychological, and economic effects on the patient. Patients may also suffer from anxiety and chronic depression.

PAIN ASSESSMENT

Assessment of pain is a crucial step when providing good pain management. A comprehensive pain evaluation should be performed by the health care provider prior to the planned surgical procedure and involving the patient and the patient's family. The evaluation will provide insight into the patient's underlying chronic pain conditions, previous experience with pain and medications used if any, the patient's attitude and beliefs regarding pain control, and expectations of the patient and family regarding pain control. Several pain intensity tools have been proposed and validated. They can be classified into tools used for cognitively intact and cognitively impaired patients.

For the cognitively intact patients, a simple scale-like verbal rating scale, which classifies pain into mild, moderate, or severe, can be used. Furthermore, a numerical rating scale can be used to assess pain. It consists of a straight horizontal line numbered at equal intervals from zero to 10 with zero denoting "no pain," 5 representing "moderate pain," and 10 implying "worst pain." The FACES scale, which can also be used, comprises of six faces showing increasing pain intensities, beginning with a smiling face and ending with a crying face. For patients who are cognitively impaired and do not have the capacity to communicate or report pain, other tools have to be used. These tools should identify the existence of pain and estimate the probable intensity. Certain patient behaviors are likely to indicate pain, and they can be assessed by behavioral assessment tools. Behavioral assessment tools are of two types: (a) pain behavior scales and (b) pain behavior checklists. An example of the pain behavior scale is the Behavior Pain Scale developed for use in critically ill patients in the intensive care unit.[7] It evaluates and scores three categories of behavior:

1. Ventilator compliance: scores range from 1 for tolerating ventilator to 4 for unable to control ventilation.
2. Upper-limb movement: scores range from 1 for no movement to 4 for permanently retracted.
3. Facial expression: scores range from 1 for relaxed to 4 for grimacing.

A score above 3 may indicate pain is present, and the score can be used to evaluate intervention but cannot be interpreted to assess pain intensity. An example of a pain behavior checklist is the Pain Assessment Checklist for Seniors with Limited Ability to Communicate (PACSLAC). The PACSLAC evaluates 60 behaviors such as facial expressions, activities, and mood. But again it cannot assess the pain intensity.[8]

TREATMENT MODALITIES

There are many ways of treating pain pharmacologically, including opioids, non-opioids, and regional anesthesia.

OPIOID ANALGESIA

Postoperative pain has been traditionally treated with opioids. Opioids exert their action by binding to the receptors (mu, delta, and kappa) in the central nervous system and peripheral nervous system. Opioids bind to the receptors at the injured tissue, which blocks signal transduction. At the dorsal root ganglion, opioids bind to the receptors of first- order and second-order neurons and block the release of neurotransmitters and hyperpolarize the cell membrane. They also bind to the receptors in the midbrain and inhibit GABAergic synaptic transmission in the descending inhibitory pathways.[9]

Among the most commonly used opioids for postoperative pain are hydromorphone, morphine, and fentanyl. They can be administered by different routes including oral, parenteral, neuraxial, and transdermal routes.

Morphine is usually titrated intravenously as 2.5 mg to 5 mg every hour to treat postoperative pain. Hydromorphone is titrated as 0.2 mg to 1 mg every hour. Fentanyl is titrated as 25 mcg to 50 mcg every hour.

Opioids have significant side effects, which include nausea, vomiting, constipation, ileus, tolerance, and respiratory depression.[10] Hence it is critical to monitor respiration in postoperative patients who are on opioids. With the introduction of enhanced recovery programs, non-opioid analgesia has been emphasized and promoted to reduce opioid consumption and hence reduce side effects associated with opioids in the postoperative period.[11]

NONOPIOID ANALGESIA

NSAIDS are the most commonly used drugs worldwide because of their analgesic, anti-inflammatory, and antipyretic effects. The therapeutic benefit of NSAIDS is believed to be mediated through the inhibition of COX-1 and COX-2 enzymes, which convert arachidonic acid to prostaglandins H2. These prostaglandins act on both peripheral and central pain pathways.

ACETAMINOPHEN

Acetaminophen can be used relatively safely to augment a multimodal approach to perioperative pain management. It has both analgesic and antipyretic properties as well as a favorable side effect profile when compared to opioids and other NSAIDs.

Derived from para-aminophenol, acetaminophen differs from NSAIDs in many respects. NSAIDs provide analgesia through the inhibition of peripherally induced COX-2. This inhibition decreases the production of prostaglandins at the site of tissue injury which would otherwise cause hyperalgesia and inflammation. Acetaminophen does not have peripheral activity on COX enzymes and therefore does not exhibit anti-inflammatory properties as compared to NSAIDs. Despite this, acetaminophen provides analgesia as evidenced by its opioid-sparing effect.[12]

Despite ongoing research, the analgesia produced by acetaminophen does not yet have a clear mechanism of action. Acetaminophen's activity is central, where it likely inhibits a different COX isoform (COX-3). Other hypotheses include modulation of descending serotonergic or NMDA pathways.[13] It is well understood that NSAIDs act through binding the COX site of the COX enzyme; however, acetaminophen appears to prevent COX activation through the peroxidase site of the enzyme. This pharmacodynamic difference likely determines its unique behavior.

Intravenous preparations of acetaminophen have only recently become available. Prior to their development, administration was limited to the oral or rectal route. Despite a relatively high oral bioavailability (80%–90%), neither enteral routes provide reliable absorption due to considerable interindividual variability.[14] Postoperative delays in gastric emptying further confound acetaminophen's enteral absorption in the small intestine. Intravenous acetaminophen (Ofirmev®) became available in the United States in 2010 and offers significant advantages to enteral administration, including faster onset of action, higher peak plasma concentrations, and increased opioid-sparing effect.

Oral/rectal dosing is typically 500 to 1000 mg every four to six hours the healthy adult. Intravenous (IV) administration for adults >50 kg is 1 g every four to six hours not to exceed 4 g/day and for adults <50kg, 15 mg/kg every four to six hours not to exceed 3 g/day.

Though the side effects of NSAIDs (gastrointestinal mucosal erosions, impaired platelet function, impaired renal perfusion) are spared with the use of acetaminophen, caution must be exercised with respect to its liver metabolism. Hepatotoxicity occurs via a metabolite N-acetyl-p-benzoquinone imine, which can cause hepatic necrosis if not bound by glutathione.[12] Although less relevant to perioperative acetaminophen use, it has been recommended to the Food and Drug Administration that oral dosing of acetaminophen be limited to less than 4 g per day in the absence of underlying liver disease.[15]

COX-2 INHIBITORS

The known platelet and gastrointestinal side effects of NSAIDs stimulated the interest in developing more specific drugs in the class. The COX enzyme was first purified in 1988, and, although its existence had been postulated, the COX-2 subtype was not isolated until 1991.[16] This opened the door to the advancement of multiple COX-2 selective agents. Celecoxib (Celebrex®) was first to be marketed and, curiously, the only remaining COX-2 specific inhibitor available in the United States for postoperative pain. Other COX-2 selective drugs, such as rofecxib (Vioxx ®) and valdecoxib (Bextra®), emerged on the market soon after. When taken long term for arthritis, these drugs were found to have reduced gastrointestinal side effects by 50% to 60% compared to traditional NSAIDs.[17] This new class of analgesic was surely compelling; however, many were recalled after trials such as the Adenomatous Polyp Prevention on Vioxx trial demonstrated increased risk of thrombotic cardiovascular events.[18] Additionally, a study of approximately 1,600 patients undergoing elective coronary artery bypass surgery showed a significant increase in thromboembolic events with short-term use of parecoxib (Dynestat®) and valdecoxib.[19]

In the United States, the remaining options for COX-2 inhibitors are somewhat limited in the perioperative context. Celecoxib is an oral preparation and may be used to augment multimodal pain management with a loading dose of 400 mg, followed by 100 to 200 mg every 12 hours. It is worth mentioning that meloxicam (Mobic®), although not a COX inhibitor-3, has been shown to be relatively specific for COX-2 and can also be used in perioperative pain management in oral doses of 7.5 to 15mg daily.[20] In Europe, multiple COX inhibitors remain in use, and, specifically, the IV preparation of parecoxib has indications for treating moderate to severe postoperative pain.

With the existing literature regarding COX-2 inhibitors and their potential adverse effects, prescribing these drugs in the postoperative setting requires attention to patient comorbidities. Certainly patients with coronary artery disease should not be treated with a COX-2 specific inhibitor. This may also extend to patients with cerebrovascular disease. As with NSAIDs, they should be avoided in patients with acute renal injury or failure. Finally, use of COX-2 selective inhibitors should not be used in patients with a sulfonamide allergy.

REGIONAL ANALGESIA

Neuraxial analgesia, which includes epidural and spinal analgesia, has been used to provide pain relief for various thoracic, abdominal, and pelvic surgeries. A continuous opioid infusion or local anesthetic infusion or combination can be used through the neuraxial route. Commonly used local anesthetics are 0.2% or 0.5% ropivacaine and 0.0625% and 0.125% bupivacaine. The commonly used opioids for neuraxial analgesia are fentanyl and morphine.

A Cochrane database review of nine randomized controlled trials comparing IV patient controlled analgesia (PCA) and continuous epidural analgesia (CEA) showed the latter achieved better pain control in the first 72 hours after abdominal surgery.[9] There was no difference in the length of hospital stay and adverse events between the two routes. There was a higher incidence of pruritus related to opioids in the CEA group.

Several other studies have revealed that neuraxial analgesia was better compared to opioids in terms of return of bowel functions, nausea/vomiting, and length of hospital stay. Complications of neuraxial blockade include injury to nerve roots, infection, and higher blockade compromising respiration.[21]

Peripheral nerve blocks, especially transversus abdominis plane block (TAP), has been used postoperatively in abdominal and pelvic surgeries for analgesia. There has been limited evidence that using TAP blocks after abdominal surgery resulted in reduced complications associated with opioids such as nausea, vomiting, and respiratory depression; reduction in the incidence of ileus; and shorter duration of hospital stay. The commonly used local anesthetics for peripheral nerve blocks include 0.5% ropivacaine and 0.125% bupivacaine. Complications of peripheral nerve block include injury to the nerves, infection, and injury to bowels and other anatomical structures. Local infiltration of anesthetics by the surgeon has been used extensively. When combined with other analgesia techniques, it has been proven to be very beneficial.

CONCLUSION

Since every patient's perception of pain is different, a multimodal pain strategy should be employed to maximize reduction in pain for patients undergoing abdominal surgery. At present, the most effective means of significantly decreasing pain is found through the combined efforts of preemptive analgesia and multimodal pain management.

Reduction of opioid intake has been primarily emphasized with the introduction of enhanced recovery programs. Preemptive analgesic techniques have been proven to be effective at reducing total opioid consumption postoperatively. NSAIDS and acetaminophen should be given for pain relief around the clock to patients if there are no contraindications. Regional analgesia, which includes epidural, spinal, and peripheral nerve blocks, should be offered to all patients if there are no contraindications to them. Without a proper and well-thought-out pain management plan, postoperative pain has the potential to cause chronic postsurgical pain in the patient, which causes significant short- and long-term negative consequences.[22,23]

REFERENCES

1. Apfelbaum JL, Chen C, Mehta SS, Gan TJ. Postoperative pain experience: results from a national survey suggest postoperative pain continues to be undermanaged. *Anesth Analg.* 2003;97(2):534–540.
2. Vadivelu N, Mitra S, Narayan D. Recent advances in postoperative pain management. *Yale J Biol Med.* 2010;83(1):11–25.
3. Harsoor S. Emerging concepts in post-operative pain management. *Indian J Anaesth.* 2011;55(2):101–103.
4. Nett MP. Postoperative pain management. *Orthopedics.* 2010;33(9 Suppl):23–26.
5. Akkaya T, Ozkan D. Chronic post-surgical pain. *Ağrı Ağrı Derneği'nin Yayın organıdır = J. Turk Soc Algol.* 2009;21(1):1–9.
6. Liu S, Carpenter RL, Neal JM. Epidural anesthesia and analgesia: their role in postoperative outcome. *Anesthesiology.* 1995;82(6):1474–1506.
7. Payen JF, Bru O, Bosson JL, et al. Assessing pain in critically ill sedated patients by using a behavioral pain scale. *Crit Care Med.* 2001;29(12):2258–2263.
8. Fuchs-Lacelle HT. Development and preliminary validation of the pain assessment checklist for seniors with limited ability to communicate (PACSLAC). *Pain Manag Nurs.* 2004;5(1):37–49.
9. Vanderah TW. Pathophysiology of pain. *Med Clin North Am.* 2007;91(1):1–12.
10. Barletta JF, Asgeirsson T, Senagore AJ. Influence of intravenous opioid dose on postoperative ileus. *Ann Pharmacother.* 2011;45(7–8):916–923.
11. Zafar N, Davies R, Greenslade GL, Dixon AR. The evolution of analgesia in an "accelerated" recovery programme for resectional laparoscopic colorectal surgery with anastomosis. *Colorectal Dis.* 2010;12(2):119–124.
12. Schilling A, Corey R, Leonard M, Eghtesad B. Acetaminophen: old drug, new warnings. *Cleve Clin J Med.* 2010;77(1):19–27.
13. Schug SA, Manopas A. Update on the role of non-opioids for postoperative pain treatment. *Best Pract Res Clin Anaesthesiol.* 2007;21(1):15–30.
14. Macario A, Royal MA. A literature review of randomized clinical trials of intravenous acetaminophen (paracetamol) for acute postoperative pain. *Pain Pract.* 2010;11(3):290–296.
15. Wróblewski T, Kobryń K, Kozieł S, et al. Acetaminophen (Paracetamol) induced acute liver failure—a social problem in an era of increasing tendency to self-treatment. *Ann Agric Environ Med.* 2015;22(4):762–7667.
16. Flower RJ. The development of COX2 inhibitors. *Nat Rev Drug Discov.* 2003;2(3):179–191.

17. Laine L. Gastrointestinal safety of coxibs and outcomes studies: what's the verdict? *J Pain Symptom Manage.* 2002;23(4):S5–S10.
18. Bresalier RS, Sandler RS, Quan H, et al. Cardiovascular events associated with rofecoxib in a colorectal adenoma chemoprevention trial. *N Engl J Med.* 2005;352(11):1092–1102.
19. Nussmeier NA, Whelton AA, Brown MT, et al. Complications of the COX-2 inhibitors parecoxib and valdecoxib after cardiac surgery. *N Engl J Med.* 2005;352(11):1081–1091.
20. Noble S, Balfour JA. Meloxicam. *Drugs.* 1996;51(3):424–430.
21. Werawatganon T, Charuluxanun S. Patient controlled intravenous opioid analgesia versus continuous epidural analgesia for pain after intra-abdominal surgery. *Cochrane Database Syst Rev.* 2005;1:CD004088.
22. Woolf CJ. Recent advances in the pathophysiology of acute pain. *Br J Anaesth.* 1989;63(2):139–146.
23. Ejlersen E, Andersen HB, Eliasen K, Mogensen T. A comparison between preincisional and postincisional lidocaine infiltration and postoperative pain. *Anesth Analg.* 1992;74(4):495–498.

7 Neuraxial Analgesia and Anesthesia in Chronic Opioid Users and Patients with Pre-existing Pain

Grace Chen and Ashley Valentine

INTRODUCTION

Pain management through neuraxial modalities includes all procedures that provide access to spinal nerves either via the subarachnoid (intrathecal) or epidural space in order to decrease or eliminate afferent nociceptor signaling. These include single injections such as a spinal (subarachnoid) block in the lumbar area, caudal (epidural) block through the sacralcoccygeal ligament, or epidural steroid injection done the thoracolumbar areas, as well as techniques with indwelling catheters such as an epidural or intrathecal pain pump. A wide range of surgeries, from toe amputation to thyroidectomy, have been performed using neuraxial analgesia.[1] A "total spinal," in which transient loss of consciousness due to complete symathectomy and hypotension, is an effective general anesthetic, though less predictable than current inhalational and intravenous (IV) techniques. While most neuraxial techniques are applied to surgeries occurring below the T4 dermatome, neuraxial blockade is indeed "indicated for any surgical procedure in which the appropriate sensory level can be accomplished without adverse patient outcomes."[2] Neuraxial techniques can be used for surgical anesthesia (i.e. surgery can be performed using a spinal or epidural without the addition of inhalational or IV anesthesia) or for analgesia to reduce pain before, during, and after surgery.

This chapter focuses first on the benefits of neuraxial modalities for general surgery with consideration of timing of the analgesic effect, then on potential adverse effects of neuraxial analgesia. Next, the use and management of the two most common neuraxial techniques for general surgery, single-injection spinals and epidural catheters, in the context of patients with a history of pre-existing pain conditions and chronic opioid or opioid substitution use are discussed.

In addition to providing perioperative pain control through synergistic local anesthetic and opioid effects superior to opioids alone, neuraxial analgesia confers nonanalgesic benefits. Although research is ongoing, epidurals may confer overall 30-day mortality benefit when epidurals replace general anesthesia in certain surgeries such as abdominal surgery, hip/knee replacement, or lower extremity revascularization.[3] Risk of perioperative pneumonia also decreases when neuraxial techniques replace, or are added to, a general anesthetic for major vascular, orthopedic, and abdominal surgeries.[3] Persistent postoperative pain may be less likely to develop when epidurals are used for thoracotomy[4] and patients undergoing curative resection of rectal adenocarcinoma.[5] Furthermore, the stress response, which contributes to postoperative immunosuppression, may be attenuated by epidural anesthesia in patients undergoing pelvic cancer[6-8] or major abdominal surgery.[9] Epidural use during certain cancer surgeries (the strongest evidence is in colorectal cancer) appears to improve overall survival but not a longer recurrence-free survival period.[10] The mechanisms underlying these immune-modulating findings are not yet known.

The timing of epidural analgesia for nonanalgesic purposes is an area of debate and ongoing investigation. The desired effect of the epidural, such as postoperative pain control, reduction of postoperative opioid use, decreased risk of persistent postsurgical pain, or decreased immunosuppression informs when analgesia or anesthesia should be achieved; preemptive (i.e., before surgical incision) versus intraoperative versus postoperative dosing, along with the required depth of analgesia. Current evidence does not support preemptive analgesia to improve postoperative pain control, reduce postoperative opioid use, attenuate opioid-induced postoperative hyperalgesia, or decrease risk of persistent postsurgical pain.[5,11-13] For these effects, it appears that intraoperative and preemptive neuraxial analgesia confer equal benefit. There are few studies that investigate the timing of analgesia delivery when the intended effect is to blunt the stress response to surgery. Research showing attenuated immune response with neuraxial techniques has been performed using preemptive analgesia.[14,15,16,17] These effects may be most clinically meaningful for surgeries where the immune system plays an important role in postoperative outcomes, such as risk of metastases after cancer surgery, but more research is needed.

ADVERSE EFFECTS OF NEURAXIAL ANALGESIA

Although there are numerous benefits, neuraxial techniques are not without risk. As with surgery, when the protective barrier of the skin is breached, there is a risk of bleeding, infection, or damage to nearby structures or tissues. Complications such as permanent nerve damage, epidural hematoma, local anesthetic toxicity, or neuraxial infection, while potentially devastating, are extremely rare. An epidural placement may result in dural puncture and postdural puncture headache. Intrathecal injection of local anesthetic intended for the epidural space can lead to a dense block that extends higher than expected. Subdural injection can result in extensive sensory block with a milder motor block, hypotension, and, in worst cases, dyspnea, bradycardia, and loss of consciousness.

In clinical practice, neuraxial analgesia must also be weighed against the risk of common side effects such as lower extremity weakness that may preclude early ambulation. Other risks include sedation, respiratory depression, pruritis, nausea, or constipation from opioid additives, urinary retention requiring maintenance of a Foley catheter (often for epidurals placed below T10), or anticipation of postoperative hypotension that may be worsened with epidural blockade (e.g., after hemorrhage or extensive fluid shifts). Patients receiving neuraxial opioids can also develop acute tolerance, which may result in an increased enteral opioid requirement when the epidural catheter is removed.

Absolute contraindications to neuraxial anesthesia include patient refusal, patient inability to cooperate in positioning or respond to abnormal sensations, and elevated intracranial pressure. Strong relative contraindications which must be weighed against the potential benefit of a neuraxial technique include infection at the site of needle insertion, systemic infection, current or anticipated coagulopathy (e.g. after major liver resection) or bleeding diathesis, afterload-dependent conditions such as severe aortic stenosis or hypertrophic cardiomyopathy, and severe hypovolemia.

Some patients are hesitant to accept, or may even refuse, neuraxial analgesia due to perceived association with postoperative back pain. Certainly, there is risk for pain or tenderness at the catheter or injection site, especially after a complicated placement. However, this type of discomfort is typically self-limited, mild, and without radicular symptoms and resolves within a few days. Bruising or tenderness from a difficult epidural placement responds well to nonsteroidal anti-inflammatory drugs (NSAIDs) and ice. Independent risk factors for developing *new* postoperative back pain include lithotomy position, immobilization during surgery greater than 2.5 hours, body mass index ≥ 32 kg/m^2, and multiple attempts for neuraxial placement.[18] There is no difference in development of new onset back pain after spinal anesthesia compared to general anesthesia, however, there may be a slight increase when epidurals are used compared to spinal anesthesia.[18]

NEURAXIAL ANESTHESIA IN CHRONIC OPIOID USERS

Neuraxial analgesia for surgical pain control in chronic opioid users is safe, provided there are no contraindications, and it is a potentially opioid-sparing technique with improved postoperative pain control. Chronic opioid users (both patients whose chronic pain is treated by opioids or recreational users of opioids including heroine) are at risk of both opioid tolerance and opioid-induced hyperalgesia. Opioid tolerance can occur after chronic opioid exposure and leads to decreased degree and duration of analgesia for a given dose of opioid. Opioid-induced hyperalgesia means that giving additional opioids increases patient sensitivity to painful stimuli. The underlying mechanism of opioid-induced hyperalgesia is not yet known, but proposed mechanisms include upregulation of pronociceptive pathways such as the N-methyl-D-aspartate (NMDA) receptor system and spinal dynorphins.[19,20] A patient with hyperalgesia experiencing heightened pain, including during injection of local anesthetic to facilitate needle placement for the epidural or spinal, may render the procedure difficult to impossible due to intolerance or inability to cooperate.

Relatively little is known about the effects of chronic opioid use on anesthetic pharmacodynamics and pharmacokinetics of neuraxial blockade. Small studies of opium abusers receiving spinal anesthesia suggest that the duration of sensory and motor blockade as well as the height of the block decrease significantly compared to non-users.[21–23] Onset of block regression after intrathecal bupivacaine for lower extremity surgery in opium abusers was half that of non-users (87 versus 162 minutes).[21] These studies, however, did not quantify daily opioid intake. It is unknown if similar effects would occur in patients taking prescribed opioids, or if there is a relationship between daily opioid dose and duration or height of blockade. Regardless, the anesthesiologist and surgeon should be aware of the potential for a shortened duration of neuraxial blockade in chronic opioid users.

Additives to neuraxial anesthesia (such as clonidine, opioids, epinephrine, or steroids) should be considered in order to prolong the block and improve analgesia in chronic opioid users. In the case of procedures amenable to spinal anesthesia, but of moderate duration, a technique that includes a catheter (i.e. combined spinal-epidural, spinal catheter, or epidural alone) may be preferred, permitting blockade to match anesthesia with surgical time. Finally, for long-duration surgeries, the patient's baseline opioid intake should be considered. It is important to meet baseline opioid intake to prevent withdrawal and worsened pre-existing pain in the immediate postoperative period.

NEURAXIAL ANESTHESIA FOR POSTOPERATIVE PAIN CONTROL IN CHRONIC OPIOID USERS

Postoperative pain management for patients with opioid tolerance is challenging. For patients with a history of chronic opioid use, the appropriateness of an epidural for postoperative pain management should always be considered. This component of multimodal analgesia is especially beneficial as it may reduce overall opioid needs postoperatively while offering more effective analgesia than supplemental opioid therapy alone. As always, epidural analgesia must be weighed against risk of unwanted side effects. In cases where side effects could be clinically significant, regional analgesia (such as femoral or sciatic blocks) may be an alternative. If epidural or regional analgesia is maintained with local anesthetic alone, postsurgical pain may be covered, but pre-existing pain unrelated to the surgical site will not. Therefore it is important to consider pre-existing pain conditions and avoid opioid withdrawal in the postoperative pain management plan.

Opioid withdrawal in a patient with an epidural for postoperative pain management can be prevented using a three-part approach. First, calculate the patient's daily dose in morphine equivalents. Second, continue the patient's daily dose via enteral, IV, or epidural routes postoperatively. Last, if the patient is to be maintained on a opioid different from his or her usual one, a dose reduction for incomplete cross-tolerance (usually about 20%–25%) is recommended.[24] There are several ways to continue a patient's baseline (maintenance) dose of opioid. It can be accomplished by simply continuing a patient's home opioid regimen with an opioid-free epidural solution. Alternatively, opioids may be added to a basal epidural infusion in sufficient quantity to cover baseline needs. Another option is that the patient could be taken off the oral opioids and given a patient-controlled analgesia or as-needed IV opioids, with access to sufficient dosage to prevent withdrawal, with an opioid-free epidural solution. Ideally, a well-functioning epidural provides sufficient analgesia such that an increase in opioids from baseline is not required. However, this is not always the case, and clinicians should not be surprised if opioid use increases postoperatively despite the presence of an epidural. Non-opioid additives to the epidural solution may improve analgesia for these patients as well. Multimodal oral or IV analgesics such as acetaminophen, NSAIDs, gabapentin/pregabalin, or ketamine can be used, pending any contraindications.[25] Finally, if additional opioids are required in an opioid-tolerant patient, expect that the intake needed to obtain satisfactory analgesia will be higher than in opioid-naïve patients. Opioids works better in the acute pain setting than in the chronic pain setting.

NEURAXIAL ANALGESIA AND OPIOID SUBSTITUTION: METHADONE AND BUPRENORPHINE

Patients being treated for a history of opioid addiction or abuse represent a unique surgical population. These patients may present in the perioperative period with considerable anxiety about pain management. Those who have chronic pain may fear inadequate postoperative pain control, while those who have successfully achieved abstinence may fear relapse with postoperative opioid exposure. Many patients will present on prescribed maintenance opioid substitution therapy such as methadone or buprenorphine. These medications are designed to prevent the euphoria associated with taking other, especially illicit, opioids and thus decrease the risk of abuse or relapse. Additionally, methadone and buprenorphine are effective analgesics and have been increasingly used to treat chronic pain conditions in patients without a substance abuse or addiction disorder.

Methadone is a full agonist of mu opioid receptors with possible antagonist activity at the NMDA receptor. (Low-dose methadone has an analgesic effect in neuropathic pain: a double-blind randomized controlled crossover trial. John S Morley John Bridson Tim P Nash John B Miles Sarah White Matthew K Makin. *Palliative Medicine*. 2003;17(7):576–587.) Methadone is associated with development of opioid tolerance and hyperalgesia. Buprenorphine is a partial agonist of mu- and antagonist of kappa-opioid receptors with effect duration of 24–72 hours. Compared to other opioids, buprenorphine is associated with less opioid tolerance and respiratory depression. However, buprenorphine has an extremely high affinity for the mu receptors. If buprenorphine is aggressively displaced by alternative opioids (as may be attempted when trying to control acute postsurgical pain), results are unpredictable due to its long duration of action. Acute respiratory depression may ensue when sufficient buprenorphine has been displaced by other long-acting opioids.

There is a paucity of literature regarding patients taking methadone or buprenorphine and postoperative pain management via epidural catheters. In general, similar to patients taking other opioids, the use of a neuraxial or regional technique as part of a multimodal analgesic plan is recommended.[26,28] Consultation with a pain medicine and/or an addiction physician starting well before surgery is also recommended. Some patients on buprenorphine may benefit from controlled dose reduction, transition to methadone, or cessation of buprenorphine over several days to weeks prior to surgery,[26] while others do best when continued on their buprenorphine therapy.[27] If a controlled de-escalation/cessation plan has not been established and monitored by a qualified practitioner prior to surgery, methadone and buprenorphine should be continued perioperatively.

There are no published recommendations or case reports for epidural solution composition for patients on methadone or buprenorphine. In general, patients taking methadone can be expected to have opioid tolerance. An opioid additive such as sufentanyl to the epidural solution is reasonable, although these patients should be monitored closely for respiratory depression. For patients taking buprenorphine, with its primary location of action in the central nervous system and spinal cord, an opioid additive to the epidural solution may cause unpredictable results and close monitoring is advised. For patients on buprenorphine, if a local anesthetic-only epidural solution plus multimodal therapy (acetaminophen/NSAID) is insufficient, it is recommended to offer short-acting IV opioids such as fentanyl via patient-controlled analgesia[26], again under very close monitoring.

NEURAXIAL ANALGESIA/ANESTHESIA IN PATIENTS WITH PRE-EXISTING CHRONIC BACK PAIN

Some practitioners avoid neuraxial techniques for patients with pre-existing chronic back pain, especially if the pain is located in the region where the injection or catheter is to be placed. While pre-existing back pain is a risk factor for persistent back pain after neuraxial anesthesia, there is little evidence to suggest epidural or spinal anesthesia worsens pre-existing back pain.[18] The exception is back pain caused by pathology that reduces spinal canal cross-sectional area such as severe spinal stenosis or epidural lipomatosis.[29]

The American Society of Regional Anesthesia and Pain Medicine (ASRA) maintains a practice advisory on neurologic complications associated with regional anesthesia which includes neuraxial techniques. While the reader is referred to the most recent update, the advisory published in 2015 encourages a risk-versus-benefit consideration for patients with specific space-occupying extradural lesions. Such lesions are "associated with temporary or permanent spinal cord injury in conjunction with neuraxial regional anesthetic techniques."[29]

NEURAXIAL ANALGESIA/ANESTHESIA IN PATIENTS WITH PRIOR BACK SURGERY

Similar to pre-existing back pain, a history of back surgery does not preclude attempting neuraxial anesthesia. Again, many practitioners will not offer epidural anesthesia to patients with a history of back surgery because placement can be difficult and analgesia may be patchy and incomplete.[18] Spinals have a higher success rate after prior back surgery compared to epidurals,[18,29] and the ASRA advisory confirms that prior spine surgery is not an absolute contraindication to neuraxial techniques. The advisory does, however, suggest reviewing imaging and possibly using fluoroscopy to guide placement in patients with previous spine surgery.[29]

PREOPERATIVE EVALUATION, LABORATORY TESTS, AND IMAGING PRIOR TO NEURAXIAL ANESTHESIA

To determine if neuraxial anesthesia or analgesia is appropriate, a thorough patient history with a review of systems that includes cardiac, pulmonary, hepatic, neurologic, hematologic, infectious, musculoskeletal, and pain histories is required. Prior surgeries, current medications, substance use, and medication allergies should also be confirmed.

Physical exam should, at a minimum, include vitals and an exam of the back, looking for scoliosis, prior surgical scars, tenderness to palpation at baseline, signs of infection at the planned site, as well as surface anatomy. For patients whose anatomy is difficult to decipher by palpation alone, or who have significant scoliosis, ultrasound or fluoroscopy for placement may be helpful.

In general, healthy patients without any comorbidities do not require specific laboratory tests or imaging prior to neuraxial anesthesia. A platelet count, hematocrit/hemoglobin, white blood cell count, blood cultures, liver function tests, and/or prothrombin time (PT) or international normalised ratio (INR) may be indicated for more complicated patients. All patients who take anticoagulants should be managed according to the most recent ASRA guidelines for the specific medication in terms of placement of neuraxial blockade and removal of catheters.

Spinal column imaging (computed tomography scan [CT] or magnetic resonance imaging [MRI]) is not routinely required but may be helpful in patients with spinal stenosis or in whom the presence of a space-occupying lesion is a concern. CT imaging may also help guide placement in patients with severe scoliosis or prior spine surgery.

If neurologic injury is suspected after a neuraxial procedure, immediate neuroimaging (typically MRI) is necessary to rule out potentially treatable conditions, such as spinal hematoma or abscess.

CONCLUSIONS

Neuraxial techniques are beneficial beyond perioperative pain control and may be a more effective way to manage perioperative pain in chronic opioid users compared to other pain control modalities. Generally, these are safe procedures for patients with prior back pain or back surgery without increasing the risk of increased chronic back pain. As with any procedure, the benefits must be balanced with the risks, and the decision to use neuraxial analgesia should be made in the context of the patient and coexisting disease, the surgery itself, and the expected perioperative course.

REFERENCES

1. Wright AD. Spinal analgesia with special reference to operations above the diaphragm. *Proc Royal Soc Med.* 1931 Mar;24:613–620.
2. Cwik J. Postoperative considerations of neuraxial anesthesia. *Anesthesiol Clin.* 2012 Sep;30:433–443.
3. Guay J, Choi P, Suresh S, Albert N, Kopp S, Pace NL. Neuraxial blockade for the prevention of postoperative mortality and major morbidity: an overview of Cochrane systematic reviews. *Cochrane Database Syst Rev.* 2014;1:CD010108.
4. Andreae MH, Andreae DA. Regional anaesthesia to prevent chronic pain after surgery: a Cochrane systematic review and meta-analysis. *Br J Anaesth.* 2013 Nov;111:711–720.
5. Lavand'homme P, De Kock M, Waterloos H. Intraoperative epidural analgesia combined with ketamine provides effective preventive analgesia in patients undergoing major digestive surgery. *Anesthesiology.* 2005 Oct;103:813–820.

6. Fant F, Tina E, Sandblom D, et al. Thoracic epidural analgesia inhibits the neuro-hormonal but not the acute inflammatory stress response after radical retropubic prostatectomy. *Br J Anaesth*. 2013 May;110:747–757.

7. Hong JY, Yang SC, Yi J, Kil HK. Epidural ropivacaine and sufentanil and the perioperative stress response after a radical retropubic prostatectomy. *Acta Anaesthesiol Scand*. 2011 Mar;55:282–289.

8. Hong JY, Lim KT. Effect of preemptive epidural analgesia on cytokine response and postoperative pain in laparoscopic radical hysterectomy for cervical cancer. *Reg Anesth Pain Med*. 2008 Jan-Feb;33:44–51.

9. Ahlers O, Nachtigall I, Lenze J, et al. Intraoperative thoracic epidural anaesthesia attenuates stress-induced immunosuppression in patients undergoing major abdominal surgery. *Br J Anaesth*. 2008 Dec;101:781–787.

10. Chen W-K, Miao C-H. The effect of anesthetic technique on survival in human cancers: a meta-analysis of retrospective and prospective studies. *PLoS One*. 2013;8:e56540.

11. Rosero EB, Joshi GP. Preemptive, preventive, multimodal analgesia: what do they really mean? *Plast Reconstruct Surg*. 2014 Oct;134:85S–93S.

12. Brennan TJ, Kehlet H. Preventive analgesia to reduce wound hyperalgesia and persistent postsurgical pain: not an easy path. *Anesthesiology*. 2005 Oct;103:681–683.

13. Katz J, Cohen L, Schmid R, Chan VW, Wowk A. Postoperative morphine use and hyperalgesia are reduced by preoperative but not intraoperative epidural analgesia: implications for preemptive analgesia and the prevention of central sensitization. *Anesthesiology*. 2003 Jun;98:1449–1460.

14. Hong J, Kim KT. Effect of preemptive epidural analgesia on cytokine response and postoperative pain in laparoscopic radical hysterectomy for cervical cancer. *Reg Anesth Pain Med*. 2008 Jan-Feb;33:44–51.

15. Ezhevskaya AA, Mlyavykh SG, Anderson DG. Effects of continuous epidural anesthesia and postoperative epidural analgesia on pain management and stress response in patients undergoing major spinal surgery. *Spine*. 2013 Jul;38:1324–1330.

16. Hadimioglu N, Ulugol H, Akbas H, Coskunfirat N, Ertug Z, Dinckan A. Combination of epidural anesthesia and general anesthesia attenuates stress response to renal transplantation surgery. *Transplant Proc*. 2012 Dec;44:2949–2954.

17. Kim C, Sakamoto A. Differences in the leukocyte response to incision during upper abdominal surgery with epidural versus general anesthesia. *J Nippon Med Sch*. 2006 Feb;73:4–9.

18. Benzon HT, Asher YG, Hartrick CT. Back pain and neuraxial anesthesia. *Anesth Analg*. 2016 Jun;122:2047–2058.

19. Stromer W, Michaeli K, Sandner-Kiesling A. Perioperative pain therapy in opioid abuse. *Eur J Anaesthesiol*. 2013 Feb;30:55–64.

20. Gordon D, Inturrisi CE, Greensmith JE, Brennan TJ, Goble L, Kerns RD. Perioperative pain management in the opioid-tolerant individual. *J Pain*. 2008 May;9:383–387.

21. Dabbagh A, Dahi-Taleghani M, Elyasi H, et al. Duration of spinal anesthesia with bupivacaine in chronic opium abusers undergoing lower extremity orthopedic surgery. *Arch Iran Med*. 2007 Jul;10:316–320.

22. Vosoughian M, Dabbagh A, Rajaei S, Maftuh H. The duration of spinal anesthesia with 5% lidocaine in chronic opium abusers compared with nonabusers. *Anesth Analg*. 2007 Aug;105:531–533.

23. Karbasy SH, Derakhshan P. Effects of opium addiction on level of sensory block in spinal anesthesia with bupivacaine for lower abdomen and limb surgery: a case-control study. *Anesthesiol Pain Med*. 2014 Dec;4:e21571.

24. Fine PG, Portenoy RK, Ad Hoc Expert Panel on Evidence Review and Guidelines for Opioid Rotation. Establishing "best practices" for opioid rotation: conclusions of an expert panel. *J Pain Symptom Manage.* 2009 Sep;38:418–425.

25. Wenzel JT, Schwenk ES, Baratta JL, Viscusi ER. Managing opioid-tolerant patients in the perioperative surgical home. *Anesthesiol Clin.* 2016 Jun;34:287–301.

26. Bryson EO. The perioperative management of patients maintained on medications used to manage opioid addiction. *Curr Opin Anaesthesiol.* 2014 Jun;27:359–364.

27. Alford DP, Compton P, Samet JH. Acute Pain Management for Patients Receiving Maintenance Methadone or Buprenorphine Therapy. *Ann Intern Med.* 2006 Mar;144:127–134.

28. Peng PW, Tumber PS, Gourlay D. Review article: perioperative pain management of patients on methadone therapy. *Can J Anaesthes.* 2005 May;52:513–523.

29. Neal JM, Barrington MJ, Brull R, et al. The Second ASRA Practice Advisory on Neurologic Complications Associated With Regional Anesthesia and Pain Medicine: executive summary 2015. *Reg Anesth Pain Med.* 2015 Sep-Oct;40:401–430.

8 Peripheral Nerve Block and Ultrasound Images

Paul K. Cheng, Tariq M. Malik,
and Magdalena Anitescu

HISTORY OF ULTRASOUND USE FOR PERIPHERAL NERVE BLOCK PROCEDURES

Peripheral nerve blocks, or regional anesthesia, can be used as the primary anesthetic for various surgical cases involving the upper extremities, lower extremities, or trunk. Nerve blocks can be used for postoperative pain control, in lieu or in addition to intravenous and oral narcotics. During a peripheral nerve block, an anesthesiologist directs a needle toward the target nerve and infuses a solution of local anesthetic (LA), such as bupivacaine, bathing the neuronal tissue and causing numbness and muscle relaxation in the corresponding nerve distribution. Historically anesthesiologists used relevant surface landmarks to infer the location of a target nerve then blindly directed the needle until a paresthesia was elicited. However, this blind technique led to inconsistent results, even with the advent of adjunctive techniques including electric nerve stimulation.[1,2]

The invention of portable ultrasound (US) machines revolutionized the field of regional anesthesia. US was first used for peripheral nerve blockade in the 1970s, with a case series describing a US-guided supraclavicular block in 1978 which highlighted the benefit of US guidance in preventing complications associated with the block, including phrenic nerve palsy, pneumothorax, spinal anesthesia, and recurrent laryngeal nerve block.[1] Use of US in clinical practice gained traction in the 1980s, and various studies in the subsequent two decades showed that US guidance was associated with faster onset of sensory block, higher quality of the block, and fewer inadvertent vascular punctures.[1]

In the 2000s, as US technology continued to improve and US use for procedures increased, low-frequency transducers began to be used for imaging for nerve blocks with deeper targets such as the sciatic nerve and blocks involving the neuraxis.

Since then more novel techniques for selective nerve blockade of both deep and superficial nerves have been developed including the transversus abdominis plane block and adductor canal block.[1] Overall US allows for direct visualization of nerves and surrounding structures and can allow for direct observation of LA deposition and spread. US guidance for nerve blocks can decrease complications, including accidental intraneural or intravascular injection, and has been shown to decrease incidence of LA systemic toxicity and be more efficacious and safer than non-US-guided techniques.[1,2] The major negative factor in US-guided nerve blocks is that US imaging is operator dependent and the image can be poor in certain areas such as axial or spinal structures where an acoustic shadow artifact can be created by the bone.[3]

THE ULTRASOUND MACHINE

There are two types of probes used for peripheral nerve blocks, each named for the layout of the echogenic crystal array. The linear probe, which, in general, has a frequency of 6 to 13 MHz and a depth of 1.8 to 6 cm, is useful for superficial blocks such as brachial plexus, abdominal wall, femoral, and popliteal nerve blocks. The curvilinear probe, with a lower frequency of 2 to 5 MHz has a greater depth of 5 to 16 cm and is useful for deep blocks including lumbar plexus/psoas compartment blocks and sciatic blocks. This probe can also be used to guide neuraxial blocks. This curvilinear probe has a decreased resolution of 2 mm axial and 3 mm lateral compared to the linear probe with a resolution of 0.5 mm axial and 1 mm lateral. Most sources recommend using the curvilinear probe when structures are anticipated to be deeper than 4 cm.[1,2]

Key US settings that can be adjusted to optimize images are depth and gain. Optimal depth is determined by the target structures. Optimal gain differs based on the area being imaged and is determined by toggling the gain buttons until the best contrast between muscles and adjacent connective tissue is obtained. Both power/sound and color Doppler is available on the majority of US and can help to identify pulsatile arterial structures as well as observe dynamically the injection of LA. An example of an US machine is shown in Figure 8.1. For ergonomic reasons, the US machine should be positioned on the opposite side of the bed as the operator and a sterile covering placed over the probe with sterile gel to allow for appropriate transmission of US waves.[4,5]

BASIC ULTRASOUND-GUIDED PERIPHERAL NERVE BLOCK TECHNIQUES

Use of the two-dimensional US requires an operator with good spacial imagination and skilled hands. There are two general techniques for nerve blocks: the out-of-plane technique and the in-plane-technique. The out-of-plane technique involves the needle passing perpendicular to the long axis of the probe while the in-plane technique involves the needle parallel to the probe face. The thin plane for the US image, which is often <1 mm, makes visualizing and advancing the needle more challenging for the in-plane technique, particularly for the inexperienced operator. However, the tip of the needle may be difficult to visualize in the out-of-plane technique.

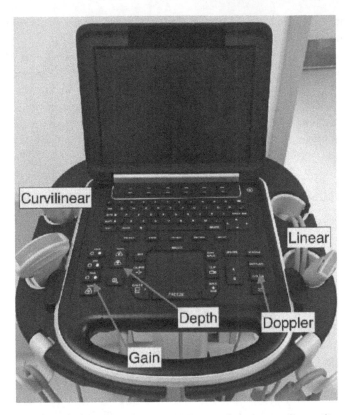

FIGURE 8.1. Ultrasound machine. A commonly used US machine showing the curvilinear probe on the left, the linear probe on the right, as well as key functions including gain, depth, and doppler.

Needle identification can be improved by various techniques including rotation of the needle, gentle in and out movements, or injection of small volumes of fluid, also called hydrodissection.[1,2]

In general vascular structures are easily identified within the US field with arteries being pulsatile and relatively noncompressible and veins being nonpulsatile and compressible. The fibrous covering of the nerve gives it a hyperechoic appearance while the neuron itself is hypoechoic; the combination of these two patterns can give a large nerve a honeycomb appearance. Muscles are typically hypoechoic with band-line striations and fascial planes appearing as hyperechoic crisp lines. Bones are intensely hyperechoic and usually have a sharp hyperechoic line where they interface with surrounding tissues.[4] When injecting LA, the operator should look for circumferential spread, which should be painless with no resistance. If LA infiltration is not seen, the operator should consider intravascular injection while resistance on injection may be a sign of intraneural needle-tip placement. After injection of LA, the nerve itself may appear brighter and more easily identified. If the nerve body itself swells, this may indicate intraneural injection.[2]

Complications of all nerve blocks irrespective of the anatomic location of the block include nerve damage, inadvertent puncture of vascular structures, bleeding or hematoma, intravascular injection of LA, and LA systemic toxicity and the related sequelae. Absolute contraindications are few and include infection in the puncture site, patient refusal, and allergy to LA. Relative contraindications include anticoagulation and pre-existing nerve damage.[6]

The choice of LA can vary between institution and individual provider. The choice of LA and the dose should be made with thorough knowledge of the pharmacology including the duration of action and toxic dose as well as the patient's comorbidities.[6] With many of these peripheral nerve blocks, a catheter can be placed to allow for continuous infusion of various mixtures of LA and opioids for longer-term pain control. However, catheter placement technique and continuous peripheral nerve infusions are outside the scope of this text and are not discussed.

ULTRASOUND-GUIDED PERIPHERAL NERVE BLOCKS

Upper Extremity

Interscalene Block (Basic)

Indication. Surgery involving the shoulder, proximal upper arm, and lateral clavicle.

Overview. The brachial plexus emerges from nerve roots C5 to C7 and runs between the anterior and medial scalene muscles in the lateral portion of the neck and are the targets for this block.

Technique. With the patient's head slightly tilted to the opposite site, place the linear probe in a transverse orientation along the lateral neck a few centimeters above the clavicle (Figure 8.2). Scan up and down along the neck until the three hypoechoic nerve roots C5 to C7 appear sandwiched between the anterior and middle scalene muscle bellies. The nerve roots should appear like stacked black circles with

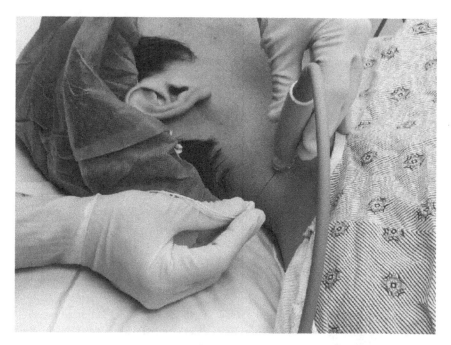

FIGURE 8.2. US probe position for interscalene block, transverse in the lateral mid-neck. Needle position corresponds to in-plane technique.

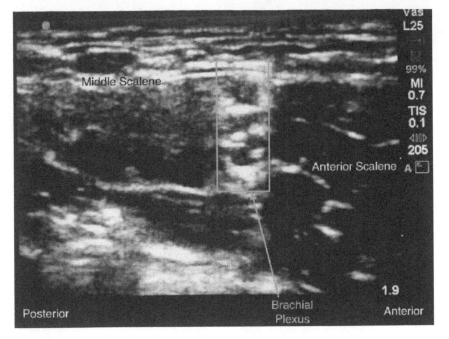

FIGURE 8.3. US image showing the brachial plexus, which appears like a stoplight sandwiched between the anterior scalene muscle and the middle scalene muscle.

hyperechoic borders, much like a stoplight (Figure 8.3). Some providers locate the brachial plexus in the supraclavicular area (see next technique) and trace the brachial plexus cephalad for ease of localization. Using the in-plane or out-of-plane approach, deposit LA around the nerve roots, ensuring circumferential spread. The ideal position of the needle tip at the time of injection is between the C6 and C7 roots.

Block success. Effective block for shoulder surgery requires blockade of C5/C6 nerve roots. Test for sensory deficit in axillary nerve distribution (numb patch of skin over the lower half of deltoid muscles) and deficit in musculocutaneous distribution (numb lateral forearm). Motor testing will reveal weak deltoid, biceps, and wrist extensors.

Key complications. Phrenic nerve paralysis, recurrent laryngeal nerve paralysis, Horner syndrome, vascular puncture of arterial structures including vertebral artery, superficial cervical artery, dorsal scapular artery, and suprascapular artery. Pronounced chronic obstructive pulmonary disease should be considered a contraindication.[6,7]

Supraclavicular Block (Intermediate)

Indication. Surgery involving the arm distal to the shoulder.

Overview. The brachial plexus runs lateral to the subclavian artery and can be easily located in the major supraclavicular fossa. The supraclavicular block has a significant risk of pneumothorax; however, US has made identification of the brachial plexus and avoidance of the pleura much easier.

Technique. With the patient's head slightly tilted to the opposite side, place the linear US probe in the major supraclavicular fossa parallel to and posterior to the

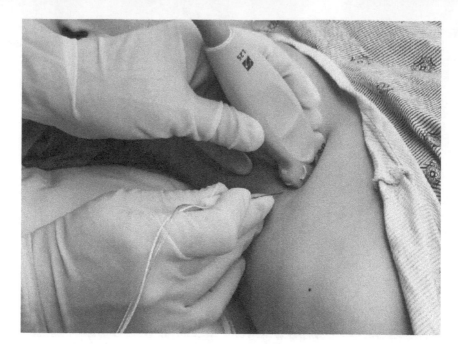

FIGURE 8.4. US probe position for supraclavicular block in the supraclavicular fossa, parallel to the clavicle and pointed caudad. Needle position corresponds to in-plane technique.

clavicle and tilt the head of the probe caudad (Figure 8.4). Identify the pulsating subclavian artery and tilt the US probe caudal or cephalad to best visualize the hyperechoic brachial plexus which is posterolateral to the subclavian artery at this level and which in the optimal position looks like a triangle with tip pointing laterally (Figure 8.5). Using an in-plane technique, advance the needle to the brachial plexus until a pop is felt corresponding to entry immediately deep to the fascia surrounding the plexus and deposit 20 to 25 mL of LA in this area. Ulnar nerve sparing can occur with the supraclavicular block; however, this can be avoided by ensuring that the LA is deposited in the inferior aspect of the brachial plexus adjacent to the subclavian artery just above the first rib. This requires careful maneuvering of needle under US to avoid any pleural puncture and resultant pneumothorax or vascular puncture. LA infiltration around the brachial plexus is expected to cause some mild compression of the subclavian artery.

Block success. The whole limb below the midhumerus should become numb. All movements in the all five digits will be weak/minimal. The ulnar nerve should be carefully tested if this block is the sole mode of anesthesia for surgery.

Key complications. Pneumothorax, phrenic nerve paralysis, vascular puncture of the subclavian artery.[6,8]

Infraclavicular Block (Intermediate)

Indication. Surgery on distal upper arm to hand.

Overview. As the brachial plexus travels below the clavicle, it runs in three cords which surround the axillary artery. Similar to the supraclavicular block, the

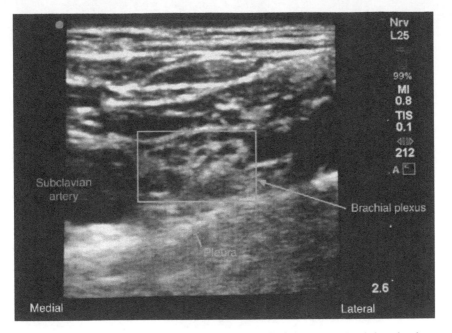

FIGURE 8.5. US image showing the triangularly shaped brachial plexus immediately lateral to the subclavian artery and superior to the hyperechoic pleura.

infraclavicular block has a significant risk of pneumothorax, so the pleura should always be clearly visualized while advancing the needle.

Technique. With the ipsilateral arm slightly abducted and the head tilted in the opposite direction, place the linear probe immediately below the clavicle just medial to the coracoid process, oriented perpendicular to the clavicle to transect the axillary artery (Figure 8.6). The pulsatile axillary artery is identified deep to the pectoralis major and minor muscles. The three cords of the brachial plexus—medial, posterior, and lateral—are located as three distinct hyperechoic bundles surrounding the artery (Figure 8.7). Using the in-plane technique, deposit 20 to 30 mL of LA around these cords in a U-shaped pattern deep to the axillary artery.

Block success. Same as the supraclavicular block

Key complications. Pneumothorax, vascular puncture of the axillary artery.[6,9]

Midhumeral/Axillary Block (Basic)

Indication. Surgery from elbow to hand.

Overview. As the brachial plexus moves to the upper arm/axillary region, it splits into three distinct nerves—median, radial, and ulnar—which surround the axillary artery. The radial nerve is located deep to the artery while the ulnar nerve is inferior/medial and median nerve is lateral/above the artery. LA is injected separately around these three nerves. The musculocutaneous nerve, which innervates the radial-side of the forearm, arises from the lateral cord of the brachial plexus and takes off more proximal in the upper arm, traveling through the coracobrachialis. It will need to be injected separately in the axillary block.

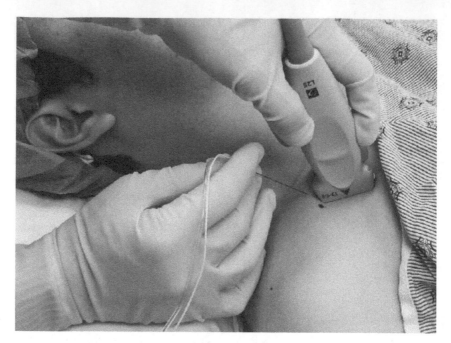

FIGURE 8.6. US probe position for infraclavicular block perpendicular to the clavicle immediately medial to the coracoid process (purple dot). Needle position corresponds to in-plane technique.

Technique. With the arm abducted at 90 degrees, place the linear probe transverse in the medial portion of the upper arm/axillary region (Figure 8.8). Scan distal and proximal until the axillary artery and the three separate nerves (radial, median, ulnar) are distinctly visualized. Using either the in-plane or out-of-plane technique, deposit 5 to 10 mL of LA around the radial nerve first, since it is deepest. Injecting LA first around the ulnar or median nerve can displace deeper structures, making subsequent deposition around the radial nerve difficult. Next infiltrate 5 to 10 mL LA around the median and ulnar nerves in no particular order (Figure 8.9). Identify the musculocutaneous nerve by scanning proximal-distal along the brachioradialis muscle just above the brachial artery, finding a hyperechoic oval structure that appears to be moving like a "wiggling worm" through the coracobrachialis muscle while scanning (Figure 8.10). Deposit a separate aliquot of 5 to 7 mL of LA around the nerve inside the muscle.

Key complications. This block avoids any respiratory compromise though inadvertent vascular puncture and intravascular injection can still occur.[6,10]

Radial/Ulnar/Median Nerve Block (Advanced)

Indication. Hand/forearm surgery, failed brachial plexus block.

Overview. The radial, ulnar, and median nerves, which are all blocked in the axillary nerve block described earlier, can be individually blocked anywhere along the course of each nerve. These blocks are commonly done in the proximal forearm and wrist for both ulnar and median nerves and the upper arm and wrist for the radial

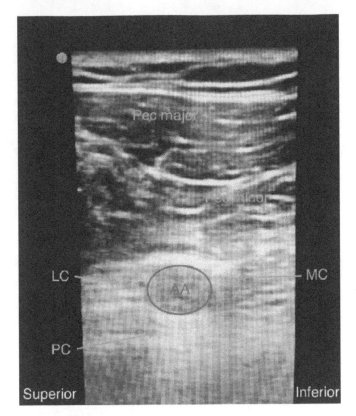

FIGURE 8.7. US image showing the cords of the brachial plexus—lateral cord (LC), posterior cord (PC), medial cord (MC)—surrounding the axillary artery (AA). Of note, the axillary artery is deep to the pectoralis major and pectoralis minor.

nerve. Care should be taken to avoid injecting LA in any tight space that can lead to nerve compression and injury. Generally the median nerve runs along the midline of the arm and travels into the carpal tunnel, the ulnar nerve travels along the course of the ulna and enters Guyons tunnel at the wrist, and the radial nerve runs in the posterior upper arm and forearm area.

Technique. With the arm abducted and supine, US is used to identify each nerve along its course and a small volume (i.e. 3–5 ml) of LA deposited. Place the linear probe perpendicular to the long axis of the arm. The nerves should be visualized as small hyperechoic oval structures. Common areas for nerve injection are as follows:

Median nerve—proximal forearm (Figure 8.11 A, B), wrist (Figure 8.12 A, B).
Ulnar nerve—proximal forearm distal to the medial epicondyle of humerus
    (Figure 8.13 A, B), ulnar aspect of the wrist (Figure 8.14 A, B).
Radial nerve—lateral aspect of the midhumerus (Fig. 8.15 A,B), radial-aspect of
    the wrist (Figure 8.16 A, B).

Key complications. Nerve damage if LA is injected into a tight space with the nerve.[6,11,12]

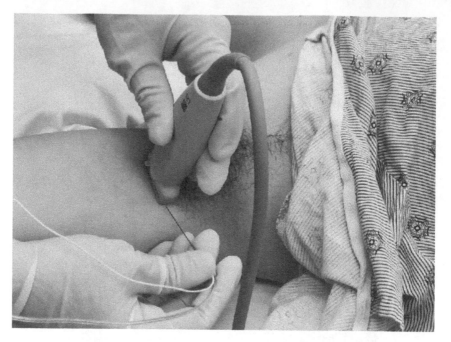

FIGURE 8.8. US probe position for axillary block transverse in the axillary area. Needle position corresponds to in-plane technique.

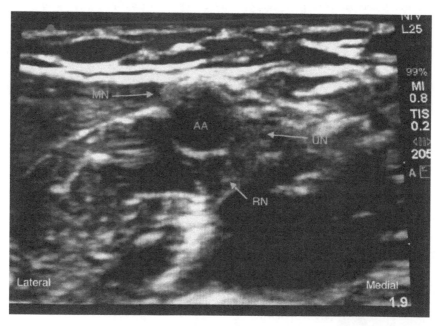

FIGURE 8.9. US image showing the medial nerve (MN), ulnar nerve (UN), and radial nerve (RN) surrounding the axillary artery (AA).

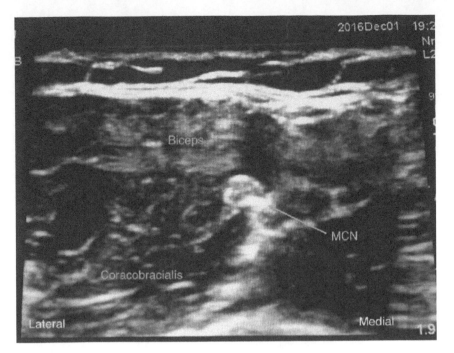

FIGURE 8.10. US image showing the oval-shaped musculocutaneous nerve (MCN) coursing between the biceps brachii and the coracobrachialis muscle.

Trunk

Intercostal Block (Advanced)

Indication. Management of acute pain after rib fractures or thoracotomy.

Overview. The goal is to place LA around the intercostal nerves, which lay between the internal and innermost intercostal muscles, tucked underneath the corresponding rib.

These nerves originate in the ventral rami of T1 to T11 nerves, with T2 to T6 forming the thoracic intercostal nerves, T7 to T11 forming the thoracoabdominal nerves, and T12 forming the subcostal nerves. The lateral cutaneous branches of these nerves supply the chest wall and the abdominal wall in their dermatomal paths of

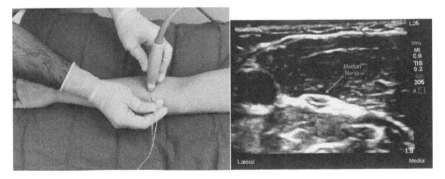

FIGURE 8.11. US probe position for forearm median nerve block and corresponding US image showing the median nerve. Needle position corresponds to in-plane technique.

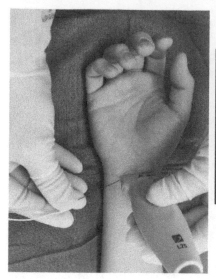

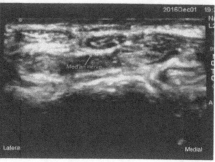

FIGURE 8.12. US probe position for median nerve block at the wrist and corresponding US image showing the median nerve. Needle position corresponds to in-plane technique.

distribution. Of note, T9 to T12 and the first lumbar nerves are widely connected and run within the transversus abdominis plane, which can be blocked separately.

Technique. With the patient prone, place the linear probe at the angle of the rib, approximately 6 to 7.5 cm lateral to the spinous process, in short axis to the ribs so two consecutive ribs are in view and the pleura is easily seen (Figure 8.17). Using either the in-plane or out of plane technique, enter the skin along the upper margin of the rib that is immediately inferior to the target intercostal nerves, advance the needle until it is between the internal intercostal and innermost intercostal muscles, and inject 3

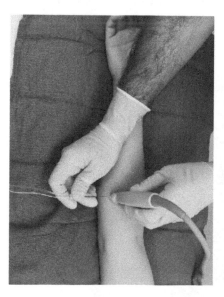

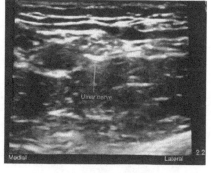

FIGURE 8.13. US probe position for forearm block of ulnar nerve and corresponding US image showing the ulnar nerve. Needle position corresponds to in-plane technique.

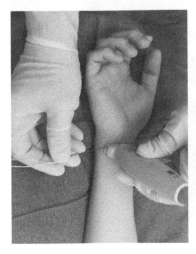
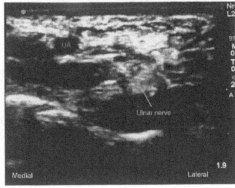

FIGURE 8.14. US probe position showing wrist block of ulnar nerve and corresponding US image showing the ulnar nerve and ulnar artery (UA). Needle position corresponds to in-plane technique.

to 5 mL of LA per level (Figure 8.18). Each targeted intercostal nerve must be injected separately. Keep in mind that the neurovascular bundle usually cannot be directly visualized as it is covered by the rib.

Key complications. Pneumothorax, as the distance between the neurovascular bundle and pleura is 0.5 cm.[3,13]

Transversus Abdominis Plane Block (Basic)

Indication. Postoperative analgesia for surgery involving incision of abdominal wall.

Overview. The nerves providing sensation to the abdominal wall originate from the ventral rami of thoracic nerves T7 to T12 as well as lumbar nerve L1 and travel parallel from posterior to anterior abdominal wall, sandwiched between the transverse abdominis and internal oblique muscles in the transversus abdominis plane.

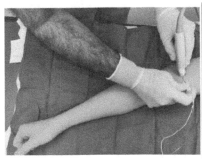
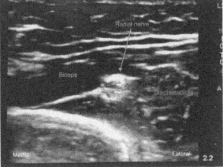

FIGURE 8.15. US probe position for upper arm radial nerve block and corresponding US image showing the radial nerve superficial to the brachialis muscle and the brachioradialis muscle. Needle position corresponds to in-plane technique.

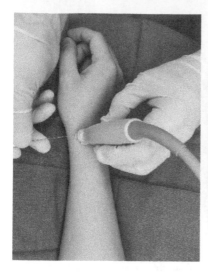
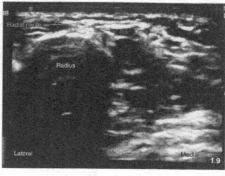

FIGURE 8.16. US probe position for wrist block of radial nerve and corresponding US image showing the radial nerve lateral to the radial artery (RA). Needle position corresponds to in-plane technique.

Technique. With the patient supine, place the linear probe transverse on the abdomen at the anterior axillary line in the area between the iliac crest and the inferior border of the rib cage (Figure 8.19). Once the three muscle layers are appreciated—external oblique, internal oblique, transverse abdominis—injected 20 to 30 mL of LA via

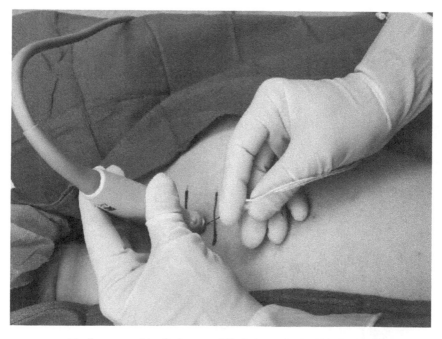

FIGURE 8.17. Needle entry position for intercostal block. US probe should be positioned perpendicular to the ribs at the angle of the ribs, approximately 6 to 7.5 cm lateral to the spinous process. Needle position corresponds to in-plane technique.

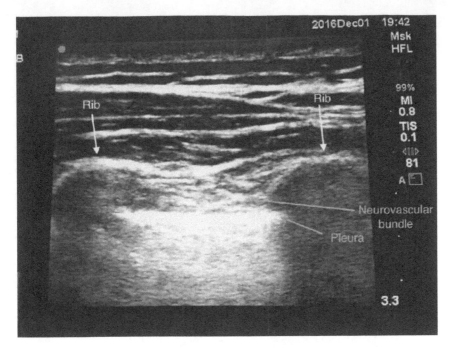

FIGURE 8.18. US image showing the intercostal area between two ribs. Above the pleura lies the neurovascular bundle between the internal intercostal and innermost intercostal muscle layers.

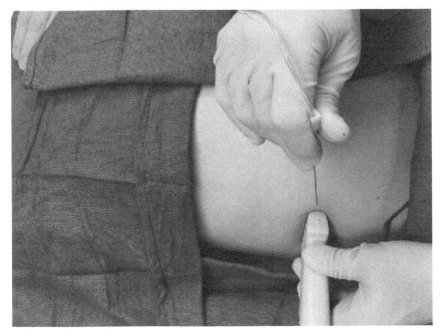

FIGURE 8.19. US probe position for transversus abdominus plane block transverse along lateral abdominal wall between the anterior superior iliac spine (purple line) and the lower costal margin. Needle position corresponds to in-plane technique.

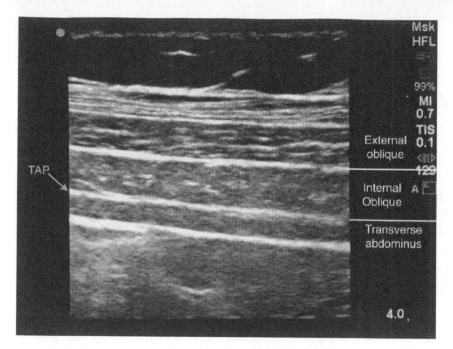

FIGURE 8.20. US image showing external oblique, internal oblique, and transverse abdominis muscle layers and transversus abdominis plane (TAP).

the out-of-plane or in-plane technique between the internal oblique, which is usually the thickest muscle layer, and transverse abdominis (Figure 8.20). The procedure is repeated on the contralateral side to obtain a bilateral block. To block the whole abdominal wall, a four-point injection technique is recommended in which each quadrant of abdominal wall is blocked by a separate injection. In such situation, a close eye is kept on the total amount of LA injected to avoid systemic LA toxicity, which can be life-threatening.

Key complications. Bowel perforation, intraperitoneal injection, systemic local anesthestic toxicity.[14]

Transversalis Fascia Plane Block

Indication. Surgery in the inguinal area and analgesia after anterior iliac crest bone graft harvesting.

Overview. The transversalis fascia plane block targets the L1 nerve branches including the ilioinguinal and iliohypogastric nerves. These nerves run between the transverse abdominis muscle and the transversalis fascia, which overlies the extraperitoneal fascia, posterior to the midaxillary line.

Technique. With the patient in a lateral decubitus or prone position, place the curvilinear probe transverse along the lateral torso immediately cephalad to the iliac crest posterior to the midaxillary line (Figure 8.21). Track the abdominal muscles back until the three muscles abut with the muscle of posterior abdominal wall, namely the quadratus lumborum. Using the in-plane technique, direct the needle immediately deep to the transverse abdominis muscle near the quadratus lumborum so that the 20 mL LA can spread out along the transversalis fascia plane (Figure 8.22).

Key complications. Intraperitoneal injection.[15]

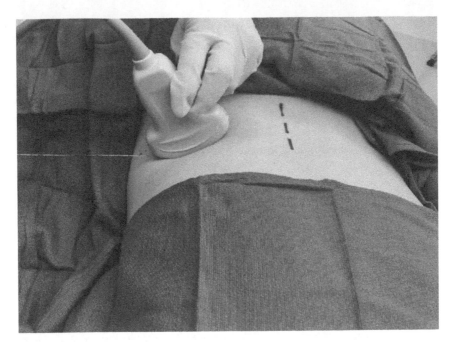

FIGURE 8.21. US probe position for transversalis fascia plane (TFP) block transverse along the lateral torso, cephalad to the iliac crest, and posterior to the midaxillary line. Needle position corresponds to in-plane technique.

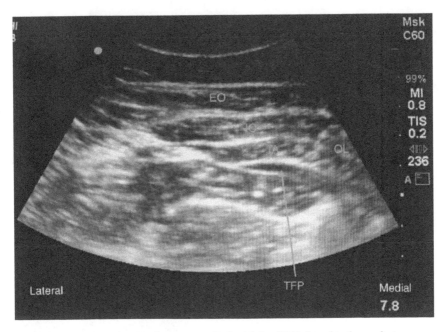

FIGURE 8.22. US image showing the transversalis fascial plan (TFP), lateral to the quadratus lumborum muscle (QL), and deep to the transverse abdominus (TA). Superior to the TA are the external and internal obliques (EO, IO).

Psoas Compartment Block (Advanced)

Indication. Surgery involving the hip, anterior thigh, and knee.

Overview. The psoas compartment block is an advanced block of the lumbar plexus, which runs within the posterior aspect of the psoas major, splitting the muscle into two halves. When combined with the sciatic nerve block, it can anesthetize the entire leg.

Technique. With the patient in a lateral decubitus or prone position, place the curvilinear probe approximately 4 cm lateral to the intersection of the midline/spinous processes and a line connecting the iliac crests, with the probe parallel to the spinous processes. This should correspond to roughly the L3 to L4 position (Figure 8.23). The US image should appear like a trident with areas of acoustic shadowing from the transverse processes of the vertebrae. In this image the hyperechoic structure between and deep to the transverse processes is the lumbar plexus, running in the posterior one-third of the psoas muscle, which is the hypoechoic striated structure around the plexus. The lumbar plexus itself is usually not well visualized with US; therefore, this block is done with nerve stimulation in conjunction with US guidance, which serves mainly to prevent excessively deep placement of the needle as well as damage to any viscera. A patellar twitch is obtained before injecting any LA. Using the in-plane or out-of-plane technique, advance the needle until the tip enters the area of the lumbar plexus and infiltrate 25 to 35 mL of LA (Figure 8.24). This block successfully blocks femoral nerves, obturator and lateral femoral cutaneous nerves more effectively than the high-volume infrainguinal three-in-one block, which is described in the femoral nerve section.

Key complications. Epidural spread of LA, intrathecal injection, intravascular injection, bowel perforation, trauma to kidneys.[16,17]

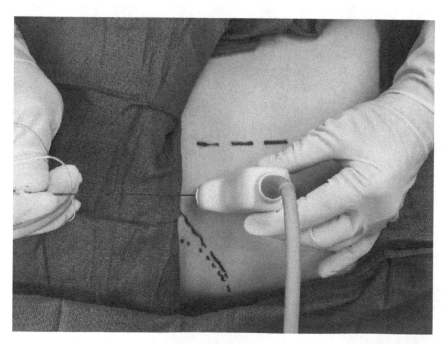

FIGURE 8.23. US probe position for psoas compartment/lumbar plexus block 4 cm lateral to the intersection of the midline/spinous processes and the iliac crests, parallel to the spinus processes. Needle position corresponds to in-plane technique.

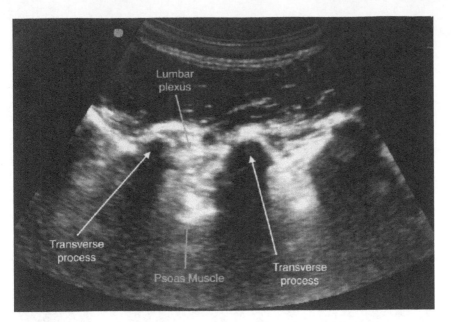

FIGURE 8.24. US image showing lumbar plexus located in the posterior one-third of the psoas muscle body, imaged between the transverse processes. This US image has the typical trident-sign appearance.

Ilioinguinal/Iliohypogastric Nerve Block (Basic)

Indication. Surgery in the inguinal area.

Overview. Ilioinguinal and iliohypogastric nerves originate from the ventral rami of L1, with some contribution of T12. They emerge from the lateral border of the psoas major and run in front of the quadratus lumborum before piercing through the transverse abdominis muscle and running in the transversus abdominus plane between the transverse abdominis and internal oblique muscles. The nerves pierce the internal oblique muscle at a variable distance from the anterior superior iliac spine (ASIS). The goal of this block is to place LA in the transversus abdominus plane to block both nerves simultaneously, though it is also possible to isolate each nerve. An important caveat is that there are many variations of sensory nerve innervation patterns to the inguinal region as there is free communication between the IL/IH and genitofemoral nerves, so results from this block are not always consistent.

Technique. In a supine patient, place the linear probe perpendicular to the inguinal line, which joins the ASIS and the pubic tubercle, with the lateral end of the probe just above or posterior to the ASIS (Figure 8.25). The probe should be tilted until the three muscle layers of the abdominal wall are visualized—external oblique, internal oblique, and transverse abdominis. The ilioinguinal and iliohypogastric nerves can sometimes be visualized as small hypoechoic ovals (Figure 8.26), though it is not necessary to identify individual nerves to perform this block successfully. The ilioinguinal nerve is often accompanied by a deep circumflex iliac artery which can be seen pulsating and is a helpful landmark to localize the correct plane and also should be avoided during an injection. Using either the in-plane or out-of-plane technique, advance the needle until the tip is between the internal oblique and the transverse abdominis and deposit 10 to 15 mL of LA.[3,14]

Key complications. Hematoma from arterial puncture.

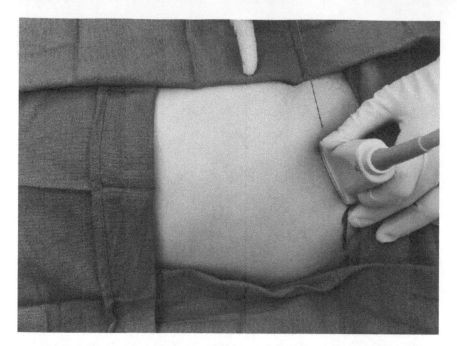

FIGURE 8.25. US probe position for ilioinguinal/iliohypogastric block perpendicular to the inguinal line with the lateral end of the probe just cephalad and posterior to the ASIS. Needle position corresponds to in-plane technique.

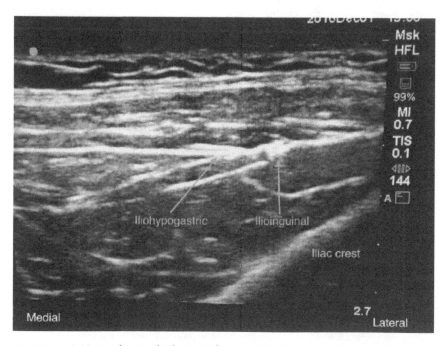

FIGURE 8.26. US image showing the ilioinguinal nerve and the iliohypogastric nerve in the transversus abdominal plane.

Lower Extremity

Obturator Nerve Block (Intermediate)

Indication. Postoperative pain relief after knee surgery usually done in conjunction with femoral nerve block.

Overview. The obturator nerve innervates the medial thigh; however, there can be interpatient variability in the specific area of innervation. It originates from the lumbar plexus and descends down the pelvis, dividing into the anterior and posterior branches before entering the thigh. The anterior branch is sandwiched between the fascia of the adductor longus and adductor brevis muscles while the posterior branch lies between the fascial planes of the adductor brevis and the adductor magnus.

Technique. With the patient supine and the leg abducted to approximately 45 degrees and slightly externally rotated, place the linear probe transverse along the medial thigh, at the inguinal line (Figure 8.27). The anterior and posterior branches of the obturator nerve are visualized between their corresponding fascial planes as described earlier (Figure 8.28). Using either the in-plane or out-of-plane techniques, deposit 5 to 7 mL of LA at each site.

Block success. Effective block of the nerve causes weakness in the adductor muscle group.

Key complications. None.[18]

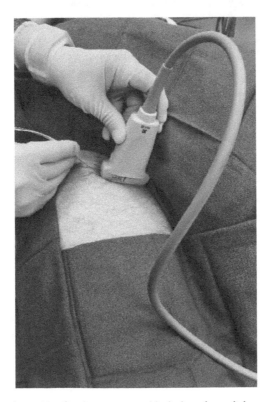

FIGURE 8.27. US probe position for obturator nerve block along the medial aspect of the inguinal crease. Needle position corresponds to in-plane technique.

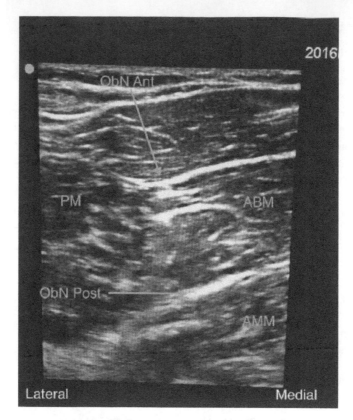

FIGURE 8.28. US image showing the obturator nerve anterior branch (ObN Ant) sandwiched between the fascia of the pectineus (PM) and adductor brevis muscle (ABM) and obturator posterior branch (ObN Post) sandwiched between the fascial planes of the adductor brevis (ABM) and the adductor magnus muscle (AMM).

Femoral Nerve Block (Basic)

Indication. Surgery involving the anterior thigh, femur, and knee.

Overview. The femoral nerve block is arguably the most straightforward block of the lower extremity, as the large femoral nerve is easily visualized lateral to the femoral artery and the inguinal crease is easy accessible, even in the most obese patients. A variation of this block exists called the three-in-one nerve block in which a larger amount (i.e., more than 30 mL) of LA is injected around the femoral nerve and during injection an assistant applies pressure 2 to 4 cm distal to the needle site for 30 seconds to cause adequate cephalic spread to block three nerves with the one injection—femoral, obturator, and lateral femoral cutaneous.

Technique. With the patient supine and the leg slightly abducted and externally rotated, place the linear probe transverse at the medial aspect of the inguinal crease and identify the femoral artery (Figure 8.29). Using either the in-plane or out-of-plane technique, advance the needle until the tip enters the fascia surrounding the femoral nerve (Figure 8.30). A "pop" sensation may be felt as the tip passes this fascia iliaca. At this point inject 10 to 20 mL of LA. The femoral nerve should be seen lifting off the surface of the iliopsoas muscle as the LA infiltrates around it. As noted, a three-in-one

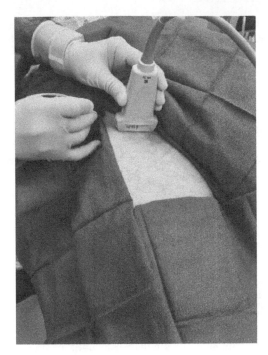

FIGURE 8.29. US probe position for femoral nerve block along the middle portion of the inguinal line. Needle position corresponds to in-plane technique.

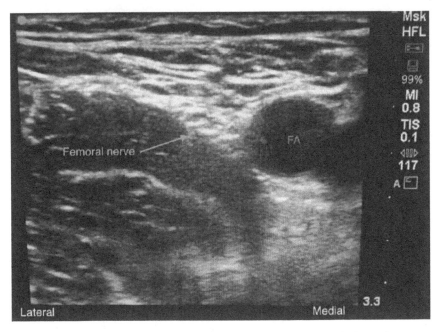

FIGURE 8.30. US image showing the triangle-shaped femoral nerve lateral to the femoral artery (FA).

block can be done by injecting 30 to 40 mL of LA around the femoral nerve while an assistant holds pressure 2 to 4 cm distal to the needle insertion site for 30 seconds.

Block success. Effective block of this nerve causes weakness in knee extensor muscle (quadriceps) muscle group.

Key complications. Inadvertent femoral artery puncture.[19]

Fascia Iliaca Block (Intermediate)

Indication. Anterior thigh and knee surgery, postoperative pain relief for hip and knee procedures.

Overview. The fascia iliac block uses a large volume of LA deposited underneath the fascia iliaca to block both the femoral nerve and the lateral femoral cutaneous nerve. The fascia is covering the sheath of iliopsoas muscle and is located anterior to the iliacus muscle on US imaging.

Technique. With the patient supine and the leg slightly abducted and externally rotated, place the linear probe transverse at the medial aspect of the inguinal crease and identify the femoral artery (Figure 8.31). This initial step is the same as for the femoral block. Once the artery and the lateral hyperechoic fascia iliaca are located, move the probe laterally until the sartorius muscle enters the US window (Figure 8.32). Using the in-plane technique, advance the needle until the tip lies deep to the fascia iliaca, medial to the sartorius muscle, and inject 30 to 40 mL of LA.

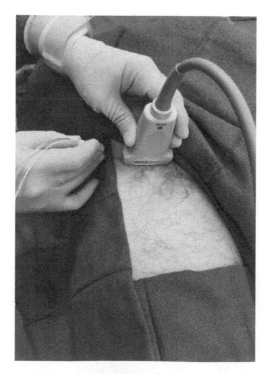

FIGURE 8.31. US probe position for fascia iliaca block along the lateral aspect of the inguinal line. Needle position corresponds to in-plane technique.

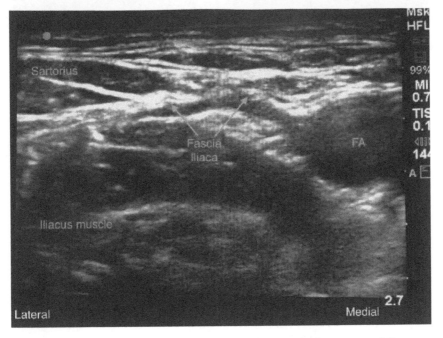

FIGURE 8.32. US image showing the fascial iliaca sandwiched between the sartorius and iliacus muscles, lateral to the femoral artery (FA).

Block success. Successful block of the femoral nerve results in weakness of quadriceps. Block of the lateral femoral cutaneous nerve is tested by weakness with hip adduction and numbness in the lateral aspect of the thigh.

Key complications. None.[20]

Sciatic Nerve Block (Basic)

Indication. Surgery involving the foot and ankle.

Overview. The sciatic nerve runs deep in the gluteal area and thigh and can be approached from multiple entry points. Here we discuss the anterior approach, which is useful in patients who cannot lie in the lateral position, and the transgluteal approach, which is somewhat more straightforward but requires lateral decubitus positioning which may be difficult based on the patient habitus and potential musculoskeletal injury. Given the depth of the nerve, the curvilinear probe should be used.

Technique. Anterior approach: With the patient supine and the leg abducted in frog-leg position, place the curvilinear US probe transverse along the anteromedial aspect of the thigh, a few centimeters below the inguinal line (Figure 8.33). The femur should be identified by its hyperechoic rim. Medial to the femur lies the hyperechoic large sciatic nerve, which is deep to the adductor magnus muscle. Using either the in-plane or out-of-plane approach, advance the needle until the tip enters the fascia surrounding the nerve and deposit 15 to 20 mL of LA. Use of nerve stimulation is recommended to confirm location of the nerve. Plantar flexion or dorsiflexion with stimulation confirms proper localization of the nerve (Figure 8.34).

Transgluteal approach: With the patient in a lateral decubitus position with the target side up and the hip flexed at 60 to 80 degrees, place a curvilinear probe

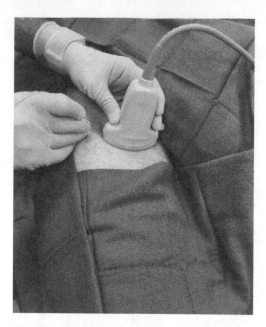

FIGURE 8.33. US probe position for sciatic nerve block anterior approach along the anteromedial thigh. Needle position corresponds to in-plane technique.

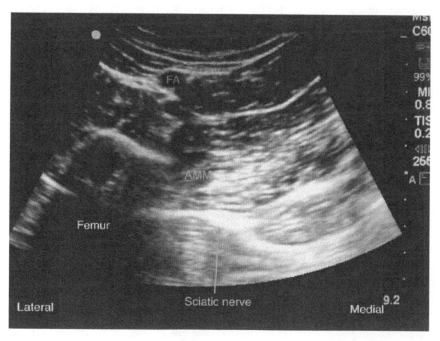

FIGURE 8.34. US image showing the sciatic nerve deep to the adductor magnus muscle (AMM) and medial/posterior to the femur in the anterior approach. The femoral artery (FA) is superficial to the femur.

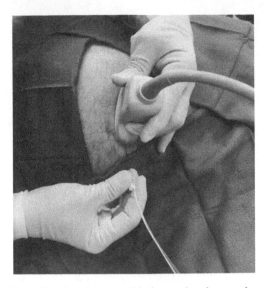

FIGURE 8.35. US probe position for sciatic nerve block transgluteal approach, transverse in the gluteal crease between the greater trochanter and the ischial tuberosity. Needle position corresponds to in-plane technique.

transverse in the gluteal crease between the greater trochanter and the ischial tuberosity (Figure 8.35). The sciatic nerve appears like a band-shaped structure on the US image and is located deep to the gluteus maximus (Figure 8.36). Nerve stimulation is recommended to confirm location of the sciatic nerve. Deposit 15 to 20 mL of LA around the nerve using either the in-plane or out-of-plane approach. This block can also be done in the prone position.

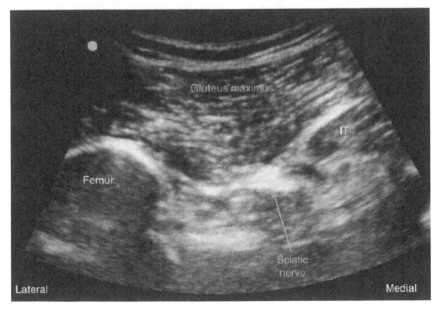

FIGURE 8.36. US image showing the sciatic nerve deep to the gluteus maximus muscle in the transgluteal approach. The sciatic nerve is located between the femur and the ischial tuberosity (IT).

Block success. Effective block of the nerve can be demonstrated with loss of all foot or toe movements.

Key complications. None.[21]

Popliteal Block (Intermediate)

Indication. Surgery involving the ankle or the foot, analgesia after knee surgery.

Overview. The sciatic nerve courses along the posterior thigh near the popliteal fossa and can be blocked at this position. It divides into the tibial and common peroneal nerve around the popliteal fossa at a variable distance from the popliteal crease, so care must be taken to appropriately infiltrate LA around each of these branches. Like the sciatic nerve block discussed earlier, the popliteal block can be done via multiple approaches, but the most common posterior approach is discussed here.

Technique. With the patient in a prone position, place the US probe transverse at the popliteal crease (Figure 8.37). The linear probe can be used in most patients due to the superficial course of the sciatic; however, a curvilinear probe may be needed for obese patients. Scanning with the probe, the posterior tibial nerve, located superficial and lateral to the popliteal artery, and common peroneal nerve are identified as hyperechoic oval or round structures (Figure 8.38). Move the US probe cephalad until the two nerves join together as the sciatic nerve (Figure 8.39). At this level, prior to the division of the sciatic nerve, infiltrate 15 to 20 mL of LA using either the in-plane or out-of-plane technique.

Key complications. Inadvertent puncture of popliteal artery.[22]

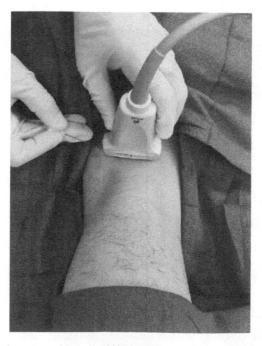

FIGURE 8.37. US probe position for popliteal block proximal to the popliteal fossa. Needle position corresponds to in-plane technique.

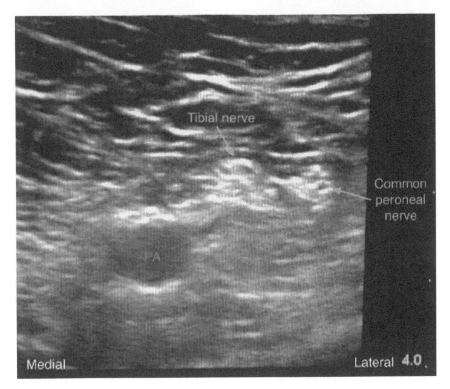

FIGURE 8.38. US image showing common peroneal nerve and tibial nerve immediately lateral to the popliteal artery (PA) in the popliteal fossa.

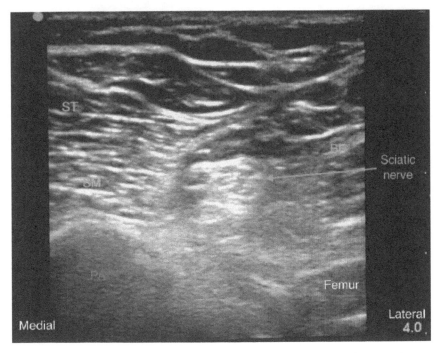

FIGURE 8.39. US image showing the combination of tibial and common peroneal nerves to form the sciatic nerve more proximal in the thigh. Also pictured are the popliteal artery (PA), the biceps femoris muscle (BF), semitendinosis (ST), and semimembranosis (SM).

Indication. Supplementation of the sciatic nerve block for medial foot and ankle surgery, anesthesia for saphenous vein stripping or harvesting.

Overview. The saphenous nerve is the terminal branch of the femoral nerve and innervates the medial aspect of the leg down to the ankle and foot. It runs in the triangular adductor canal which is surrounded superiorly by the sartorius, medially by the adductor longus and magnus, and laterally by the vastus medialis. Though the hyperechoic nerve sometimes cannot be well visualized by US, it runs lateral to the artery in the upper half of the canal and then crosses over to the medial side of the femoral artery in the lower half of the canal. The goal is to infiltrate LA around the lateral or medial aspect of the femoral artery in the adductor canal depending upon the site of block. The technique described here corresponds to a block at the lower half of the adductor canal, where the saphenous nerve is medial to the artery.

Technique. With the patient supine, place the linear probe transverse in the anteromedial aspect of the mid-thigh (Figure 8.40). Visualize the femoral artery in the adductor canal. Superior and lateral to the artery lies the saphenous nerve (Figure 8.41). If the operator places the probe more distal and images the lower half of the adductor canal, the nerve will be medial to the artery. Deposit 5 to 10 mL of LA around the nerve in the adductor canal using either the in-plane or out-of-plane technique.

Key complications. None.[23]

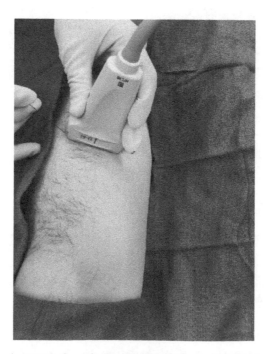

FIGURE 8.40. US probe position for saphenous nerve/adductor canal block in the anteromedial aspect of mid-thigh. Needle position corresponds to in-plane technique.

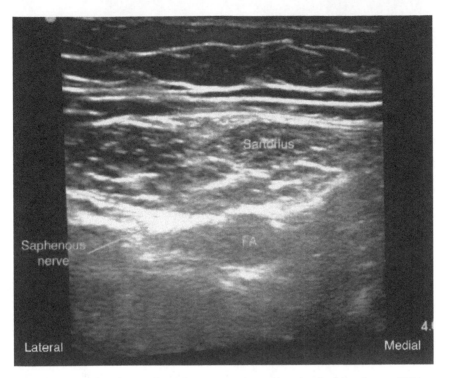

FIGURE 8.41. US image showing the saphenous nerve located lateral to the femoral artery (FA) in the upper half of the adductor canal. Superior to the canal is the sartorius muscle.

REFERENCES

1. Mariano ER, Marshall ZJ, Urman RD, Kaye AD. Ultrasound and its evolution in perioperative regional anesthesia and analgesia. *Best Pract Res Clin Anaesthesiol.* 2014;28(1):29–39. doi:10.1016/j.bpa.2013.11.001

2. Griffin J, Nicholls B. Ultrasound in regional anaesthesia. *Anaesthesia.* 2010;65:1–12. doi:10.1111/j.1365-2044.2009.06200.x

3. Peng PWH, Narouze S. Ultrasound-guided interventional procedures in pain medicine: a review of anatomy, sonoanatomy, and procedures. Part I: non-axial structures. *Reg Anesth Pain Med.* 2009;34(5):458–474. doi:10.1097/aap.0b013e3181aea16f

4. Xu D. Optimizing an ultrasound image. New York School of Regional Anesthesia. http://www.nysora.com/regional-anesthesia/foundations-of-us-guided-nerve-blocks-techniques/3085-optimizing-an-ultrasound-image.html. Accessed November 20, 2016.

5. Regional Anesthesia Ultrasound Equipment. Ultrasound for regional anesthesia. http://www.usra.ca/machine.php Accessed November 20, 2016.

6. Steinfeldt T, Volk T, Kessler P, et al. Peripheral nerve blocks on the upper extremity. *Der Anaesthesist.* 2015;64(11):846–854. doi:10.1007/s00101-015-0091-x

7. Ultrasound-guided interscalene brachial plexus block. New York School of Regional Anesthesia. http://www.nysora.com/techniques/ultrasound-guided-techniques/upper-extremity/3014-ultrasound-guided-interscalene-brachial-plexus-block.html. Accessed November 20, 2016.

8. Ultrasound-guided supraclavicular brachial plexus block. New York School of Regional Anesthesia. http://www.nysora.com/techniques/ultrasound-guided-techniques/upper-

extremity/3220-ultrasound-guided-supraclavicular-brachial-plexus-block.html. Accessed November 20, 2016.

9. Ultrasound-guided infraclavicular brachial plexus block. New York School of Regional Anesthesia. http://www.nysora.com/techniques/ultrasound-guided-techniques/upper-extremity/3016-ultrasound-guided-infraclavicular-brachial-plexus-block.html. Accessed November 20, 2016.

10. Ultrasound-guided axillary brachial plexus block. New York School of Regional Anesthesia. http://www.nysora.com/techniques/ultrasound-guided-techniques/upper-extremity/3017-ultrasound-guided-axillary-brachial-plexus-block.html. Accessed November, 2016.

11. Ultrasound-guided wrist block. New York School of Regional Anesthesia. http://www.nysora.com/techniques/ultrasound-guided-techniques/upper-extremity/3067-ultrasound-guided-wrist-block.html. Accessed November 20, 2016.

12. Ultrasound-guided forearm block. New York School of Regional Anesthesia. http://www.nysora.com/techniques/ultrasound-guided-techniques/upper-extremity/3066-ultrasound-guided-forearm-block.html. Accessed November 20, 2016.

13. Intercostal block. New York School of Regional Anesthesia. http://www.nysora.com/techniques/neuraxial-and-perineuraxial-techniques/landmark-based/3072-intercostal-block.html. Accessed November 20, 2016.

14. Truncal and cutaneous blocks. New York School of Regional Anesthesia. http://www.nysora.com/techniques/ultrasound-guided-techniques/3253-truncal-and-cutaneous-blocks.html. Accessed November 20, 2016.

15. Transversalis fascia plane block. Ultrasound for Regional Anesthesia. http://www.usra.ca/tfpanatomy.php. Accessed November 20, 2016

16. Lumbar plexus block. New York School of Regional Anesthesia. http://www.nysora.com/techniques/neuraxial-and-perineuraxial-techniques/ultrasound-guided/3279-lumbar-plexus-block.html. Accessed November 20, 2016.

17. Psoas compartment block. Ultrasound for Regional Anesthesia. http://www.usra.ca/psoanatomy.php. Accessed November 20, 2016

18. Ultrasound-guided obturator nerve block. New York School of Regional Anesthesia. http://www.nysora.com/techniques/ultrasound-guided-techniques/lower-extremity/3058-ultrasound-guided-obturator-nerve-block.html. Accessed November 20, 2016.

19. Ultrasound-guided femoral nerve block. New York School of Regional Anesthesia. http://www.nysora.com/techniques/ultrasound-guided-techniques/lower-extremity/3056-ultrasound-guided-femoral-nerve-block.html. Accessed November 20, 2016.

20. Ultrasound-guided fascia iliaca block. New York School of Regional Anesthesia. http://www.nysora.com/techniques/ultrasound-guided-techniques/lower-extremity/3057-ultrasound-guided-fascia-iliaca-block.html. Accessed November 20, 2016.

21. Sciatic nerve block: anterior/transgluteal/subgluteal approach. New York School of Regional Anesthesia. http://www.nysora.com/techniques/ultrasound-guided-techniques/lower-extremity/3482-sciatic-nerve-block-anterior-transgluteal-subgluteal-approach.html. Accessed November 20, 2016.

22. Ultrasound-guided popliteal sciatic block. New York School of Regional Anesthesia. http://www.nysora.com/techniques/ultrasound-guided-techniques/lower-extremity/3418-ultrasound-guided-popliteal-sciatic-block.html. Accessed November 20, 2016.

23. Ultrasound-guided saphenous nerve block. New York School of Regional Anesthesia. http://www.nysora.com/techniques/ultrasound-guided-techniques/lower-extremity/3059-ultrasound-guided-saphenous-nerve-block.html. Accessed November 20, 2016.

9 Long-Acting Perioperative Opioids

Kenneth D. Candido and Teresa M. Kusper

INTRODUCTION

Opioid medications are extensively utilized in the management of acute and chronic pain in the outpatient and inpatient clinical settings, as well as being used worldwide during both routine and complex surgeries. They have a long-standing, proven history of providing pain control during the perioperative period and have become an indispensable element of postsurgical analgesia. Opioid prescriptions in the operating room account for about 40% of surgical analgesics.[1] Despite their widespread utilization and excellent analgesic benefits, opioid use is not without significant potential risks. This chapter describes perioperative application of opioid medications, with a special focus on the long-acting opioids, morphine and hydromorphone. Most common side effects engendered using these agents and the remedies available for the treatment of those side effects are briefly discussed. Finally, the chapter provides a concise summery of various factors influencing the effectiveness of opioid analgesics, as well as analgesic considerations for special patient populations.

OPIOID CHARACTERISTICS

Opioid Classification

Opioids are divided into four separate groups based on their actions at the opioid receptors: full opioid agonists, partial opioid agonists, mixed agonists-antagonists, and opioid antagonists. Full opioid agonists (morphine, codeine, hydrocodone, oxycodone, meperidine, methadone, fentanyl, sufentanil) bind opioid receptors eliciting specific clinical effects. Partial opioid agonists, such as buprenorphine, produce a limited response upon binding to the opioid receptor. Opioid antagonists, naloxone and naltrexone, bind to opioid receptors without activating them while blocking the activity of other agonists. Mixed agonist-antagonists (buprenorphine, nalbuphine, pentazocine) behave as agonists at low doses and as antagonists at higher doses.

Opioid Receptors and Analgesic Action

The nociceptive network is comprised of peripheral efferent sensory neurons, the dorsal horn of the spinal cord, ascending spinal tracts, reticular formation of the brainstem, midbrain (periaqueductal gray matter), thalamus, and the cortex. Mu (μ), kappa (κ), delta (Δ), and sigma (σ) receptors are widely distributed at the peripheral, spinal, and supraspinal levels and bind endogenous opioid peptides endorphins, enkephalins, and dynorphins, as well as the exogenous opiates, thereby producing clinically significant effects. Opioid receptors belong to the group of G-protein coupled receptors. Binding of an opiate to the receptor causes dissociation of the G-protein, which triggers a chain of intracellular events, including diminished conductance through the voltage-gated calcium channels, stimulation of the inward potassium rectifying channels, inhibition of adenylyl cyclase, reduction of cAMP production, prevention of substance P release from the afferent sensory neurons, and ultimately hyperpolarization of the neuronal cell membrane, preventing transmission of painful nerve impulses. Analgesic response is achieved after the stimulation of the μ-receptors, although some activity is present at the κ-receptors.[2,3]

Opioid Pharmacokinetics

Absorption and bioavailability of opioid medications varies between different agents and routes of administration. Opioids undergo extensive first-pass metabolism following oral administration. Physiochemical properties (pKa, partition coefficient) determine onset and duration of analgesia derived from opioid medications (Table 9.1). The octanol/water partition coefficient is a measure of lipid solubility, which determines the efficiency of absorption and diffusion of the medications from

Table 9.1. Physiochemical Properties of Opioid Medications

Opioid	MW	pKa	Partition Coefficient
Morphine	285	7.9	1.42
Hydromorphone	285	8.2	2.0
Remifentanil	376	7.2	17.9
Meperidine	247	8.5	38.8
Methadone	309	9.3	116.0
Alfentanil	416	6.5	145.0
Fentanyl	336	8.4	813.0
Sufentanil	386	8.0	1778.0

MW = molecular weight of the compound; pKa = acid/base ionization constant; partition coefficient = determinant of lipid solubility.

Table 9.2. Comparison of Characteristics of Hydrophilic and Lipophilic Opioid Medications

Hydrophilic	*Lipophilic*
Morphine, Hydromorphone	Fentanyl, Sufentanil
Spinal side of action	Spinal +/− systemic side of action
Slower to cross CSF: delayed onset	Rapid access to CSF: quick onset
Slower to clear from CSF: delayed elimination, longer duration of action	Greater vascular uptake: shorter duration; higher serum concentration
Extensive CSF spread; does not penetrate fat	Penetrates fat
Rostral spread: both early and delayed respiratory depression, nausea and vomiting, pruritus	Primarily early respiratory depression; sedation mainly due to the systemic effects
	Lower incidence of nausea and pruritus

CSF = cerebrospinal fluid.

peripheral sites. Lipophilic agents, such as fentanyl and sufentanil, are readily absorbed after intranasal, intrabuccal, and transdermal applications and rapidly redistribute between fat and blood compartments after intravenous (IV) administration, therefore having a fast onset and offset and a short duration of analgesia. Epidural and intrathecal (IT) administration of lipophilic fentanyl or sufentanil results in a rapid absorption of the drugs from the cerebrospinal fluid (CSF) via the arachnoid granulations into the dorsal horn of the spinal cord and equally rapid offset after redistribution into the azygous venous system. In contrast, hydrophilic drugs, such as morphine and hydromorphone, are characterized by slow absorption into the CNS and slow redistribution, accounting for their delayed onset and offset and longer duration of action (Table 9.2).

Opioid medications, except for remifentanil, which is hydrolyzed by plasma esterase, undergo hepatic biotransformation into molecules excreted by the kidneys. A majority of opioid drugs undergo oxidation by the cytochrome P450 system. Meperidine is metabolized by N-demethylation into the normeperidine metabolite with analgesic yet inherent epileptic properties. Hepatic glucuronidation is responsible for the breakdown of hydrophilic morphine and hydromorphone medications. Morphine is broken down into two main metabolites: morphine-3-glucuronide (M3G) and morphine-6-glucuronide (M6G). M3G is produced in higher quantities, and while it lacks analgesic efficacy, it is known for its central nervous system (CNS) toxicity.[4] M6G is the minor metabolite possessing some analgesic activity and contributing to side effects in patients with decreased renal clearance. Metabolism of hydromorphone gives rise to an active metabolite, hydromorphone-3-glucuronide (H3G), devoid of analgesic properties but capable of producing neurologic side effects; myoclonus, allodynia, and seizures.[5]

PERIOPERATIVE USE OF LONG-ACTING OPIOIDS

Long-acting opioids, morphine and hydromorphone, are considered the cornerstone of surgical pain control. During the perioperative period, they are usually administered via IV and intraspinal routes and may be continued orally in those tolerating oral intake, for postoperative pain relief as tolerated by the patient, in immediate release or extended-release formulations. The IV route is the preferred and most commonly used mode of delivery due to the convenience of use, easy titration, and faster onset of action compared to oral opioid medications. Additionally, the IV route bypasses first-pass metabolism thereby resulting in a lower concentration of glucuronide metabolites and reduced risk of side effects.[6] Patient-controlled analgesia (PCA) provides continuous delivery of preprogrammed dosages of opioid medication and sustained pain control on an as-needed basis while allowing the patient's engagement and ultimately increasing patient satisfaction.[7] Both morphine and hydromorphone can be used with IV-PCA. Hong et al. assessed the efficacy and safety profile of PCA morphine (1 mg/ml) and hydromorphone (0.2 mg/ml) in a prospective randomized double-blind study ($n = 50$) during the first eight hours following general and gynecological surgeries and found no significant differences in analgesic efficacy and opioid-related adverse effects between the two agents.[8] Addition of ketamine to morphine or hydromorphone PCA resulted in improved postoperative analgesia, reduction of opioid usage by 5 to 20 mg at 24 to 72 hours, and decreased nausea and vomiting without any added ketamine-related side effects.[9] The addition of buprenorphine to morphine PCA did not confer additional analgesic benefit or reduce the incidence of side effects in 120 patients after abdominal surgery.[10]

The presence of μ- and κ- opioid receptors in the Rexed's laminae I, II, and V of the dorsal horn enables IT application of opioid medications for a wide variety of surgical procedures. With the IT route, it is possible to achieve a profound analgesia with much smaller opioid doses than those required for comparable pain relief via the IV or epidural routes, thereby limiting a chance of adverse reactions. The success of IT therapy has been documented in numerous reports describing surgical pain control after various surgical procedures, including orthopedic,[11] spinal,[12,13] obstetric,[14,15] abdominal,[16,17] and cardiac surgeries,[18,19] among others. There is substantial evidence showing superiority of IT morphine to IV opioid administration for analgesia in a variety of circumstances.[17,18] IT opioids can be used alone or in conjunction with other adjuvant agents. A concomitant IV naloxone infusion was administered with IT opioids without diminishing pain control yet while reducing the risk of adverse events.[20] Likewise, an addition of ketamine (0.1 mg/kg) to IT or epidural morphine improved postsurgical pain control without producing additional side effects.[21,22]

Epidural analgesia is accomplished by the interaction of opioid drugs with opioid receptors present in Rexed's lamina II of the dorsal horn via spinal and supraspinal/systemic mechanisms. Opioids can be delivered into the epidural space as a single bolus injection or via continuous infusions through preplaced catheters. Single-shot injections of morphine or hydromorphone provide pain relief lasting approximately 18 hours. Epidural administration of morphine or hydromorphone results in lower postsurgical analgesic requirements compared to IV opioids.[23,24] Epidural opioids can also be combined with IV-PCA to achieve improved therapeutic outcomes and reduce postoperative opioid consumption after select surgical procedures.[25,26] Patient-controlled epidural analgesia (PCEA) with morphine offers greater pain control than IV opioids alone.[26,27] Moreover, PCEA with bupivacaine and hydromorphone was compared to a multimodal pain regimen consisting of periarticular injection, clonidine patch, and sustained-release oxycodone in 41 patients after total hip arthroplasty.[28] The patients treated with PCEA demonstrated lower pain scores, lower opioid consumption, and faster discharge but higher rates of opioid-related nausea, vomiting, and itchiness.

OPIOID-RELATED ADVERSE EFFECTS

Opioid-related side effects are a serious concern limiting the therapeutic benefits of opioid analgesics or prohibiting the use of this therapy in susceptible patients. A possibility of adverse reactions must be taken into account before the initiation and throughout the maintenance of the therapy. According to a meta-analysis of randomized controlled trials, approximately 80% of noncancer patients on chronic opioids experience at least one adverse reaction from opioids, and the most common side effects are constipation (41%), nausea (32%), and somnolence (29%).[29] Some adverse effects might have life-threatening consequences; therefore, patients need to be continuously evaluated for signs and symptoms of opioid toxicity. Naloxone, an opioid-receptor antagonist, is the agent of choice used to reverse the deleterious effects of opioid administration and prevent patient morbidity and mortality. Possible side effects and available treatment options used in the clinical practice to counteract these effects are listed in Table 9.3.

Table 9.3. Most Common Opioid-Related Side Effects and Available Treatment Options

Nausea and Vomiting	**Prevention:**
	Preoperative: gabapentin 300–600 mg PO 1 hr before surgery
	Intraoperative: ondansetron 4mg IV + dexamethasone 4–8 mg IV; propofol 30 mg IV
	Rescue:
	Dopamine receptor antagonists:
	Metoclopromide 5–10 mg PO or IV every 6 hr
	Prochlorperazine 5–10 mg PO or IV every 8 hr
	Promethazine 12.5–25 mg PO or IV every 6 hr
	Serotonin receptor antagonist:
	Ondansetron 4 mg IV every 6 hr
Pruritus	**Antihistamines:**
Sedation	Benadryl 25–50 mg IV or PO; repeat 12.5–25 mg IM
Urinary Retention	**Opioid antagonists:**
	Naloxone 100 μg bolus; followed by 1μg/kg/hr IV infusion
	Mixed opioid agonist/antagonist:
	- Nalbuphine 2.5–10 mg IV or IM
	- Butorphanol 0.5–1 mg IV or IM
Respiratory Depression	**Opioid antagonist:**
	Naloxone 100 μg bolus until RR >10
	Followed by 5 μg/kg/hr IV infusion

PO = by mouth; IV = intravenous; IM = intramuscular; RR = respiratory rate.

Gastrointestinal (GI) issues such as nausea and vomiting or constipation are frequently reported symptoms by patients on opioid therapy. Long-term administration of opioid medications increases the risk of GI dysfunction.[30] Nausea and vomiting occur secondary to the rostral migration of the hydrophilic agents or systemic effects from the lipophilic opioids. The symptoms are induced by the stimulation of various receptors within the chemoreceptor trigger zone located in the medulla: μ- and Δ- opioid receptors, dopamine, serotonin, histamine, neurokinin-1, cannabinoid receptor-1, and acetylcholine receptors.[31] Constipation results from the activation of the enteric μ- receptors, which reduces GI tract motility; decreases secretion of gastric, pancreatic, and biliary juices; increases intestinal fluid absorption; and tightens the tone of the sphincters.[32] Nausea and vomiting can be prevented with a combination of intraoperative corticosteroids and serotonin receptor antagonists, which administered together are more effective than either of the agents given alone.[33-35] A subhypnotic dose of propofol given 15 minutes prior to skin closure has found to be equally efficacious in postoperative nausea and vomiting prevention to 10 mg of metoclopramide.[36] Additional parenteral antiemetic agents that can be used postoperatively include dopamine receptor antagonists (prochlorperazine, metoclopramide, promethazine) and substance P and the neurokinin receptor antagonist, aprepitant. Preoperative administration of oral gabapentin either alone or in combination with a serotonin receptor inhibitor or corticosteroid has shown promise in preventing and reducing the incidence of postoperative nausea and vomiting.[37-39]

Sedation is a frequently encountered adverse reaction to opioid therapy during the postoperative course. Cognitive impairment, psychomotor dysfunction, memory deficits, and sleep disturbances are other possible neuropsychological effects related to opioid analgesic use.[40] Cognitive decline, delirium, and dementia have been documented in the geriatric population.[41,42] These effects are mainly attributed to neurotoxic metabolites liberated during the breakdown of morphine, codeine, hydromorphone, fentanyl, and meperidine and possibly due to the inhibition of cholinergic activity.[40] Mild to moderate sedation is usually addressed by decreasing the rate of a continuous opioid infusion, whereas severe sedation is treated as potential respiratory depression and requires naloxone administration. It is important to note that cognitive impairment might herald impending respiratory depression.

Respiratory depression is a well-recognized and likely the most dangerous side effect associated with perioperative use of opioid analgesics. The onset of respiratory depression varies between the lipophilic and hydrophilic opioid medications and their respective routes of administration. Lipophilic agents such as fentanyl produce a rapid onset of respiratory depression within minutes to hours after absorption into the vascular system. Conversely, administration of a hydrophilic agent, such as morphine, might produce early- and late-onset (biphasic) respiratory depression, with a peak onset between 3 and 12 hours.[43] A review of data collected from 1,524 patients treated with either IV or neuraxial morphine demonstrated the occurrence of respiratory depression between 2 to 31 and 2 to 12 hours, respectively, after the last morphine administration.[44] The use of extended-release epidural morphine is associated with a higher risk of respiratory depression compared to IV-PCA morphine.[45] Rostral spread of the hydrophilic medication from the epidural space, into the CSF and then into the brainstem results in binding to the μ- and Δ- opioid receptors in the ventral medullary respiratory centers, potentially depressing respiratory rate and depth, increasing pulmonary resistance and chest wall rigidity, suppressing hypercarbic and hypoxic ventilatory responses, and precipitating apnea and respiratory failure.[46,47] More specifically, opioid-related respiratory depression is induced by opioid binding to neurokinin-1 receptors expressed by neurons in the medullary pre-Botzinger complex.[48] The opioid-receptor antagonist naloxone is the main therapeutic option used to reverse respiratory depression.[49] Use of the opioid antagonist, however, may also reverse the analgesic effect produced by lipophilic opioid medications.

Pruritus is most commonly seen after neuraxial opioid analgesia, specifically IT opioid administration. The symptom is usually mild in intensity and might either be generalized or segmental, limited to the area of the injection, or noted on the face, neck, or torso. The pathophysiology of opioid-induced pruritus is still poorly understood but might involve activation of the μ- opioid and serotonergic receptors in the dorsal horn and in the nucleus of the spinal tract of the trigeminal nerve in the medulla.[50] The prevailing thought process is that the symptom is not related to histamine release but rather due to the facilitation of protective spinal cord reflexes and enhanced "cross-talk" between interneurons located in laminae II to V of the dorsal horn of the spinal cord.[51] Though histamine liberation is not the culprit, antihistamines remain the first-line treatment option, while other therapeutic options include serotonin-receptor antagonists, propofol, and opioid antagonists (naloxone) or mixed opioid agonist/antagonists (nalbuphine and butorphanol).

Urinary retention is more frequent after IT and epidural techniques than after IV opioid delivery. Opioid binding inhibits the sacral parasympathetic nervous system causing relaxation of the detrusor muscle[52] and stimulates sympathetic outflow, increasing sphincter tone of the bladder and inhibiting the micturition reflex.[53] Urinary retention might require catheterization and in severe cases naloxone reversal.

ANESTHETIC CONSIDERATIONS IN SPECIAL PATIENT POPULATIONS

A significant degree of interpatient variability exists relating to opioid requirements and propensity for adverse reactions. Analgesic efficacy and safety profiles appear to be influenced by number of different factors, including age, gender, ethnicity, comorbidities, and illness severity in the patients treated with opioid medications. Age is the main factor affecting opioid requirements and postsurgical pain management. It also appears to be the most significant predictor of opioid requirements in the initial 24 hours after surgery as shown by a retrospective chart review of 1,010 patients <70 years of age with postsurgical pain treated with PCA morphine.[54] There are important age-related physiological changes in different body systems influencing the pharmacokinetics of analgesic drugs and predisposing the geriatric patient to increased sensitivity to opioids and increased vulnerability to adverse effects related to the opioid therapy, most significantly the renal, hepatic, and metabolic changes. Changes involving the renal system include decrease in renal cortical mass, renal blood flow, and glomerular filtration rate, which results in reduced clearance and accumulation of the opioid drug or its active metabolites and increased risk of morphine toxicity. Accumulation of active M3G and M6G metabolites after morphine administration may lead to respiratory depression and neurologic side effects in patients with renal insufficiency.[4,55] The H3G metabolite may accumulate after hydromorphone use in patients with renal dysfunction, resulting in neuroexcitatory effects, such as agitation, tremor, and myoclonus.[56] Similarly, with aging specific physiological changes ensue within the hepatobiliary system, such as reduced blood flow and decreased production of important enzymes and proteins, leading to reductions in hepatic metabolism of opioid drugs.[57] Additionally, the aging process is associated with an increase in body fat and a decrease in total body water, which reduce the volume of distribution and increases plasma concentrations of the hydrophilic drugs, such as morphine.[58] It is recommended to implement opioid therapy using a 50% dose reduction and prolonged dosing intervals to prevent the build-up of toxic metabolites and to reduce the likelihood of potential complications.[59] There was no difference in efficacy and incidence of adverse events between morphine and hydromorphone medications in elderly patients.[60] Undoubtedly, age-related changes combined with possible organ dysfunction and/or cognitive impairment increase the complexity of perioperative pain management; nevertheless they should not preclude proper assessment of pain and delivery of an adequate analgesic therapy in the elderly population.

Significant organ changes might be precipitated or escalated during an acute illness. Pharmacokinetics of opiate narcotics were evaluated in a group of intensive care patients to determine variations in drug metabolism and elimination compared to healthy counterparts. One such study analyzed concentrations of morphine and M3G collected from 135 intensive care unit (ICU) patients on continuous morphine infusions and 20 healthy volunteers given an IV bolus of morphine and a one-hour infusion.[61] The study showed reduced elimination and elevated levels of M3G metabolite in ICU patients with both normal and decreased creatinine levels compared to the healthy volunteers. Consequently, a reduction of 33% in the maintenance dose was recommended in ICU patients with renal failure.[61]

Gender-related differences in pain perception and sensitivity to opioid analgesics have been examined extensively and continue to be the subject of great debate. Higher analgesic efficacy, slower onset and offset of action, and lower morphine requirements in those of female gender have been documented in various reports.[62–64] Doses of opioid analgesics may need to be increased by 30% to 40% in male patients for a similar pain score compared to female patients.[63] These results are challenged by other reports, which show higher pain scores and greater opioid consumption in female patient populations and consider that the female gender is a predictor of worse postoperative pain compared to males.[65,66] The differences in pain reactivity and responsiveness to opioid medications are primarily attributed to variations in the gonadal hormones (estrogens and androgens), as well as stress-induced changes in the cortisol level between the two genders.[67]

Interethnic differences appear to influence the metabolic clearance and responsiveness of an individual to morphine therapy. A cohort study of 66 young healthy males (Caucasians, native Americans, and Latinos; $n = 22$ in each group) demonstrated an 18% increase in blunting of the hypercapnic ventilatory response after morphine administration in Native Americans compared to Caucasians and Latinos, despite higher levels of the M6G metabolite in the Caucasian participants.[68] No significant differences in postsurgical pain scores, morphine requirements, or adverse effects from the opioid therapy were noted between Asian and Caucasian females ($n = 60$ each group) treated with IV morphine after total abdominal hysterectomy,[69] although previous studies suggested possible differences in these variables between the two ethnic groups.[70] African Americans demonstrated lower Visual Analog Scale scores and lower morphine requirements compared to white patients at 12 hours, at the first and third day postoperatively, but not at the second day, after scoliosis surgery.[71]

CONCLUSION

Opioid medications are a mainstay treatment option for acute severe postsurgical pain. Morphine and hydromorphone are suitable choices for managing postoperative pain due to their great analgesic potency and efficacy, thereby permitting the administration of prolonged analgesia compared to more lipophilic opioids. With many routes of administration available, the use of these opioid agents can be tailored to various specific clinical scenarios. Specific factors might influence the level of analgesia and risks of side effects and help predict the severity of postsurgical pain. Knowledge of these factors carries important implications related to provision of optimal, safe, and quality pain management treatment with a propensity to induce numerous side effects. Because of the significant side-effect profile of opioid medications, it is imperative to balance the delivery of an adequate postoperative pain control with cautious and responsible prescribing practices in the surgical patient population.

REFERENCES

1. Levy B, Paulozzi L, Mack KA, Jones CM. Trends in opioid analgesic-prescribing rates by specialty, U.S., 2007-2012. *Am J Prev Med.* 2015;49(3):409–413.
2. Pasternak GW. The pharmacology of mu analgesics: from patients to genes. *Neuroscientist.* 2001;7(3):220–231.
3. McDonald JLD. Opioid receptors. *Contin Educ Anaesthes Crit Care Pain.* 2005;5(1): 22–25.
4. Smith MT. Neuroexcitatory effects of morphine and hydromorphone: evidence implicating the 3-glucuronide metabolites. *Clin Exp Pharmacol Physiol.* 2000;27(7):524–528.
5. Paramanandam G, Prommer E, Schwenke DC. Adverse effects in hospice patients with chronic kidney disease receiving hydromorphone. *J Palliat Med.* 2011;14(9):1029–1033.
6. Osborne R, Joel S, Trew D, Slevin M. Morphine and metabolite behavior after different routes of morphine administration: demonstration of the importance of the active metabolite morphine-6-glucuronide. *Clin Pharmacol Ther.* 1990;47(1):12–19.
7. Walder B, Schafer M, Henzi I, Tramer MR. Efficacy and safety of patient-controlled opioid analgesia for acute postoperative pain: a quantitative systematic review. *Acta Anaesthesiol Scand.* 2001;45(7):795–804.
8. Hong D, Flood P, Diaz G. The side effects of morphine and hydromorphone patient-controlled analgesia. *Anesth Analg.* 2008;107(4):1384–1389.
9. Wang L, Johnston B, Kaushal A, Cheng D, Zhu F, Martin J. Ketamine added to morphine or hydromorphone patient-controlled analgesia for acute postoperative pain in adults: a systematic review and meta-analysis of randomized trials. *Can J Anaesth.* 2016;63(3):311–325.
10. Oifa S, Sydoruk T, White I, et al. Effects of intravenous patient-controlled analgesia with buprenorphine and morphine alone and in combination during the first 12 postoperative hours: a randomized, double-blind, four-arm trial in adults undergoing abdominal surgery. *Clin Ther.* 2009;31(3):527–541.

11. Cole PJ, Craske DA, Wheatley RG. Efficacy and respiratory effects of low-dose spinal morphine for postoperative analgesia following knee arthroplasty. *Br J Anaesth.* 2000;85(2):233–237.

12. Li Y, Hong RA, Robbins CB, et al. Intrathecal morphine and oral analgesics provide safe and effective pain control after posterior spinal fusion for adolescent idiopathic scoliosis. *Spine.* 2017;43(2).

13. Hong RA, Gibbons KM, Li GY, Holman A, Voepel-Lewis T. A retrospective comparison of intrathecal morphine and epidural hydromorphone for analgesia following posterior spinal fusion in adolescents with idiopathic scoliosis. *Paediatr Anaesth.* 2017;27(1):91–97.

14. Milner AR, Bogod DG, Harwood RJ. Intrathecal administration of morphine for elective Caesarean section: a comparison between 0.1 mg and 0.2 mg. *Anaesthesia.* 1996;51(9):871–873.

15. Beatty NC, Arendt KW, Niesen AD, Wittwer ED, Jacob AK. Analgesia after Cesarean delivery: a retrospective comparison of intrathecal hydromorphone and morphine. *J Clin Anesth.* 2013;25(5):379–383.

16. Yamaguchi H, Watanabe S, Motokawa K, Ishizawa Y. Intrathecal morphine dose-response data for pain relief after cholecystectomy. *Anesth Analg.* 1990;70(2):168–171.

17. Dichtwald S, Ben-Haim M, Papismedov L, Hazan S, Cattan A, Matot I. Intrathecal morphine versus intravenous opioid administration to impact postoperative analgesia in hepato-pancreatic surgery: a randomized controlled trial. *J Anesth.* 2017;31(2):237–245.

18. Jara FM, Klush J, Kilaru V. Intrathecal morphine for off-pump coronary artery bypass patients. *Heart Surg Forum.* 2001;4(1):57–60.

19. Zarate E, Latham P, White PF, et al. Fast-track cardiac anesthesia: use of remifentanil combined with intrathecal morphine as an alternative to sufentanil during desflurane anesthesia. *Anesth Analg.* 2000;91(2):283–287.

20. Rebel A, Sloan P, Andrykowski M. Postoperative analgesia after radical prostatectomy with high-dose intrathecal morphine and intravenous naloxone: a retrospective review. *J Opioid Manag.* 2009;5(6):331–339.

21. Abd El-Rahman AM, Mohamed AA, Mohamed SA, Mostafa MAM. Effect of intrathecally administered ketamine, morphine, and their combination added to bupivacaine in patients undergoing major abdominal cancer surgery a randomized, double-blind study. *Pain Med.* 2018;19(3):561–568.

22. Subramaniam K, Subramaniam B, Pawar DK, Kumar L. Evaluation of the safety and efficacy of epidural ketamine combined with morphine for postoperative analgesia after major upper abdominal surgery. *J Clin Anesth.* 2001;13(5):339–344.

23. Liu S, Carpenter RL, Mulroy MF, et al. Intravenous versus epidural administration of hydromorphone: effects on analgesia and recovery after radical retropubic prostatectomy. *Anesthesiology.* 1995;82(3):682–688.

24. Weller R, Rosenblum M, Conard P, Gross JB. Comparison of epidural and patient-controlled intravenous morphine following joint replacement surgery. *Can J Anaesth.* 1991;38(5):582–586.

25. Ko JS, Choi SJ, Gwak MS, et al. Intrathecal morphine combined with intravenous patient-controlled analgesia is an effective and safe method for immediate postoperative pain control in live liver donors. *Liver Transpl.* 2009;15(4):381–389.

26. Aydogan MS, Bicakcioglu M, Sayan H, Durmus M, Yilmaz S. Effects of two different techniques of postoperative analgesia management in liver transplant donors: a prospective, randomized, double-blind study. *Transplant Proc.* 2015;47(4):1204–1206.

27. Loper KA, Ready LB, Nessly M, Rapp SE. Epidural morphine provides greater pain relief than patient-controlled intravenous morphine following cholecystectomy. *Anesth Analg*. 1989;69(6):826–828.

28. Jules-Elysee KM, Goon AK, Westrich GH, et al. Patient-controlled epidural analgesia or multimodal pain regimen with periarticular injection after total hip arthroplasty: a randomized, double-blind, placebo-controlled study. *J Bone Joint Surg Am*. 2015;97(10):789–798.

29. Kalso E, Edwards JE, Moore RA, McQuay HJ. Opioids in chronic non-cancer pain: systematic review of efficacy and safety. *Pain*. 2004;112(3):372–380.

30. Tuteja AK, Biskupiak J, Stoddard GJ, Lipman AG. Opioid-induced bowel disorders and narcotic bowel syndrome in patients with chronic non-cancer pain. *Neurogastroenterol Motil*. 2010;22(4):424–430, e96.

31. Smith HS, Laufer A. Opioid induced nausea and vomiting. *Eur J Pharmacol*. 2014;722:67–78.

32. Nelson AD, Camilleri M. Opioid-induced constipation: advances and clinical guidance. *Ther Adv Chronic Dis*. 2016;7(2):121–134.

33. Bano F, Zafar S, Aftab S, Haider S. Dexamethasone plus ondansetron for prevention of postoperative nausea and vomiting in patients undergoing laparoscopic cholecystectomy: a comparison with dexamethasone alone. *J Coll Physicians Surg Pak*. 2008;18(5):265–269.

34. Gautam B, Shrestha BR, Lama P, Rai S. Antiemetic prophylaxis against postoperative nausea and vomiting with ondansetron-dexamethasone combination compared to ondansetron or dexamethasone alone for patients undergoing laparoscopic cholecystectomy. *Kathmandu Univ Med J*. 2008;6(23):319–328.

35. Elhakim M, Nafie M, Mahmoud K, Atef A. Dexamethasone 8 mg in combination with ondansetron 4 mg appears to be the optimal dose for the prevention of nausea and vomiting after laparoscopic cholecystectomy. *Can J Anaesth*. 2002;49(9):922–926.

36. Naghibi K, Kashefi P, Azarnoush H, Zabihi P. Prevention of postoperative nausea and vomiting with a subhypnotic dose of propofol in patients undergoing lower abdominal surgery: a prospective, randomized, double-blind study. *Adv Biomed Res*. 2015;4:35.

37. Grant MC, Lee H, Page AJ, Hobson D, Wick E, Wu CL. The effect of preoperative gabapentin on postoperative nausea and vomiting: a meta-analysis. *Anesth Analg*. 2016;122(4):976–985.

38. Kim KM, Huh J, Lee SK, Park EY, Lee JM, Kim HJ. Combination of gabapentin and ramosetron for the prevention of postoperative nausea and vomiting after gynecologic laparoscopic surgery: a prospective randomized comparative study. *BMC Anesthesiol*. 2017;17(1):65.

39. Agrawal N, Chatterjee C, Khandelwal M, Chatterjee R, Gupta MM. Comparative study of preoperative use of oral gabapentin, intravenous dexamethasone and their combination in gynaecological procedure. *Saudi J Anaesth*. 2015;9(4):413–417.

40. Dhingra L, Ahmed E, Shin J, Scharaga E, Magun M. Cognitive effects and sedation. *Pain Med*. 2015;16(Suppl 1):S37–S43.

41. Pisani MA, Murphy TE, Araujo KL, Van Ness PH. Factors associated with persistent delirium after intensive care unit admission in an older medical patient population. *J Crit Care*. 2010;25(3):540 e1–e7.

42. Dublin S, Walker RL, Gray SL, et al. prescription opioids and risk of dementia or cognitive decline: a prospective cohort study. *J Am Geriatr Soc*. 2015;63(8):1519–1526.

43. Kafer ER, Brown JT, Scott D, et al. Biphasic depression of ventilatory responses to CO_2 following epidural morphine. *Anesthesiology*. 1983;58(5):418–427.

44. Shapiro A, Zohar E, Zaslansky R, Hoppenstein D, Shabat S, Fredman B. The frequency and timing of respiratory depression in 1524 postoperative patients treated with systemic or neuraxial morphine. *J Clin Anesth.* 2005;17(7):537–542.

45. Sumida S, Lesley MR, Hanna MN, Murphy JD, Kumar K, Wu CL. Meta-analysis of the effect of extended-release epidural morphine versus intravenous patient-controlled analgesia on respiratory depression. *J Opioid Manag.* 2009;5(5):301–305.

46. Lalley PM. Opioidergic and dopaminergic modulation of respiration. *Respir Physiol Neurobiol.* 2008;164(1-2):160–167.

47. Weil JV, McCullough RE, Kline JS, Sodal IE. Diminished ventilatory response to hypoxia and hypercapnia after morphine in normal man. *N Engl J Med.* 1975;292(21):1103–1106.

48. Montandon G, Qin W, Liu H, Ren J, Greer JJ, Horner RL. Pre-Botzinger complex neurokinin-1 receptor-expressing neurons mediate opioid-induced respiratory depression. *J Neurosci.* 2011;31(4):1292–1301.

49. Longnecker DE, Grazis PA, Eggers GW Jr. Naloxone for antagonism of morphine-induced respiratory depression. *Anesth Analg.* 1973;52(3):447–453.

50. Kumar K, Singh SI. Neuraxial opioid-induced pruritus: an update. *J Anaesthesiol Clin Pharmacol.* 2013;29(3):303–307.

51. Ballantyne JC, Loach AB, Carr DB. Itching after epidural and spinal opiates. *Pain.* 1988;33(2):149–160.

52. Chaney MA. Intrathecal and epidural anesthesia and analgesia for cardiac surgery. *Anesth Analg.* 2006;102(1):45–64.

53. Durant PA, Yaksh TL. Drug effects on urinary bladder tone during spinal morphine-induced inhibition of the micturition reflex in unanesthetized rats. *Anesthesiology.* 1988;68(3):325–334.

54. Macintyre PE, Jarvis DA. Age is the best predictor of postoperative morphine requirements. *Pain.* 1996;64(2):357–364.

55. Osborne R, Joel S, Slevin M. Morphine intoxication in renal failure: the role of morphine-6-glucuronide. *Br Med J (Clin Res Ed).* 1986;293(6554):1101.

56. Gagnon DJ, Jwo K. Tremors and agitation following low-dose intravenous hydromorphone administration in a patient with kidney dysfunction. *Ann Pharmacother.* 2013;47(7-8):e34.

57. Schmucker DL. Age-related changes in liver structure and function: implications for disease? *Exp Gerontol.* 2005;40(8-9):650–659.

58. Glare PA, Walsh TD. Clinical pharmacokinetics of morphine. *Ther Drug Monit.* 1991;13(1):1–23.

59. Pergolizzi J, Boger RH, Budd K, et al. Opioids and the management of chronic severe pain in the elderly: consensus statement of an International Expert Panel with focus on the six clinically most often used World Health Organization Step III opioids (buprenorphine, fentanyl, hydromorphone, methadone, morphine, oxycodone). *Pain Pract.* 2008;8(4):287–313.

60. Chang AK, Bijur PE, Baccelieri A, Gallagher EJ. Efficacy and safety profile of a single dose of hydromorphone compared with morphine in older adults with acute, severe pain: a prospective, randomized, double-blind clinical trial. *Am J Geriatr Pharmacother.* 2009;7(1):1–10.

61. Ahlers SJ, Valitalo PA, Peeters MY, et al. Morphine glucuronidation and elimination in intensive care patients: a comparison with healthy volunteers. *Anesth Analg.* 2015;121(5):1261–1273.

62. Chia YY, Chow LH, Hung CC, Liu K, Ger LP, Wang PN. Gender and pain upon movement are associated with the requirements for postoperative patient-controlled

IV analgesia: a prospective survey of 2,298 Chinese patients. *Can J Anaesth.* 2002;49(3):249–255.

63. Pleym H, Spigset O, Kharasch ED, Dale O. Gender differences in drug effects: implications for anesthesiologists. *Acta Anaesthesiol Scand.* 2003;47(3):241–259.

64. Sarton E, Olofsen E, Romberg R, et al. Sex differences in morphine analgesia: an experimental study in healthy volunteers. *Anesthesiology.* 2000;93(5):1245–1254; discussion 6A.

65. Aubrun F, Salvi N, Coriat P, Riou B. Sex- and age-related differences in morphine requirements for postoperative pain relief. *Anesthesiology.* 2005;103(1):156–160.

66. Zheng H, Schnabel A, Yahiaoui-Doktor M, et al. Age and preoperative pain are major confounders for sex differences in postoperative pain outcome: a prospective database analysis. *PLoS One.* 2017;12(6):e0178659.

67. Rollman GB. Introduction: sex makes a difference: experimental and clinical pain responses. *Clin J Pain.* 2003;19(4):204–207.

68. Cepeda MS, Farrar JT, Roa JH, et al. Ethnicity influences morphine pharmacokinetics and pharmacodynamics. *Clin Pharmacol Ther.* 2001;70(4):351–361.

69. Al-Hashimi M, Scott S, Griffin-Teall N, Thompson J. Influence of ethnicity on the perception and treatment of early post-operative pain. *Br J Pain.* 2015;9(3):167–172.

70. Konstantatos AH, Imberger G, Angliss M, Cheng CH, Meng AZ, Chan MT. A prospective cohort study comparing early opioid requirement between Chinese from Hong Kong and Caucasian Australians after major abdominal surgery. *Br J Anaesth.* 2012;109(5):797–803.

71. Son-Hing JP, Poe-Kochert C, Thompson GH, Potzman J, Tripi PA. Intrathecal morphine analgesia in idiopathic scoliosis surgery: does sex or racial group affect optimal dosing? *J Pediatr Orthop.* 2011;31(5):489–495.

10 Pain Management in Breast Surgery

Jarrod T. Bogue and Christine H. Rohde

INTRODUCTION

Breast surgeries commonly performed by plastic surgeons include breast reductions, breast augmentations, implant-based and autologous breast reconstructions, as well as cosmetic and reconstructive breast revisions. Pain after breast surgery can be a significant issue as its management can impact postoperative recovery and overall patient experience.

Opioid medications are standard for postoperative pain control. However, their use is associated with side effects of nausea/vomiting, constipation, as well as addiction and overdose potential. The opioid epidemic in the United States is growing, with an estimated 90 people dying each day from opioid overdose.[1] The Centers for Disease Control and Prevention has labeled this a crisis with its estimated economic impact of $78.5 billion dollars per year.[2] In order to understand how these addictions begin, it has been shown that 21% to 29% of patients prescribed opioids for the treatment of chronic pain misuse these medicines. Subsequently, between 8% and 12% of these patients go on to develop an opioid use disorder.[3,4] It has also been shown that 80% of individuals who use heroin first misused prescription opioids.[4] With prescriptions for opioid pain medications commonplace in surgical and postsurgical care, the potential for exposing patients to these risks is high. Novel non-opioid options for postoperative pain control have the potential to decrease the use of opioids and their associated risks.

Breast surgery patients all experience acute pain as part of their postoperative course, but it is important to note that up to two-thirds of these patients go on to experience chronic pain.[5] Studies have shown that one important risk factor for developing chronic pain after breast surgery is experiencing severe acute postoperative pain.[6] Therefore, postoperative pain control is imperative for all breast surgery patients.

Previous work has shown that patients at risk for greater acute postoperative pain have been found to have a certain constellation of risk factors which include younger age, greater surgical invasiveness, and emotional distress.[6] Katz et al. sought to further elucidate risk factors for the persistence of acute pain in patients undergoing breast surgery. The presence of persistent pain in this study correlated most strongly with anxiety. It also confirmed that patients who are of younger age, are unmarried, are undergoing more invasive surgery, and have greater preoperative emotional distress had the presence of more significant postoperative pain.[6]

Studies then focused on elucidating risk factors for developing chronic pain after breast surgery in order to further shed light on what subset of breast surgery patients are at higher risk. Poleshuck et al. prospectively followed 95 breast surgery patients in order to establish which patients developed chronic pain three months postoperatively and analyzed risk factors that were common among those patients. Only age less than 50 was associated with the development of chronic pain.[7] Risk factors associated with more severe pain included more invasive surgery, radiation therapy after surgery, and clinically meaningful acute postoperative pain. Interestingly, this study did not show that the presence or intensity of chronic postoperative pain was correlated with preoperative emotional distress.[7]

Due to the risk of developing chronic postoperative pain resulting from breast surgery, a comprehensive postoperative pain management strategy is encouraged. A systematic review published by Chang et al. encourages a multimodal approach in order to reduce the incidence of chronic pain in this population. The authors do not endorse a specific multimodal approach but do support the use of paravertebral block as a component·of a well-balanced and managed protocol.[8] The literature includes many published articles concerning approaches to treating patients undergoing breast surgery without opioids. Options range from tailored use of local analgesia to external devices and cognitive-behavioral therapies. Multiple alternative modalities are available to treat patients in ways that minimize opioid use.

LOCAL ANESTHETICS AND REGIONAL BLOCKS

Local anesthetics are commonplace in plastic surgical practice and are used in a wide range of applications from emergency department procedures to aesthetic surgeries and beyond. They act by inhibiting local neuron pain signaling and come in many varieties. Local anesthetics as perioperative analgesia in breast surgery have been shown to be effective in decreasing narcotic consumption. Bupivacaine, a longer-acting local anesthetic, has been studied in the setting of breast reduction. When used perioperatively in breast reduction patients, bupivacaine significantly lowered postoperative visual analog pain scores and opioid consumption upon discharge.[9] Bupivacaine has also been instilled via drains after mastectomy. This method has also been found to be effective for controlling pain postoperatively and decreasing narcotic requirement.[10]

It is also important to note the differing and evolving formulations of local analgesics. Liposomal bupivacaine is now available to physicians. It is a much longer-acting form of bupivacaine which utilizes microvesicular liposomal delivery. Liposomal bupivacaine has been validated in its effectiveness for controlling pain and decreasing opioid consumption. Due to its long duration of action, it can be used in place of more invasive methods of pain control.[11] Incorporating local anesthetics into perioperative planning has been shown to effectively decrease the opioid requirement of patients undergoing breast surgery.

Transversus Abdominis Plane Blocks

Transversus abdominis plane blocks instill local analgesia to the plane between the internal oblique and transversus abdominis muscles. This is the plane where the neurovascular bundles which provide sensation to the abdominal wall are located. This therapy can be used in abdominally based breast reconstruction to provide analgesia for the donor site. Its utility has been investigated in patients undergoing abdominally based microsurgical breast reconstruction and has been found in several studies to result in less opioid-containing medication use and shorter hospital stays.[12,13]

Pain Pumps

Continuous local analgesic infusions via pump have also been used as adjunctive postoperative therapies to decrease opioid consumption. Using this modality, a catheter is placed into the breast surgical site typically via stab incision. The catheter tip is then draped over the pectoralis fascia, and local anesthetic is slowly infused through it. It has been shown that the use of such pumps decreases both postoperative nausea and vomiting as well as the use of opioids in patients undergoing breast reduction.[14,15] Pain pumps provide a novel way for continuous use of local analgesia extending through the perioperative period to the postoperative period.

Paravertebral Blocks

Local anesthetic delivered as a paravertebral block (PVB) has been studied in the setting of breast surgery as an effective alternative to general anesthesia (GA). Regional anesthesia in the form of a paravertebral block utilizes local anesthetic infiltration surrounding the spinal nerves as they exit the intervertebral foramen.[16] This in turn causes sensory, motor, and sympathetic blockade. When utilized in the upper thoracic region, it can provide analgesia for breast surgery. Figure 10.1 demonstrates the ultrasound image that guides infiltration, with the arrow showing the plane of local anesthetic infiltration.

A recent systematic review analyzed eight randomized controlled trials, which investigated the effectiveness and safety of PVBs.[17] Six of these studies focused on the use of PVBs in breast surgery. Parameters measured included effectiveness, postoperative pain, postoperative nausea and vomiting, length of hospital stay, and overall patient satisfaction. It was noted that the complete or partial failure of PVBs in grouped analysis was no greater than 13%. Patients who received PVBs compared to GA were found to have significantly less pain in the early postoperative period with some evidence pointing toward longer-lasting pain relief up to five days after surgery. However, the authors concluded that the strongest evidence for pain relief difference is in the early postoperative period. In terms of length of hospital stays in PVBs versus GA, data analyzed showed significantly shorter hospital stays in patients who received PVBs. The systematic review also investigated overall patient satisfaction with PVBs, finding increased satisfaction in the PVB groups. Postoperative nausea and vomiting

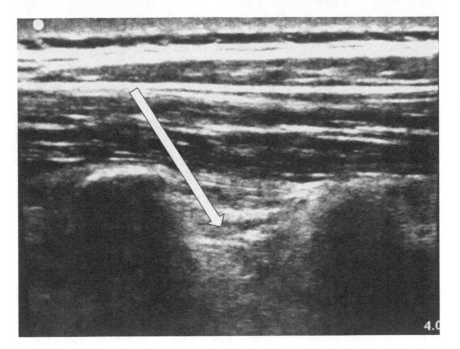

FIGURE 10.1. Ultrasound image for paravertebral block with arrow denoting the plane for local anesthetic infiltration.

was investigated in six studies with varied overall findings. The complication rates of PVBs in these studies ranged between 2% and 6%. The most commonly observed complications of PVBs included pleural puncture seen in one patient in one study, hypotension, and epidural spread.[17]

Pectoralis Block

An alternative to PVB is the use of local anesthetic in the form of pectoralis and pectoralis-serratus fascial blocks. They have been investigated in the setting of both reconstructive and cosmetic breast surgery as an adjunct to GA in order to control postoperative pain and limit narcotic use. The pectoralis block or "pecs block" was first described by Blanco et al. in 2011.[18] In this paper, the group put forth a novel block technique utilizing a pectoralis interfascial plane block. Local anesthetic is infiltrated in the interfascial plane between the pectoralis major and minor to block the lateral and medial pectoral nerves. This is performed via ultrasound guidance and was first described in a case series of 50 patients undergoing breast reconstruction with subpectoral tissue expanders.[18] Figure 10.2 shows the ultrasound image that guides infiltration, with the arrow showing the plane of local anesthetic infiltration for a pectoralis block. A serratus block is an adjunct to the pectoralis block and Figure 10.3 shows the plane for infiltration.

The pectoralis block and serratus block were studied in a retrospective cohort study in which mastectomy patients who underwent pectoralis block or serratus blocks preoperatively were compared with patients who did not receive blocks.[19] The study aimed to analyze two outcome measures: postoperative opioid usage and postoperative

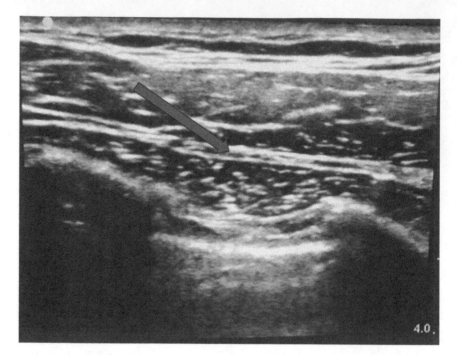

FIGURE 10.2. Ultrasound image for pectoralis block with arrow demonstrating the plane for local anesthetic infiltration.

opioid-induced side effects, namely nausea and vomiting.[19] The pectoralis block and serratus block cohorts had significantly less postoperative pain, nausea and vomiting, intraoperative opioid total dosage, and time in the postanesthesia care unit compared with the no block cohort.

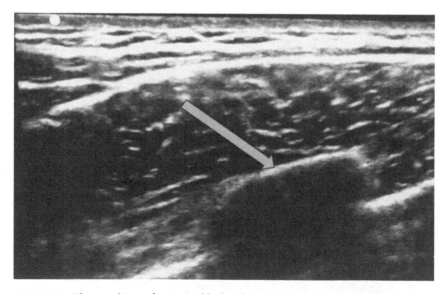

FIGURE 10.3. Ultrasound image for serratus block with arrow denoting the plane for local anesthetic infiltration.

PVBs have been compared to pectoralis block in order to evaluate the efficacy and safety of these two modalities against each other. A randomized trial was carried out with 64 patients undergoing unilateral mastectomy with axillary dissection to compare pectoralis serratus interfascial blocks (PSB) to PVB. The primary endpoint was the first postoperative 24-hour morphine consumption. Patients in the PSB group had significantly more morphine consumption in the first 24 hours ($p < .001$) when compared to the PVB group. However, the study authors noted that overall the pain scores postoperatively were low in both groups.[20] No complications were reported in either group, and the authors concluded that both PSB and PVB are safe options but PVBs are more efficacious.

Pectoralis blocks have also been studied in the setting of cosmetic breast surgery and are utilized by some practitioners in the setting of submuscular breast augmentation. One group, Nasr et al., published a pilot study of intercostal nerve block versus pectoralis block and did not find any statistically significant difference in pain score postoperatively.[21] Leiman et al. published a case report in which they used liposomal bupivacaine to selectively block the lateral and medial pectoral nerves in a patient undergoing submuscular breast augmentation. In this case, their patient did not utilize narcotics in the first 10 days postoperatively and reported no pectoralis muscle spasm during this time period.[22]

Outside of pharmacotherapies, there exist alternative modalities that may be beneficial in reducing postoperative pain in breast surgery.

PULSED ELECTROMAGNETIC FIELD THERAPY DEVICE

A nonpharmacologic option for pain control in breast surgery is the pulsed electromagnetic field device (PEMF). Figure 10.4 shows a device in place after breast reduction surgery. PEMF devices are portable, lightweight, disposable devices that have been approved by the Food and Drug Administration for use in treating pain and edema. Additionally, they have previously been shown to aid in wound and fracture healing.[23-25] PEMF devices have also been implicated in modulating the inflammatory cascade postoperatively which may contribute to some of its positive end effects. Specifically, PEMF devices have been associated with changes in calcium binding to calmodulin in injured tissues, modulating the NO/cGMP signaling pathway.[23] There exists now a significant amount of literature indicating their positive effect in the setting of breast surgery recovery. Lifei et al. reviewed the used of PEMF devices in a meta-analysis and found statistically significant reductions in postoperative pain and edema as well as positive effects on wound healing.[25] This meta-analysis included 25 controlled studies and concluded that there is strong evidence for the use of PEMF devices for postoperative recovery.

PEMF devices have been studied for use in the setting of cosmetic breast augmentation. In order to assess the efficacy of PEMF in this setting, Heden et al. in 2008 published a randomized, placebo-controlled trial that sought to answer the question of utility.[24] Forty-two patients undergoing cosmetic breast augmentation were randomized into three groups: bilateral breasts treated with PEMF devices, bilateral breasts treated with sham devices, and one breast treated with a PEMF device and one breast with a sham device. A difference in postoperative pain was demonstrated by a 2.7 times decrease in postoperative pain on postoperative day 3 in the PEMF-treated

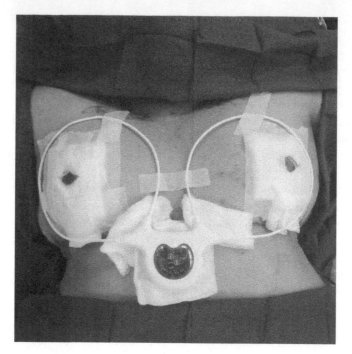

FIGURE 10.4. Immediate postoperative view of PEMF device in place after a breast reduction. The device is placed over surgical dressings and underneath the surgical bra.

breasts compared to sham device treated breasts. Actively treated patients also utilized less prescription pain medicines than patients treated with sham therapies.[25]

Cosmetic breast augmentation and the efficacy of PEMF devices were again studied by in 2012 by Rawe et al., who published a randomized placebo-controlled trial including 18 patients.[26] This group studied visual analog scales and narcotic usage for seven days postoperatively in order to determine pain and opioid usage among patients treated with PEMF devices. Rawe et al. found that pain scores and pain medication usage were both significantly lower in patients treated with PEMF devices.[26]

PEMF device use has also been studied in cases of breast reduction. Rohde et al. investigated the use of PEMF devices in breast reduction patients in a randomized placebo-controlled trial with outcome measures including visual analog pain scores, narcotic usage, and wound exudate IL-1β levels.[27,28] These outcome measures were chosen in order to both evaluate the utility of PEMF devices for pain control and investigate the physiologic effect of PEMF devices on the calcium-calmodulin signaling pathway. Patients in the active treated group were found to have a three-fold decrease in pain scores and a two-fold decrease in narcotic pain usage. Wound exudate IL-1β levels (a cytokine associated with inflammatory pain hypersensitivity) were also significantly decreased in the actively treated group.

Similar significant findings were made in patients undergoing more extensive transverse rectus abdominis (TRAM) flap breast reconstructions with use of the PEMF device on both breast and abdominal sites. In a randomized, double-blind, placebo-controlled study, patients in the PEMF-treated group had significantly lower pain scores postoperatively as well as lower narcotic usage and wound exudate IL-1β levels.[28]

TUMESCENT MASTECTOMY

Tumescent mastectomy has been described in the breast surgery literature as a technique with the potential impact to lower narcotic pain medication usage. Previously, tumescent mastectomy has been utilized in sicker, elderly patients, but, notably in these cases, minimal opioid medications are needed. Tumescent technique has been utilized for liposuction in order to deliver both local anesthesia for pain control and epinephrine in order to facilitate vasoconstriction and decreased blood loss.[29] However, this technique is not only applicable to liposuction. Khater et al. performed a prospective study on the tumescent mastectomy in 20 patients who required total mastectomy and axillary nodal dissection and were American Society of Anesthesiologists score III to IV patients. The study determined this to be a safe and effective alternative to GA, and no patient required traditional opioid pain medication. Instead, the postoperative pain management regimen included doses of ketorolac and paracetamol and incremental doses of nalbuphine, which were given until pain was in better control. This non-opioid combination merits further study in breast surgery patients.[30]

ENHANCED RECOVERY PATHWAYS AND MULTIMODAL PAIN MANAGEMENT REGIMENS

Enhanced recovery pathways have been developed and implemented in order to guide postoperative management of patients and avoid complications.[31,32] They are algorithms designed to promote evidence-based care surrounding perioperative and postoperative management. These algorithms tend to be multidisciplinary and multimodal in their approach to these care elements and may serve a role in the care of breast surgery patients. Dumestre et al. sought to apply an enhanced recovery after surgery (ERAS) model to patients undergoing implant-based breast reconstruction.[33] A prospective study comprised of three groups of breast surgery patients were assessed in order to determine differences among recovery. The three groups were comprised of patients treated in the traditional fashion, those treated in a transitional fashion incorporating some ERAS elements, and those treated according to ERAS. ERAS patients were treated with a combination of opioid and non-opioid medications pre- and postoperatively, as well as a local nerve block.[33] ERAS patients had significantly less pain and nausea when compared with the other groups. Further studies are needed in other varieties of breast surgery, but this may be an emerging technique to decrease pain in breast surgery.

Multimodal pain management regimens are another aspect of templated care that could potentially be implemented in order to decrease both opioid usage and pain experienced after breast surgery. Wick et al. published a review of literature concerning many modes of analgesia including opioid medications and examined the evidence in support of their efficacy and safety. Medications examined included opioids, nonsteroidal anti-inflammatory drugs, specifically ketorolac, N-methyl-D-aspartate receptor modulators, tramadol, local infiltration of anesthetics, and acetaminophen among other non-opioids. The data supported a well-thought-out multimodal approach in order to minimize opioid usage. This approach fits with more modern ERAS approaches and may be coupled with them in order to address pain control postoperatively.[34] ERAS protocols are an evolving modality in the armamentarium of plastic surgeons performing breast surgery. Consensus guidelines for their use are being developed and analyzed currently.[35] These protocols address a need for a designed and thoughtful evidence-based approach to caring for breast surgery patients.

OPIOID-FREE BREAST REDUCTION

Opioid-free approaches have been trialed in breast reduction surgery as well. Parsa et al. aimed to investigate differences in need for opioids, hospital stay, and unplanned hospital admissions in patients undergoing breast reduction.[36] Study participants were split into three groups: patients undergoing breast reduction via traditional GA and adjunctive opioids, patients treated with intravenous sedation and local anesthesia, and patients undergoing GA with use of local anesthesia intraoperatively. Patients in the second two groups received gabapentin and celecoxib preoperatively and bupivacaine infiltration before closure and were prescribed Tylenol postoperatively. The two groups treated in an opioid-free manner when compared to traditional opioid-treated patients had a significantly shorter time from the end of operation to discharge, less postoperative opioid use, and fewer unplanned hospital admissions. It was also found that patients treated without opioids utilized less antiemetic medication due to less postoperative nausea.[36] Parsa et al. demonstrates the safety and benefits of avoiding opioid medications in this patient population.

COGNITIVE-BEHAVIORAL THERAPY

One etiological component of pain that has been underaddressed is its emotional underpinnings. Cognitive-behavioral therapy (CBT) has been put forward as an adjunctive treatment for chronic pain in order to better deal with its emotional component. Tang et al. explain that CBT is talk therapy that explores our behavior and thoughts and their implications on our emotions.[37] Previous work has shown that pain is not an isolated biological phenomenon but is also an emotional response, and their study aims to advocate for the inclusion of CBT to treat this component of the perception of pain. Current evidence suggests that CBT in can be useful in the treatment of chronic pain as part of a hybrid approach.

CONCLUSIONS

Breast surgeries are some of the most common procedures performed by plastic surgeons. The opioid epidemic is far-reaching and impacts the approach of surgeons to postoperative pain control. Opioids are effective pain medications but have significant side effects and risks. Designing pain management plans for patients to address expected postoperative pain in a multimodal fashion that limits opioid exposure is vital to decreasing the potential for addiction and untoward side effects of opioids. This process begins preoperatively and extends through the perioperative and postoperative period. Including a discussion of pain expectations with patients and forming relationships with anesthesiology are key features for designing and implementing opioid-reducing strategies. Ultimately, the surgeon should design an approach that maximizes patient pain control and recovery while minimizing the risks from traditional pain control modalities.

REFERENCES

1. Rudd RA, Seth P, David F, Scholl L. Increases in drug and opioid-involved overdose deaths—United States, 2010–2015. *MMWR Morb Mortal Wkly Rep.* 2016;65: 1445–1452.

2. Florence CS, Zhou C, Luo F, Xu L. The economic burden of prescription opioid overdose, abuse, and dependence in the United States, 2013. *Med Care.* 2016;54(10):901–906.

3. Vowles KE, McEntee ML, Julnes PS, Frohe T, Ney JP, van der Goes DN. Rates of opioid misuse, abuse, and addiction in chronic pain: a systematic review and data synthesis. *Pain.* 2015;156(4):569–576.

4. Muhuri PK, Gfroerer JC, Davies MC. Associations of nonmedical pain reliever use and initiation of heroin use in the United States. *CBHSQ Data Rev.* Aug 2013.

5. Jung BF, Ahrendt GM, Oaklander AL, Dworkin RH. Neuropathic pain following breast cancer surgery: proposed classification and research update. *Pain.* 2003;104:1–13.

6. Katz J, Poleshuck EL, Andrus CH, Hogan LA, Jung BF, Kulick DI, Dworkin RH. Risk factors for acute pain and its persistence following breast cancer surgery. *Pain.* 2005 Dec 15;119(1–3):16–25.

7. Poleshuck EL, Katz J, Andrus CH, et al. Risk factors for chronic pain following breast cancer surgery: a prospective study. *J Pain.* 2006 Sep;7(9):626–634.

8. Chang SH, Mehta V, Langford R. Acute and chronic pain following breast surgery. *Acute Pain.* 2009;11:1–14.

9. Culliford AT 4th, Spector JA, Flores RL, Louie O, Choi M, Karp NS. Intraoperative Sensorcaine significantly improves postoperative pain management in outpatient reduction mammaplasty. *Plast Reconstr Surg.* 2007 Sep15;120(4):840–844.

10. Jonnavithula N, Khandelia H, Durga P, Ramachandran G. Role of wound instillation with bupivacaine through surgical drains for postoperative analgesia in modified radical mastectomy. *Indian J Anaesth.* 2015 Jan;59(1):15–20.

11. Vyas KS, Rajendran S, Morrison SD, et al. Systematic review of liposomal bupivacaine (Exparel) for postoperative analgesia. *Plast Reconstr Surg.* 2016 Oct;138(4):748e–756e.

12. Jablonka EM, Lamelas AM, Kim JN, et al. Transversus abdominis plane blocks with single-dose liposomal bupivacaine in conjunction with a nonnarcotic pain regimen help reduce length of stay following abdominally based microsurgical breast reconstruction. *Plast Reconstr Surg.* 2017 Aug;140(2):240–251.

13. Zhong T, Ojha M, Bagher S, et al. Transversus abdominis plane block reduces morphine consumption in the early postoperative period following microsurgical abdominal tissue breast reconstruction: a double-blind, placebo-controlled, randomized trial. *Plast Reconstr Surg.* 2014 Nov;134(5):870–878.

14. Rawlani V, Kryger ZB, Lu L, Fine NA. A local anesthetic pump reduces postoperative pain and narcotic and antiemetic use in breast reconstruction surgery: a randomized controlled trial. *Plast Reconstr Surg.* 2008 Jul;122(1):39–52.

15. Kryger ZB, Rawlani V, Lu L, Fine NA. Decreased postoperative pain, narcotic and antiemetic use after breast reduction using a local anesthetic pain pump. *Ann Plast Surg.* 2008 Aug;61(2):147–152.

16. Coveney E, Weltz CR, Greengrass R, et al. Use of paravertebral block anesthesia in the surgical management of breast cancer: experience in 156 cases. *Ann Surg.* 1998 Apr;227(4):496–501.

17. Thavaneswaran P, Rudkin GE, Cooter RD, Moyes DG, Perera CL, Maddern GJ. Brief reports: paravertebral block for anesthesia: a systematic review. *Anesth Analg.* 2010;110(6):1740–1744.

18. Blanco R. The "pecs block": a novel technique for providing analgesia after breast surgery. *Anaesthesia.* 2011 Sep;66(9):847–848.

19. Abdallah FW, MacLean D, Madjdpour C, Cil T, Bhatia A, Brull R. Pectoralis and serratus fascial plane blocks each provide early analgesic benefits following ambulatory breast cancer surgery: a retrospective propensity-matched cohort study. *Anesth Analg.* 2017 Mar 21;125(1):294–302.

20. Hetta DF, Rezk KM. Pectoralis-serratus interfascial plane block vs thoracic paravertebral block for unilateral radical mastectomy with axillary evacuation. *J Clin Anesth.* 2016 Nov;34:91–97.

21. Nasr MW, Habre SB, Jabbour H, Baradhi A, El Asmar Z. A randomized controlled trial of postoperative pain control after subpectoral breast augmentation using intercostal nerve block versus bupivacaine pectoralis major infiltration: a pilot study. *J Plast Reconstr Aesthet Surg.* 2015 Apr;68(4):e83–e84.

22. Leiman D, Barlow M, Carpin K, Piña EM, Casso D. Medial and lateral pectoral nerve block with liposomal bupivacaine for the management of postsurgical pain after submuscular breast augmentation. *Plast Reconstr Surg Glob Open.* 2015 Jan 8;2(12):e282.

23. Markov MS, Pilla AA. Weak static magnetic field modulation of myosin phosphyorylation in a cell-free preparation: calcium dependence. *Bioelectrochem Bioenergetics.* 1997;43:235–240.

24. Hedén P, Pilla AA. Effects of pulsed electromagnetic fields on postoperative pain: a double-blind randomized pilot study in breast augmentation patients. *Aesthet Plast Surg.* 2008;32:660–666.

25. Lifei G, Kubat NJ, Nelson TR, Isenberg RA. Meta-analysis of clinical efficacy of pulsed radio frequency energy treatment. *Ann Surgery.* 2012 March;255(3):457–467.

26. Rawe IM, Lowenstein A, Barcelo CR, Genecov DG. Control of postoperative pain with a wearable continuously operating pulsed radio frequency energy device: a preliminary study. *Aesthet Plast Surg.* 2012;36:458–463.

27. Rohde C, Chiang A, Adipojou O, Casper D, Pilla AA. Effects of pulsed electromagnetic fields on IL-1β and post-operative pain: a double-blind, placebo-controlled pilot study in breast reduction patients. *Plast Reconstr Surg.* 2010;125:1620–1629.

28. Rohde CH, Taylor EM, Alonso A, Ascherman JA, Hardy KL, Pilla AA. Pulsed electromagnetic fields reduce postoperative interleukin-1β, pain, and inflammation: a double-blind, placebo-controlled study in TRAM flap breast reconstruction patients. *Plast Reconstr Surg.* 2015 May;135(5):808e–817e.

29. Beck-Schimmer B, Pasch T. Tumescent technique for local anesthesia. *Anasthesiol Intensivmed Notfallmed Schmerzther.* 2002;37(2):84–88.

30. Khater A, Mazy A, Gad M, Taha Abd Eldayem O, Hegazy M. Tumescent mastectomy: the current indications and operative tips and tricks. *Breast Cancer.* 2017 Mar 30;9:237–243.

31. Ansari D, Gianotti L, Schröder J, Andersson R. Fast-track surgery: procedure-specific aspects and future direction. *Langenbecks Arch Surg.* 2013;398:29–37.

32. Varadhan KK, Neal KR, Dejong CH, Fearon KC, Ljungqvist O, Lobo DN. The enhanced recovery after surgery (ERAS) pathway for patients undergoing major elective open colorectal surgery: a meta-analysis of randomized controlled trials. *Clin Nutr.* 2010;29:434–440.

33. Dumestre DO, Webb CE, Temple-Oberle C. Improved recovery experience achieved for women undergoing implant-based breast reconstruction using an enhanced recovery after surgery model. *Plast Reconstr Surg.* 2017 Mar;139(3):550–559.

34. Wick EC, Grant MC, Wu CL. Postoperative multimodal analgesia pain management with nonopioid analgesics and techniques: a review. *JAMA Surg.* 2017 Jul 1;152(7):691–697.

35. Temple-Oberle C, Shea-Budgell MA, Tan M, et al. Consensus review of optimal perioperative care in breast reconstruction: Enhanced Recovery after Surgery (ERAS) Society Recommendations. *Plast Reconstr Surg.* 2017 May;139(5):1056e–1071e.

36. Parsa FD, Cheng J, Stephan B, et al. Bilateral breast reduction without opioid analgesics: a comparative study. *Aesthet Surg J.* 2017;37(8):892–899.

37. Tang NK. Cognitive behavioural therapy in pain and psychological disorders: towards a hybrid future. *Prog Neuropsychopharmacol Biol Psychiatry.* 2017 Mar 8.pii: S0278–5846(17)30083–0.

11 Pain Management in Body Contouring Procedures

Cyril S. Gary, Samuel Kim, and Deepak Narayan

INTRODUCTION

Body contouring refers to any surgical intervention that reshapes areas of the body to improve form and appearance. Body contouring procedures include, but are not limited to, abdominoplasty, liposuction, contouring following bariatric surgery, implant placement (e.g. calf, gluteal, pectoral), and gluteal augmentation with autologous fat grafting. This chapter addresses general perioperative pain management considerations for common body contouring procedures and also highlights special considerations associated with each specific procedure.

PREOPERATIVE CONSIDERATIONS

It is important to remember that preoperative pain management plans affect postoperative recovery. Successful planning can improve postoperative pain control, decrease opioid consumption, and shorten recovery times. Investigators have looked to analgesics such as cyclooxygenase-2 (COX-2) inhibitors and acetaminophen for these purposes.

COX-2 Inhibitors

Though not exclusive to plastic surgery procedures, a review of preoperative administration of COX-2 inhibitors by Straube et al. found a significant reduction in postoperative pain scores and postoperative analgesic consumption in 15 of 20 trials evaluated when compared to placebo.[1] They also reported increased patient satisfaction in all studies that reported this metric, further highlighting the perioperative benefits of COX-2 inhibitor administration. Their use, however, is not without controversy.

Rofecoxib, a once-promising COX-2 inhibitor, was found to increase the risk of myocardial infarction in the VIGOR trial and was subsequently pulled from the market in 2004.[2] Celecoxib, the only remaining approved COX-2 inhibitor, was allowed to be marketed with a black box warning by the Food and Drug Administration under the condition that a clinical trial—the Prospective Randomized Evaluation of Celecoxib Integrated Safety versus Ibuprofen or Naproxen (PRECISION) trial—evaluate its cardiovascular safety. The results of this trial, published in 2016, found that celecoxib did not increase the risk of cardiovascular events compared to naproxen or ibuprofen. Moreover, celecoxib had significantly lower rates of major gastrointestinal events compared to naproxen or ibuprofen.[3] The trial concluded that celecoxib was safe at moderate doses and noninferior to naproxen and ibuprofen. Despite these encouraging findings, plastic surgeons are reluctant to use COX-2 inhibitors for their potential effects of increase in bleeding, especially in procedures that involve large areas of subcutaneous dissection.

Acetaminophen

Acetaminophen is a strong analgesic and antipyretic agent. Similar to nonsteroidal anti-inflammatory drugs (NSAIDs), it is thought to work through inhibiting COX-1 and COX-2 driven prostaglandin synthesis, though its exact mechanism is unknown. Several studies have supported the use of preoperative acetaminophen for postoperative pain control. Murray et al. examined outcomes for 12 patients who underwent abdominoplasty and received a standard postoperative pain regimen including fentanyl, morphine, and/or Demerol and compared them to 15 patients who received 1 g of intravenous (IV) acetaminophen preoperatively along with the same postoperative pain regimen.[4] The study found a significant reduction in discharge time (117 minutes vs. 83 minutes) for patients who received both IV acetaminophen and the standard postoperative pain management versus patients who just received the standard postoperative pain management alone and found no complications in either group. Though not specific to plastic surgery procedures, a 2011 randomized controlled trial by Moon et al. examined the effects of administering 2 g IV acetaminophen preoperatively to women undergoing abdominal hysterectomy.[5] This study found a 30% reduction in postoperative hydromorphone consumption in women who had received IV acetaminophen along with a lower incidence of postoperative nausea and vomiting. Based upon studies such as these and consideration for postoperative bleeding, preoperative acetaminophen administration has been advocated for postoperative pain control in patients undergoing body contouring procedures.

INTRAOPERATIVE CONSIDERATIONS

General Anesthesia and Sedation

Body contouring procedures are performed in either the inpatient or outpatient setting and are done under general anesthesia, conscious sedation, or deep sedation.[6,7] The surgeon should be aware of the different considerations for anesthesia in order to optimize pain management, recovery times, outcomes, and patient satisfaction. Important considerations for postoperative pain are procedure specific. For example, patients undergoing abdominoplasty under general anesthesia may experience nausea, retching, or vomiting during emergence from general anesthesia or during the postoperative recovery period. The act of retching or vomiting may lead to complications such as seroma, clot release leading to hematoma, or even frank disruption of sutures. Astute choice of induction agent such as the use of propofol over thiopental[8] and careful consideration for the administration and reduction of drugs during emergence from anesthesia may help reduce such incidences. General anesthesia may be avoided altogether for deep sedation or conscious sedation as multiple studies have shown their efficacy and safety during abdominoplasty.[9-12] The choice ultimately remains at the discretion of the patient and the surgeon. The specifics of general anesthesia and sedation are further discussed in other chapters.

Liposomal Bupivacaine

Liposomal bupivacaine (Exparel®) administration intraoperatively is one potential strategy to reduce pain, reduce opioid consumption, and decrease recovery time. Bupivacaine, like lidocaine, functions by blocking voltage-gated sodium channels on neurons, preventing depolarization, transmission of action potentials, and ultimately transmission of pain sensation. Liposomes are small, biodegradable, nonimmunogenic, double-layered phospholipid microparticles that are used to form spheres around molecules of bupivacaine. The gradual dissolution of these spheres allows for a slow release and more effective delivery of bupivacaine into target tissues.[13] Liposomal formulations of bupivacaine provide a gradual release and, therefore, greater control over drug concentration in target tissues than bupivacaine alone. Furthermore, while the analgesic duration of bupivacaine alone is typically less than 12 hours, liposomal bupivacaine can last between 72 to 96 hours after administration, emphasizing its potential for longer-term anesthesia.[14]

POSTOPERATIVE CONSIDERATIONS

Ketorolac is a first generation NSAID that has been used as part of a multimodal approach to pain management following surgery. Ketorolac represents an attractive alternative to opioid medications because of its excellent pain control properties without the opioid-related side effects including postoperative nausea and vomiting. Furthermore, ketorolac does not have the hepatotoxic properties of acetaminophen, further underlying its clinical utility. However, postoperative bleeding risk has largely precluded the use of ketorolac in body contouring procedures.

PROCEDURE-SPECIFIC CONSIDERATIONS

Abdominoplasty

Abdominoplasty, or "tummy tuck," is one of the most popular aesthetic plastic surgery procedures, with more than 120,000 operations performed in the United States in 2016.[15] Common causes of abdominal deformity leading to abdominoplasty requests include pregnancy, obesity-associated pannus, and extreme weight loss. Abdominoplasty after extreme weight loss is particularly relevant given the advances of and increased demand for bariatric surgery over the last decade.[16] Abdominoplasty involves excision of excess skin and adipose tissue from the abdomen along with fascial plication to tighten the rectus abdominis muscles and may be performed as a standalone procedure or with concurrent liposuction.[17,18] Given the large amount of undermining, extensive resection of excess skin and adipose tissue, and large surface area typically covered, pain is an obvious and pertinent concern to patients undergoing abdominoplasty, and optimizing pain management is crucial.[7]

Regional Blocks

Regional blocks, which involve the injection of local anesthetic near a specific nerve or bundle of nerves to anesthetize the entire region of innervation, may be used intraoperatively to reduce pain and need for opioids following abdominoplasty. Several types of regional blocks have been described in the plastic surgery literature, including the combined ilioinguinal, iliohypogastric, and pararectus blocks, and the transversus abdominis plane (TAP) block. Feng first described a "painless abdominoplasty" regional block technique that involved a combination of intraoperative ilioinguinal, iliohypogastric, and pararectus blocks achieved with buvicaine, tetracaine, and Depo-Medrol. This retrospective study reported that patients who received the combined nerve blocks intraoperatively had significantly lower pain scores, lower opioid consumption, less time spent in the recovery room, less postoperative nausea, and a faster return to normal activities than patients who did not receive the nerve blocks.[6] Thus, the combined regional block described by Feng represents one potential technique to better manage postoperative pain in abdominoplasty patients. Sensory innervation to the anterior abdominal wall is provided by afferent neurons that run between the transversus abdominis and internal oblique muscles, and a TAP block consists of injecting a bolus of local anesthetic into this plane in a space bordered by the inguinal ligament inferiorly, the costal margin superiorly, and the lateral border of the rectus abdominis anteriorly. Multiple approaches to access this plane have been described, including the lateral approach through the lumbar Petit triangle which effectively blocks the T10 to T12 dermatomes, and the subcostal approach which blocks the T7 to T10 dermatomes.[19] Multiple studies have demonstrated the efficacy of a TAP block for postoperative pain control in patients undergoing abdominoplasty. Sforza et al., in a prospective randomized clinical trial, examined pain and narcotic consumption in 14 patients undergoing abdominoplasty who received an intraoperative TAP block and a standard multimodal pain regimen compared to 14 patients who received just a standard multimodal pain regimen. They found a significant reduction in pain and need for morphine postoperatively for patients who received the TAP block.[20] Fiala, in a retrospective study, determined that 16 patients undergoing abdominoplasty who received an intraoperative TAP block had significantly lower postoperative opioid consumption and an increased time to first pro re nata narcotic than 16 patients undergoing abdominoplasty who received a combination of pararectus, ilioinguinal, and iliohypogastric nerve blocks as described by Feng.[6,19] Thus, the TAP block represents another potential nerve block technique to better control postoperative pain in abdominoplasty patients. Though regional blocks are effective, some caveats must be mentioned. Regional blocks are more technically challenging to perform than other methods of pain control, and though no data has been published to date, the TAP block in particular carries a risk of peritoneal puncture given the adjacent anatomy. Furthermore, it appears that the TAP block may be more effective than the Feng combined nerve block, though the only study that has compared them to date is small and retrospective in nature.

Pain Pumps

Like formulations of liposomal bupivacaine, pain pumps provide pain relief by delivering a local anesthetic (typically bupivacaine) at a steady rate to the surgical site and effectively function as a continuous nerve block. Theoretically, pain pumps should reduce postoperative pain and need for opioids, but evidence regarding pain pump use in abdominoplasty is mixed with contradictory studies plagued by small patient cohort sizes. In a 2005 study, Mentz et al. determined that a postoperative pain pump significantly reduced pain and opioid consumption and shortened time to ambulation in 10 abdominoplasty patients.[8] Conversely, Bray et al., in a retrospective study, examined pain outcomes in 38 abdominoplasty patients who received postoperative analgesia and 35 patients who did not and found no difference in postoperative opioid consumption, pain scores, hospital length of stay, or antiemetic use between the two groups.[21] In the most recent study to date, Chavez-Abraham et al. demonstrated that a pain pump significantly decreased pain and opioid consumption in 215 abdominoplasty patients compared to 200 abdominoplasty patients who were not provided a pain pump.[22] Thus, though a consensus regarding the efficacy of pain pumps in abdominoplasty has not been reached, it is nevertheless reassuring that the largest study to date has found positive effects on reducing postoperative pain and opioid consumption. Pain pump use has also been controversial in plastic surgery because of a perceived increase in complications, including seroma formation and infection.[23] Recent evidence, however, has largely mitigated these fears.[24,25] Still, concerns regarding pain pump use exist, especially in comparison to intraoperative liposomal bupivacaine, as the pump and associated catheters are bulky, expensive, and inconvenient for the patient.

Complications

Abdominoplasty is associated with higher complication rates than other aesthetic plastic surgery procedures (Winocour et al. report a 4.0% complication rate for abdominoplasties and a 1.9% complication rate for all aesthetic procedures). It is, therefore, critical for the plastic surgeon to be aware of complications that can either exacerbate postoperative pain or, perhaps more importantly, be masked by pain medication consumption.[26] Although a review of all complications associated with abdominoplasty is beyond the scope of this chapter, the following are infrequently mentioned but nonetheless important complications. Abdominal compartment syndrome (ACS) following abdominoplasty is a rare but potentially fatal complication that is sparsely reported in the plastic surgery literature.[27,28] ACS is defined as a sustained intra-abdominal pressure >20 mmHg that is concurrent with new-onset organ dysfunction or failure. Symptoms of ACS are often nonspecific and can include malaise, weakness, lightheadedness, and dyspnea, along with abdominal pain and distention. Its nonspecific presentation may make it difficult to differentiate from expected postoperative pain, especially if the patient is consuming opioid medications. If ACS is suspected (either from clinical exam or through blood laboratory derangements), a diagnosis can be made by indirectly measuring intra-abdominal pressure through measuring the bladder pressure. Once the diagnosis is confirmed, a decompressive laparotomy should be performed without delay to prevent irreversible organ damage. Abdominal hernias are also rare complications that can follow abdominoplasty and may result from iatrogenic damage to the abdominal wall during the operation. Though not as emergent as ACS, untreated herniation may cause significant pain, cosmetic dissatisfaction, and, in the most serious cases, bowel strangulation necessitating resection and surgical repair. Pain resulting from abdominal herniation may be masked by pain medication consumption, and thus the postoperative physical examination, particularly if the surgeon has a high suspicion for iatrogenic injury, may help prevent disastrous sequelae.

Liposuction

Liposuction remains one of the most common body contouring procedures in the world and involves the removal of adipocytes via a suction cannula with simultaneous preservation of surrounding non-adipose tissue, including nerves and vasculature. Liposuction may be performed as a standalone procedure or in combination with other body contouring surgeries, such as an abdominoplasty (i.e., lipoabdominoplasty). The procedure can be done using a variety of techniques including suction-assisted liposuction, ultrasound-assisted liposuction, laser-assisted liposuction, power-assisted liposuction, or radiofrequency-associated liposuction.[29] Given the inherent vascularity of adipose tissue and the large amount of body surface area typically covered by liposuction, postoperative bruising, bleeding, and pain are well-known problems for patients following liposuction, and optimizing pain management is important for both patient satisfaction and cosmetically desired outcomes.

Tumescent Solution

Klein first introduced the preoperative use of a tumescent wetting solution to improve perioperative bleeding and pain control for patients undergoing liposuction. The use of tumescent solution soon replaced "dry" liposuction as the preferred technique.[30] Klein's original formulation described infiltrating large volumes of dilute lidocaine (.1% or .05%) and epinephrine (1:1,000,000) in normal saline directly into the subcutaneous tissue to produce regional anesthesia and to induce swelling and firmness of areas targeted for liposuction. Since then, many variations of tumescent solution have been described with maximal doses of lidocaine administered ranging from 35 to 55 mg/kg.[31-33] Advantages of utilizing tumescent solution include prolonged analgesic effects (Klein estimated that analgesic effects of tumescent solution may last for up to 18 hours following administration), decreasing the need for postoperative pain medication, vasoconstriction leading to decreased blood loss, and, most importantly, sufficient pain control to perform the entirety of the procedure without general anesthesia or sedation, which has subsequently revolutionized liposuction. Clinical studies have supported the use of tumescent solution over dry liposuction. Triana et al., in a retrospective review of 26,259 patients undergoing dry liposuction or liposuction with tumescent solution, found a remarkable difference between postoperative incidence of anemia between dry and tumescent groups (60% vs. 12%), suggesting that tumescent solution was vastly superior in achieving hemostasis.[34] Numerous studies have also demonstrated that the preoperative use of tumescent solution can be safely performed under local anesthesia, thereby avoiding the risks associated with general anesthesia or IV sedation.[35-37] However, though tumescent liposuction has been shown to be superior to dry liposuction with regards to bleeding and avoiding general anesthesia and sedation, the effects on postoperative pain have been less well characterized in the literature. The same study by Triana et al. found identical rates of postoperative pain (90% and 90%) reported by patients in both groups, though the pain was not quantified and instead reported on a binary scale. Thus, while the use of tumescent solution before liposuction remains advantageous with regards to reducing blood loss and avoiding the risks associated with general anesthesia and IV sedation, the postoperative analgesic properties, while theoretically sound, remain unproven in clinical data.

Body Contouring Following Bariatric Surgery

The popularity and incidence of bariatric surgery in the United States has continued to increase over the last decade. Per the American Society for Metabolic and Bariatric Surgery, an estimated 196,000 bariatric surgeries were performed in 2015, up from 158,000 in 2011.[38] Though patients achieve sustained weight loss, improved control of diabetes, and improvement of joint pain following surgical intervention, the remnant excess skin does not contract in response to the massive weight loss, leading many patients to seek body contouring procedures to improve aesthetic appearances.[39] Recent evidence has demonstrated that 74% to 95% of bariatric surgery patients desire body contouring surgery following weight loss with the most frequently requested procedures being abdominoplasty, followed by lower body lift, breast lift, thigh lift, and upper arm lift.[40,41] Given this rise in demand for plastic surgery procedures following bariatric surgery, it is vital that plastic surgeons are aware of specific considerations for this challenging patient population.

Psychopathology

Bariatric surgery patients have significantly higher rates of preoperative psychopathological disturbances than the general population. Strikingly, Mitchell et al. reported a 68.6% lifetime prevalence of any psychiatric disorder, a 35.7% lifetime prevalence of any substance use disorder, and a 44.2% prevalence of any mood disorder in such patients, and other studies have reported similar rates.[42-44] The effects of bariatric surgery and subsequent massive weight loss on psychopathology following surgical intervention have been shown to be largely positive, with particularly noted decreases in depression incidence.[45,46] However, postbariatric surgery patients still have significantly higher rates of postoperative depression than the general obese population, and bariatric surgery seems to have no effect on reducing postoperative anxiety.[46] Furthermore, Kitzinger et al. report that 96% of patients develop problematic excess skin following massive weight loss, leading to subsequent body image issues and contributing to the desire for corrective body contouring surgery.[47] Numerous studies have reported positive effects on body image, quality of life, and patient satisfaction following bariatric surgery and subsequent body contouring.[48-50] However, the effects of body contouring on psychiatric disturbances, including depression and anxiety, have been conflicting in the literature. De Swaan et al. reported no difference in anxiety and depression between patients who underwent body contouring after bariatric surgery versus bariatric surgery alone, while Azin et al. reported significantly improved anxiety and depression for patients who underwent body contouring following bariatric surgery versus bariatric surgery alone.[41,49] While body contouring after bariatric surgery has positive effects on life and function, patients likely will still suffer from high postoperative rates of depression and anxiety. The high rates of postoperative psychiatric disturbances in body contouring following bariatric surgery patients are particularly relevant to questions regarding pain management, as depression and anxiety are known to modulate the perception of pain and can induce hyperalgesia to certain stimuli.[51,52] Thus, pain management for these patients may require not just multimodal treatments involving opioids, NSAIDs, and other anesthetic medications but also psychiatric drugs, with a particular emphasis on antidepressants and antianxiety medications. A multidisciplinary approach utilizing input from psychiatrists can help diagnose and manage both pre- and postoperative depression and anxiety, which should ultimately improve pain management for these patients.

Implants

Synthetic implants (e.g., calf, gluteal, pectoral) are typically silicone based and may be utilized for the purpose of aesthetic enhancement or augmentation following certain disease processes. Though not nearly as popular as the aforementioned procedures (abdominoplasty, liposuction, and body contouring following bariatric surgery and massive weight loss), implants remain an important part of the plastic surgery repertoire, and surgeons should be aware of special considerations regarding pain management for such patients. Breast implants, which vastly outnumber all other types of implants combined, deserve a more in-depth discussion and are addressed in a subsequent chapter.

Anesthesia Consideration and Ropivacaine

Though general anesthesia may be implemented for such procedures, calf implants can be performed using either a spinal block or IV sedation with local anesthesia, along with ropivacaine for pain management. Niechajev, in a series of 18 patients, reported using a spinal block, 1% lidocaine with 5 μg/mL epinephrine as local anesthetic, and 2 mg/mL ropivicaine in 15 to 20 mL flushes intraoperatively to the peri-implant space. An epidural catheter provided intermittent, 10 mL flushes of 2 mg/mL ropivacaine to the surgical site for pain management on the first postoperative day.[53] Niechajev reported that the use of ropivacaine, particularly during the first postoperative day, helped to significantly reduce postoperative pain and narcotic requirements though cited no data to support this statement in his article. Nevertheless, ropivacaine, in combination with a spinal block or with IV sedation with local anesthesia, may be a beneficial strategy to help patients avoid having to undergo general anesthesia. Like calf implants, gluteal implants may be safely performed using general anesthesia, spinal anesthesia, or epidural anesthesia, and pectoral implants may be performed using general anesthesia or IV sedation with either epidural or local anesthesia.[54,55] Strategies to avoid general anesthesia may be of particular importance in reducing incidence of postoperative nausea and vomiting in such patients.

Complications and Other Considerations

Body contouring procedures that utilize silicone-based implants have been associated with relatively high rates of complications, especially for implants that are placed in subcutaneous pockets. Calf implants have been reported to have a 4.0% rate of seroma formation, a 4.8% rate of capsular contraction, a 4.8% rate of infection, a 2.4% rate of cosmetic dissatisfaction, and a <2% rate of persistent numbness at the ankle; gluteal implants have been associated with up to a 14% rate of wound dehiscence, and pectoral implants have been associated with up to a 30% rate of seroma formation.[56] Given these rates, it is particularly important for plastic surgeons to be vigilant in monitoring for these complications, especially those that present with pain or pain masked by postoperative pain medication consumption. As a final thought, patients should avoid pressure to the implants postoperatively in order to avoid implant dislodgement and prevent seroma formation. Patients with gluteal implants should avoid sitting on their buttocks in the postoperative period, and patients with calf implants should avoid similar positionally dependent compression to their lower legs (i.e., sitting with their legs crossed). Likewise, patients with pectoral implants should be instructed to sleep on their back postoperatively for similar considerations.

Gluteal Augmentation with Fat Grafting

Fat grafting is a commonly utilized technique in plastic surgery for the treatment of contour and volume deficits and for soft tissue augmentation. The use of autologous fat for gluteal augmentation, with or without concurrent liposuction, has been gaining popularity as a safe and effective procedure for aesthetic enhancement and an alternative to implant-based augmentation.[57] Given the necessity of harvesting fat from a donor site for grafting, along with the sensitive nature of the recipient site, the treating surgeon must be aware of the following considerations for optimal pain management and patient satisfaction.

Site-Specific Considerations

Adipose tissue for grafting is typically harvested from areas of the body with a high fat content, including the abdomen and thigh, though the final choice of donor site is determined by the patient's individual body habitus. Given the extensive body surface area perturbed by fat harvesting along with proximity to the large muscles of the abdominal wall and thigh, pain at the donor site remains a significant problem for such patients postoperatively. The injection of tumescent solution to the donor site preoperatively, as described earlier in the chapter, can help both reduce postoperative bleeding and improve postoperative pain management.[58] Patients may also experience painful muscle spasms at the donor site following fat harvesting (depending on the degree of muscular trauma caused by the suction cannula) and may require a benzodiazepine muscle relaxant (e.g., diazepam) for optimal postoperative pain management. Patients undergoing gluteal augmentation with autologous fat have high rates of postoperative infection. Bruner et al. reported a 7% infection rate for such patients, and posited that this may be due to a number of factors, including (a) proximity of the recipient site incisions to the anus, (b) increased risk of contaminating extracted fat given multiple steps in procedure (i.e. harvesting, processing, injecting), (c) lack of a vascular supply to the grafted fat until at least four to seven days following injection (promoting an excellent bacterial growth media with minimal immune system access during this time frame), and (d) trauma to the injection site skin which subverts its antibacterial barrier properties.[59] These aforementioned problems can be mitigated by administering preoperative antibiotics, minimizing handling of harvested fat, coating the cannula used for grafting with iodine, and washing the grafted fat with triple antibiotic (e.g., ampicillin/sulbactam, gentamicin, cefazolin) before injection. Finally, patients undergoing gluteal augmentation with fat grafting should be instructed to avoid sitting on their buttocks postoperatively to avoid strangulating the graft and inducing fat necrosis and oil cysts. The inability of patients to sit may add to their postoperative discomfort and pain, especially if the patients are uncomfortable in the lateral or prone positions. Finding a comfortable resting position that avoids pressure and shearing forces on the gluteal region is crucial to both graft survival and patient satisfaction.

REFERENCES

1. Straube S, Derry S, McQuay HJ, Moore RA. Effect of preoperative Cox-II-selective NSAIDs (coxibs) on postoperative outcomes: a systematic review of randomized studies. *Acta Anaesthesiol Scand.* 2005;49:601–613.
2. Karha J, Topol EJ. The sad story of Vioxx, and what we should learn from it. *Cleve Clin J Med.* 2004;71:933–934, 936, 938–939.
3. Nissen SE, Yeomans ND, Solomon DH, et al. Cardiovascular safety of celecoxib, naproxen, or ibuprofen for arthritis. *N Engl J Med.* 2016;375:2519–2529.
4. Murray M, Haiavy J. Preoperative intravenous acetaminophen improves recovery time after abdominoplasty. *Am J Cosmetic Surg.* 2015;32:144–148.
5. Moon YE, Lee YK, Lee J, Moon DE. The effects of preoperative intravenous acetaminophen in patients undergoing abdominal hysterectomy. *Arch Gynecol Obstet.* 2011;284:1455–1460.
6. Feng LJ. Painless abdominoplasty: the efficacy of combined intercostal and pararectus blocks in reducing postoperative pain and recovery time. *Plast Reconstr Surg.* 2010;126:1723–1732.
7. Constantine FC, Matarasso A. Putting it all together: recommendations for improving pain management in body contouring. *Plast Reconstr Surg.* 2014;134:113S–119S.
8. Mentz HA, Ruiz-Razura A, Newall G, Patronella CK. Use of a regional infusion pump to control postoperative pain after an abdominoplasty. *Aesthetic Plast Surg.* 2005;29:415–421; discussion 422.
9. Rosenberg MH, Palaia DA, Bonanno PC. Abdominoplasty with procedural sedation and analgesia. *Ann Plast Surg.* 2001;46:485–487.
10. Mustoe TA, Kim P, Schierle CF. Outpatient abdominoplasty under conscious sedation. *Aesthet Surg J.* 2007;27:442–449.
11. Kryger ZB, Fine NA, Mustoe TA. The outcome of abdominoplasty performed under conscious sedation: six-year experience in 153 consecutive cases. *Plast Reconstr Surg.* 2004;113:1807–1817; discussion 1818–1809.

12. Byun MY, Fine NA, Lee JY, Mustoe TA. The clinical outcome of abdominoplasty performed under conscious sedation: increased use of fentanyl correlated with longer stay in outpatient unit. *Plast Reconstr Surg.* 1999;103:1260–1266.

13. Beiranvand S, Eatemadi A, Karimi A. New updates pertaining to drug delivery of local anesthetics in particular bupivacaine using lipid nanoparticles. *Nanoscale Res Lett.* 2016;11:307.

14. Vyas KS, Rajendran S, Morrison SD, et al. Systematic review of liposomal bupivacaine (Exparel) for postoperative analgesia. *Plast Reconstr Surg.* 2016;138:748e–756e.

15. 2016 Plastic surgery statistics report. https://www.plasticsurgery.org/documents/News/Statistics/2016/plastic-surgery-statistics-full-report-2016.pdf. Accessed July 18, 2017.

16. Spiegelman JI, Levine RH. Abdominoplasty: a comparison of outpatient and inpatient procedures shows that it is a safe and effective procedure for outpatients in an office-based surgery clinic. *Plast Reconstr Surg.* 2006;118:517–522; discussion 523–514.

17. Matarasso A. Liposuction as an adjunct to a full abdominoplasty. *Plast Reconstr Surg.* 1995;95:829–836.

18. Brauman D, Capocci J. Liposuction abdominoplasty: an advanced body contouring technique. *Plast Reconstr Surg.* 2009;124:1685–1695.

19. Fiala T. Tranversus abdominis plane block during abdominoplasty to improve postoperative patient comfort. *Aesthet Surg J.* 2015;35:72–80.

20. Sforza M, Andjelkov K, Zaccheddu R, Nagi H, Colic M. Transversus abdominis plane block anesthesia in abdominoplasties. *Plast Reconstr Surg.* 2011;128:529–535.

21. Bray DA Jr, Nguyen J, Craig J, Cohen BE, Collins DR Jr. Efficacy of a local anesthetic pain pump in abdominoplasty. *Plast Reconstr Surg.* 2007;119:1054–1059.

22. Chavez-Abraham V, Barr JS, Zwiebel PC. The efficacy of a lidocaine-infused pain pump for postoperative analgesia following elective augmentation mammaplasty or abdominoplasty. *Aesthetic Plast Surg.* 2011;35:463–469.

23. Morales R Jr, Mentz H 3rd, Newall G, Patronella C, Masters O 3rd. Use of abdominal field block injections with liposomal bupivicaine to control postoperative pain after abdominoplasty. *Aesthet Surg J.* 2013;33:1148–1153.

24. Smith MM, Hovsepian RV, Markarian MK, et al. Continuous-infusion local anesthetic pain pump use and seroma formation with abdominal procedures: is there a correlation? *Plast Reconstr Surg.* 2008;122:1425–1430.

25. Hovsepian RV, Smith MM, Markarian MK, et al. Infection risk from the use of continuous local-anesthetic infusion pain pumps in aesthetic and reconstructive abdominal procedures. *Ann Plast Surg.* 2009;62:237–239.

26. Winocour J, Gupta V, Ramirez JR, Shack RB, Grotting JC, Higdon KK. Abdominoplasty: risk factors, complication rates, and safety of combined procedures. *Plast Reconstr Surg.* 2015;136:597e–606e.

27. Izadpanah A, Izadpanah A, Karunanayake M, Petropolis C, Deckelbaum DL, Luc M. Abdominal compartment syndrome following abdominoplasty: a case report and review. *Indian J Plast Surg.* 2014;47:263–266.

28. Shen GX, Gu B, Xie F, et al. [Three case reports of abdominal compartment syndrome after full abdominoplasty]. *Zhonghua Zheng Xing Wai Ke Za Zhi.* 2007;23:226–228.

29. Berry MG, Davies D. Liposuction: a review of principles and techniques. *J Plast Reconstr Aesthet Surg.* 2011;64:985–992.

30. Klein JA. Tumescent technique for regional anesthesia permits lidocaine doses of 35 mg/kg for liposuction. *J Dermatol Surg Oncol.* 1990;16:248–263.

31. Klein JA. Anesthetic formulation of tumescent solutions. *Dermatol Clin.* 1999;17:751–759, v–vi.

32. Ostad A, Kageyama N, Moy RL. Tumescent anesthesia with a lidocaine dose of 55 mg/kg is safe for liposuction. *Dermatol Surg.* 1996;22:921–927.

33. Habbema L. Efficacy of tumescent local anesthesia with variable lidocaine concentration in 3430 consecutive cases of liposuction. *J Am Acad Dermatol.* 2010;62:988–994.

34. Triana L, Triana C, Barbato C, Zambrano M. Liposuction: 25 years of experience in 26,259 patients using different devices. *Aesthet Surg J.* 2009;29:509–512.

35. Hanke CW, Bernstein G, Bullock S. Safety of tumescent liposuction in 15,336 patients: national survey results. *Dermatol Surg.* 1995;21:459–462.

36. Klein JA. Tumescent technique for local anesthesia improves safety in large-volume liposuction. *Plast Reconstr Surg.* 1993;92:1085-1098; discussion 1099–1100.

37. Boeni R. Safety of tumescent liposuction under local anesthesia in a series of 4,380 patients. *Dermatology.* 2011;222:278–281.

38. Estimate of bariatric surgery numbers, 2011-2015. http://asmbs.org/resources/estimate-of-bariatric-surgery-numbers. Accessed July 18, 2017.

39. Colwell AS. Current concepts in post-bariatric body contouring. *Obes Surg.* 2010;20:1178–1182.

40. Kitzinger HB, Abayev S, Pittermann A, et al. The prevalence of body contouring surgery after gastric bypass surgery. *Obes Surg.* 2012;22:8–12.

41. Azin A, Zhou C, Jackson T, Cassin S, Sockalingam S, Hawa R. Body contouring surgery after bariatric surgery: a study of cost as a barrier and impact on psychological well-being. *Plast Reconstr Surg.* 2014;133:776e–782e.

42. Mitchell JE, Selzer F, Kalarchian MA, et al. Psychopathology before surgery in the longitudinal assessment of bariatric surgery-3 (LABS-3) psychosocial study. *Surg Obes Relat Dis.* 2012;8:533–541.

43. Kalarchian MA, Marcus MD, Levine MD, et al. Psychiatric disorders among bariatric surgery candidates: relationship to obesity and functional health status. *Am J Psychiatry.* 2007;164:328–334; quiz 374.

44. Muhlhans B, Horbach T, de Zwaan M. Psychiatric disorders in bariatric surgery candidates: a review of the literature and results of a German prebariatric surgery sample. *Gen Hosp Psychiatry.* 2009;31:414–421.

45. Dymek MP, le Grange D, Neven K, Alverdy J. Quality of life and psychosocial adjustment in patients after Roux-en-Y gastric bypass: a brief report. *Obes Surg.* 2001;11:32–39.

46. de Zwaan M, Enderle J, Wagner S, et al. Anxiety and depression in bariatric surgery patients: a prospective, follow-up study using structured clinical interviews. *J Affect Disord.* 2011;133:61–68.

47. Kitzinger HB, Abayev S, Pittermann A, et al. After massive weight loss: patients' expectations of body contouring surgery. *Obes Surg.* 2012;22:544–548.

48. Tremp M, Delko T, Kraljevic M, et al. Outcome in body-contouring surgery after massive weight loss: a prospective matched single-blind study. *J Plast Reconstr Aesthet Surg.* 2015;68:1410–1416.

49. de Zwaan M, Georgiadou E, Stroh CE, et al. Body image and quality of life in patients with and without body contouring surgery following bariatric surgery: a comparison of pre- and post-surgery groups. *Front Psychol.* 2014;5:1310.

50. Modarressi A, Balague N, Huber O, Chilcott M, Pittet-Cuenod B. Plastic surgery after gastric bypass improves long-term quality of life. *Obes Surg.* 2013;23:24–30.

51. Bar KJ, Brehm S, Boettger MK, Boettger S, Wagner G, Sauer H. Pain perception in major depression depends on pain modality. *Pain.* 2005;117:97–103.

52. Woo AK. Depression and anxiety in pain. *Rev Pain.* 2010;4:8–12.

53. Niechajev I. Calf augmentation and restoration. *Plast Reconstr Surg.* 2005;116:295–305; discussion 306–297.

54. Senderoff DM. Aesthetic surgery of the buttocks using implants: practice-based recommendations. *Aesthet Surg J.* 2016;36:559–576.

55. Pereira LH, Sabatovich O, Santana KP, Picanco R. Pectoral muscle implant: approach and procedure. *Aesthet Plast Surg.* 2006;30:412–416.

56. Flores-Lima G, Eppley BL. Body contouring with solid silicone implants. *Aesthet Plast Surg.* 2009;33:140–146.

57. Harrison D, Selvaggi G. Gluteal augmentation surgery: indications and surgical management. *J Plast Reconstr Aesthet Surg.* 2007;60:922–928.

58. Peren PA, Gomez JB, Guerrerosantos J, Salazar CA. Gluteus augmentation with fat grafting. *Aesthet Plast Surg.* 2000;24:412–417.

59. Bruner TW, Roberts TL 3rd, Nguyen K. Complications of buttocks augmentation: diagnosis, management, and prevention. *Clin Plast Surg.* 2006;33:449–466.

12 Pain Management and Urinary Retention

Sophia Delpe, Amanda Norwich, and Toby C. Chai

LOWER URINARY TRACT (BLADDER AND URETHRA) ANATOMY

The lower urinary tract is comprised of the bladder and the urethra. It functions to store and empty urine. These functions require the bladder and urethra have opposite roles. During urinary storage, the bladder must accommodate a wide range of volumes without increasing the intravesical pressure (e.g., compliant bladder) with the urethral sphincter contracted to prevent urinary leakage. During urinary emptying, the bladder must contract to expel the urine while the urethral sphincter must relax so that the bladder can empty unimpeded.[1]

The urinary bladder is a hollow viscous which is situated in the pelvis anterior to the rectum, inferior to the symphysis pubis. The adult bladder is considered an extraperitoneal pelvic organ. Its purpose is for storage and emptying of urine, which is created by the kidneys proximally and delivered into the bladder via the ureters. The most distal portion of the bladder (bladder neck) connects to the urethra, which allows for evacuation of urine. In males, the most proximal portion of the urethra (the portion of the urethra that is connected to the bladder neck) is encircled by the prostate. The prostate can be enlarged in older men or associated with increased urinary outlet resistance leading to urinary retention. Both sexes have an external urethral sphincter that provides the primary continence mechanism preventing urinary incontinence. The external urethral sphincter can be voluntarily contracted as part of the pelvic skeletal muscular apparatus which includes the external anal sphincter.[1]

Anatomically, the bladder is divided into the fundus/dome and the trigone. The trigone contains the ureteral orifices. Just caudal to the trigone is the bladder neck which funnels into the urethra.

The bladder is comprised of three layers which are, from outer to innermost: serosa, muscularis mucosa (detrusor muscle), and mucosa transitional epithelium or urothelium and lamina propria). The peritoneum overlies the fundus or dome of the bladder. The detrusor smooth muscle layer is the thickest layer and contracts to evacuate urine. The mucosal layer is the layer that protects the bladder from urine and microorganisms.

The main arterial supply to the bladder is the superior and inferior vesical pedicles, which are branches of the internal iliac artery. There is a rich venous plexus surrounding the bladder which ultimately empties into the internal iliac veins. Lymphatic drainage is mainly via the external iliac lymph nodes; however, drainage also occurs via obturator and internal iliac nodes and at times up to the common iliac nodes.

NEURAL CONSIDERATIONS IN BLADDER FUNCTION

Neuroanatomy and Neuropharmacology

The motor innervation of the detrusor smooth muscle is from the parasympathetic nervous system (PNS). The motor nuclei of the parasympathetic preganglionic neurons reside in the interomedial lateral cell column (IMLCC) of the gray matter within S2 to S4 spinal cord.[1] Efferent fibers exit through the ventral horn of the spinal cord and then travel as the pelvic nerves, along blood vessels where they synapse within ganglia in the pelvis, as well as ganglia within the bladder wall. Postganglionic motor neurons send axons to the detrusor smooth muscle cell where the neuroeffector (neuromuscular) junctions are formed. The preganglionic neurons release acetylcholine (ACh) at the ganglia; the postganglionic neurons release ACh at the neuromuscular junction. Muscarinic receptor subtypes M2 and M3 on the smooth muscle membrane respond to the ACh released by the postganglionic motor nerves.[2] The excitation-coupling of the detrusor smooth muscle in generating a contraction is beyond the scope of this chapter. The agonist effect of ACh on detrusor smooth muscle contraction is why use of medications with anticholinergic effects increase the risk of urinary retention. The nuclei for the cholinergic motor neurons innervating the external urethral sphincter reside in Onuf's nucleus in the anterior horn of the gray matter in S2 to S4 spinal cord. These somatic motor nerve fibers exit the ventral horn and are contained in the pudendal nerve and ultimately synapse on the skeletal muscle fibers of the external urethral sphincter. The neurotransmitter released by the pudendal nerve is ACh, which then acts on nicotinic receptors on the external urethral sphincter.[2]

The role of the autonomic sympathetic nervous system (SNS) in the lower urinary tract is not as well understood. The preganglionic motor neurons of the SNS reside in the IMLCC of the thoracolumbar spinal cord. The preganglionic nerve fibers exit the ventral horn and travel through the sympathetic chain ganglia to the inferior mesenteric ganglia and then to the hypogastric nerve. Preganglionic nerves synapse in the inferior mesenteric, paravertebral, and pelvic ganglia where they release ACh.[3] SNS ganglia typically are located further away from the effector organ, compared to PNS ganglia located closer to effector organs (or within the effector organs). Postganglionic SNS fibers travel to the neuromuscular junction and release adrenergic neurotransmitters (nor-, epinephrine). The SNS postganglionic nerve fibers release adrenergic neurotransmitters (norepinephrine, epinephrine) at the neuromuscular junction. The presumed role for the SNS in the lower urinary tract is for bladder neck closure since there are α_1-adrenoceptors at the bladder neck. The bladder neck closure mechanism is important in men to prevent retrograde ejaculation and promotes urinary continence. Conversely, medications having α_1-adrenoceptor agonism (such as cold medications with pseudoephedrine) increase the risk of urinary retention. This is why α_1-blockers such as tamsulosin are used to treat urinary retention—with the mechanism of action of relaxing the bladder neck to facilitate urinary emptying. The role of SNS in suppressing detrusor smooth muscle contractility has been shown by the clinical use of a β_3-adrenorecptor agonist (mirabegron) in treating an overactive bladder or detrusor smooth muscle overactivity (uninhibited contractions of the detrusor smooth muscle).[4]

Afferent or sensory activity of the bladder is initiated in the mucosal layer. Mucosal stretch activates sensory fibers within the lamina propria and these sensory signals travel via the afferent nerve fibers from the bladder with sympathetic and parasympathetic nerves and arrive at the dorsal root ganglia (DRG) at thoracolumbar and sacral spinal levels. The DRG neurons have bipolar processes and send fibers through the dorsal portion of the spinal cord and into the dorsal horn of the gray matter in the spinal cord. Higher order neurons synapse with the sensory afferents at the dorsal horn, and, ultimately, sensory signals terminate at the cerebral cortex where sensory signals are processed.

Neural Reflexes

During filling of the bladder, distension of the bladder causes low-level afferent firing. This stimulates SNS outflow and pudendal nerve outflow promoting bladder relaxation, preventing unintended smooth muscle contractions and external urethral sphincter contractions.[1]

As the bladder distends, stretch receptors send afferent signals are relayed by myelinated Aδ-delta fibers in the pelvic nerves to the spinal cord. Sympathetic nervous system activation then occurs from L1 to L3, which inhibit parasympathetic inputs to the bladder at the periphery. Postganglionic sympathetic neuronal action via the β_3-adrenoceptors on the detrusor smooth muscle also relax the smooth muscle.

The somatic storage reflex or "guarding reflex" allows for preservation of continence during Valsalva with a full bladder. During normal storage this reflex is tonically active and becomes dynamically active with Valsalva to contract the external urethral sphincter.[1]

The bladder and external urethral sphincter have to work in synchrony to allow for normal urinary storage and emptying. Storage of urine in a normal individual does not increase intravesical pressures. The bladder has high compliance during filling to allow for low pressures. Emptying requires that the bladder neck and the striated sphincter of the urethra relax while the bladder contracts. This requires great coordination by multiple areas in the brain. The main area in the brain that coordinates bladder reflexes is the pontine micturition center (PMC) or Barrington's nucleus. The PMC is connected to multiple different areas of the brain. Because of these connections, diseases, conditions, and drugs that affect the brain can also affect continence and micturition, which includes urinary retention.[1] Furthermore, because the brain is involved in other functions such as awareness, emotion, executive function, cognition, and behavior, any perturbations of these functions can lead to urinary retention also. It is beyond the scope of this chapter to go into details related to brain control of continence and micturition.

POSTOPERATIVE URINARY RETENTION

While the term "urinary retention" implies an "all or none" situation—that is, a patient with urinary retention cannot void at all when there is a sufficient volume in the bladder—the term "urinary retention" has been many times also utilized to describe an individual who has "incomplete bladder emptying." "Incomplete bladder emptying" means that a person can voluntarily void but cannot sufficiently empty the bladder. These two conditions are not necessarily linearly associated—urinary retention does not have to be preceded by incomplete bladder emptying, and incomplete bladder emptying does not necessarily result in urinary retention. It also should be noted that incomplete bladder emptying is purely an objectively measured phenomenon that does not yet have well-studied clinical endpoints. An individual who does not completely empty his or her bladder does not necessarily have bladder symptoms and will not necessarily develop other pathologies. Urinary retention is defined by complete inability to voluntarily void despite an adequate volume in the bladder. Even with this seemingly straightforward definition, an "adequate volume" at which a patient cannot voluntarily void has no accepted standard. So, if a patient has 300 cc in his or her bladder and cannot void, is this urinary retention? How about if the volume is 400 cc, 500 cc, 600 cc, or 700 cc? The point here is that there is no "cut-off" value that has been validated to state that a patient is in urinary retention or is pathologic. Obviously, as the volume becomes greater, there is more concern that this represents a pathological condition. As discussed previously, normal bladder function relies on complex brain functions such as executive function, emotion, and awareness. Other individual factors also come into play such as local pathology, medications, compensatory abilities of the bladder, and age/size of the patient, all of which can impact the "adequate volume" that would trigger the diagnosis of "urinary retention." However, most would consider 500 cc in the bladder as the volume at which intervention should be instituted in a postoperative patient (see algorithm figure).

Postoperative urinary retention (POUR) is not an uncommon occurrence following surgical procedures and requires both the anesthesia and surgical team to be aware of this possibility. The diagnosis of POUR in the past typically required the clinician to incorporate history and physical exam to arrive at this diagnosis. The typical historical information gathered would include patient's age, medication use, past medical and surgical history, type of surgical procedure, duration of surgical procedure, and type of anesthetic used during the surgical procedure. The physical exam would focus on whether a palpable bladder could be detected. However, with the advent of an accurate, reliable, low-cost point-of-care bladder volume determination using an ultrasound bladder scanner, reliance on history and physical to diagnose POUR is diminishing. While clinical index of suspicion for POUR is still required, the use of bladder scanner has supplanted the physical exam. One should realize that there are limitations also to the reliability of a volume determination by a bladder scanner. Bladder scanners do not work well in morbidly obese patients. Female patients with pelvic cysts or uterine fibroids may cause the bladder scanner to overestimate the bladder volume. Bladder volumes <200 cc may be inaccurate, though with POUR, inaccuracies of smaller volumes are not as much of a concern. Nevertheless, the bladder scanner has changed how POUR is diagnosed. A bladder scan should be utilized in all cases in which POUR is suspected.

TREATMENT OF POUR

If a patient does not void four hours after surgery or four hours after the urethral catheter is removed in the postanesthesia recovery area, the algorithm for POUR should be instituted (see algorithm figure). A bladder scan volume of 500 cc is the upper limit in which in-and-out catheterization should be performed. If a patient is to be going be discharged (outpatient surgery), a Foley indwelling urethral catheter can be placed instead of performing an in-and-out catheterization. If a patient does not wish to go home with an indwelling urethral catheter, a longer time period for attempts at spontaneous voiding can be attempted.

When a patient voids, the voided volume is typically not measured, with only the post-void volume being measured. However, post-void volume is just one measure of bladder-emptying function. Another measure is voiding efficiency, which is similar to the concept of cardiac functional measure of left ventricular ejection fraction. Voiding efficiency may be a better indicator of bladder emptying function than a post-void residual volume. Voiding efficiency is the ratio of the voided volume divided by voided volume plus post-void residual volume (total bladder volume). The cut-off value for voiding efficiency is 66%; this minimum acceptable value (see algorithm figure) is based on the authors' personal experience in managing patients with urinary retention. Some would substitute a post-void residual volume cutoff of 200 cc in place of the 66% voiding efficiency cut-off.

MANAGEMENT OF POUR ALGORITHM

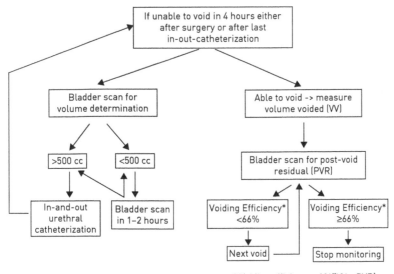

* Voiding efficiency = VV/(VV + PVR)

REFERENCES

1. Chai TC, Birder M, Lory AP. Physiology and pharmacology of the bladder and ure-thra. In: Wein AJ, ed. *Campbell-Walsh Urology*, 11th ed. Philadelphia: Elsevier; 2015:1631–1699.

2. Birder L, De Groat W, Mills I, Morrison J, Thor K, Drake M. Neural control of the lower urinary tract: peripheral and spinal mechanisms. *Neurourol Urodyn*. 2010;29(1):128–139. doi:10.1002/nau.20837

3. Yoshimura N, Chancellor MB. Neurophysiology of lower urinary tract function and dysfunction. *Rev Urol*. 2003;5(Suppl 8):S3–S10. http://www.ncbi.nlm.nih.gov/pmc/arti-cles/PMC1502389/%5Cnhttp://www.ncbi.nlm.nih.gov/pmc/articles/PMC1502389/pdf/RIU005008_00S3.pdf

4. Wagg A, Cardozo L, Nitti VW, et al. The efficacy and tolerability of the 3-adrenoceptor agonist mirabegron for the treatment of symptoms of overactive bladder in older patients. *Age Ageing*. 2014;43(5):666–675. doi:10.1093/ageing/afu017

13 Pain Management for General Pediatric Surgery

Jodi-Ann Oliver, Lori-Ann Oliver,
Michael Casimir, and Caroline Walker

INTRODUCTION

The management of pain is an essential part of patient care, especially in the postoperative period, since adequate pain control has been shown to improve patient outcome measures such as faster recovery times and decreased hospital length of stay.[1] Most patients undergoing surgery endorse some degree of postoperative pain, but retrospective studies demonstrate that fewer than half of these patients received adequate postoperative pain relief.[2] Pain has been defined by the International Association for the Study of Pain as "an unpleasant and emotional experience associated with actual or potential tissue damage, or described in terms of such damage."[3] Pain is indeed subjective with individual experiences associated with injury in early life, especially during periods of neuronal development and maturation, serving as framework for what is ultimately perceived as pain. The clinician must realize that a lack of ability to effectively communicate verbally or otherwise express feelings of pain does not negate its existence.[4] This concept applies particularly to children, who usually lack the ability to describe the feelings they subjectively perceive or experience as pain.

There are various ways to classify pain and types of pain, but in the most simplistic terms, pain can be broadly divided into two major categories: acute and chronic pain. Acute pain is defined as pain limited in duration and can last between three and six months or less.[5] Acute pain is often described as sharp and severe in nature and usually resolves with healing of tissue injury.[5] Chronic pain, therefore, is defined as pain that persists beyond the usual prescribed healing time and can be debilitating in nature.[5] It is important to note that, while chronic pain may arise from a physical disease state, it may also develop as a result of certain psychological states. These painful perceptions serve no biological purpose, and there is commonly no discernable endpoint.[5] Some patients develop pain syndromes associated with chronic pain. Despite the general division of pain into acute and chronic, there exists quite a bit of overlap, which may be referred to as acute on chronic pain. This concept is especially true in certain disease states such as sickle cell disease, where an acute vasoocclusive crisis has an initial presentation consistent with acute pain but often occurs in a patient who has been on chronic opioid therapy. Recognizing both of these components is critical to providing the best care possible. However, before we can tackle the issue of pain management in children, we must first address the issues associated with recognizing pain in this patient population. In order to correctly assess pain in the pediatric patients, some knowledge of the complex neurophysiologic and neurocognitive developments in children must be addressed.[4]

NEUROPHYSIOLOGY AND COGNITIVE DEVELOPMENT IN CHILDREN

Pain management is particularly challenging when caring for infants in the early stages of development. These patients have no verbal language, and therefore reliable and quantitative pain measurement is particularly challenging. The fact that the nervous system is not fully developed at birth has led to the misconception that neonates and infants do not have the neurocognitive capabilities needed to perceive pain. However, a review of literature has indicated that neonates have considerable maturation of pain transmission pathways by as early as 26 weeks of gestation.[4] There is an increasing body of evidence to suggest that both the neurotransmitters and the central and peripheral pathways necessary for the transmission of pain are intact and functional by late gestation. These pathways continue to mature following birth.[4] The clinician must be aware of the unique issues in this age group, because improper or ineffective management of pain may have long-term consequences lasting well into adulthood.[4] It is for these reasons that a neurophysiological and neuropharmacological approach must be adopted to address the problem of quantifying and then appropriately treating pain in infants.[4]

Studies have shown that the nervous system following birth is hypersensitive to sensory stimuli when compared to the adult nervous system. As a result, infants have lower threshold responses for mechanical and thermal stimulation, which can result in sensitization following repetitive noxious stimuli. This process of sensitization eventually results in the development of pain and the perception of pain, which vary dramatically based on the age and mental development of each patient. In fact, severe pain experienced by neonates may have long-term adverse effects, and some studies have indicated that younger children experience more distress and pain after surgery than older children. One such study showed that infants following heel lancing developed behavioral changes consistent with the development of pain that remained for hours after the stimuli had dissipated.[6] Taddio et al. also noted a similar phenomenon in male infants following circumcision with the use of distraction compared to those who received appropriate analgesia prior to undergoing the procedure.[7]

During the postnatal period, sensory and motor pathways in the infant central nervous system (CNS) are undergoing both functional and structural maturation, and significant transition is occurring.[8] Postnatal development pertaining to nociceptive processing is dependent upon an appropriate balance of neural sensory activity.[8] Tissue injury in early life can thus interfere with normal neural development, resulting in long-term alterations in somato-sensory processing and sensitivity to painful stimuli.[9] Proper understanding of these developmental pathways and appropriate targeting of analgesics early on may be helpful in preventing these changes from happening.

Further complicating the matter, analgesic targets are still developing in infants, and the same analgesic protocols applied to older patients may not have the safe clinical effect.[9] Changes are occurring in the distribution and function of the transmitters and receptors involved in analgesia, and, as a result, the same analgesic agent may have a drastically different pharmacodynamic profile in infants. Additional research is necessary to develop more evidence-directed analgesia protocols for early life.[9]

PAIN ASSESSMENT IN CHILDREN: HOW TO DIFFERENTIATE PAIN FROM OTHER CAUSES IN CHILDREN FOLLOWING SURGERY

Having briefly reviewed the complex neurophysiologic and neurocognitive developments in children, the importance of developing and utilizing objective pain assessment measures cannot be overstated. Children are at an increased risk of inadequate pain management, due to the inability of medical practitioners and parents/caregivers to properly recognize pain. Failure to recognize and treat pain has been associated with increased morbidity and worsening medical outcomes in children. Poorly managed postsurgical pain in children has been associated with elevated levels of stress hormones, resulting in catabolism, immunosuppression, and hemodynamic instability.[10] Other hospital metrics such as prolonged hospital stay and poor patient and parent satisfaction scoring has also been documented in patients with inadequately managed pain. It is important to modify the approach and assessment of pain based on the age and neurocognitive developmental stage of each patient. Older children will be able to express and quantify their pain verbally, while younger children may express their pain behaviorally.

Developmental differences in pain expression have been well documented.[11] For example, according to Pawar and Garten, pain in infants may expressed as body rigidity (such as arching), facial expressions (such as brows lowered and drawn together), in addition to intense crying, increased irritability, inability to sleep, and poor oral intake. Some of these behaviors may be mistaken for hunger and not pain, resulting in the infant receiving a bottle instead of pain medications. Toddlers may become more verbally aggressive with intense crying or may appear withdrawn, with guarding of the painful area. Preschool children may be able to verbalize the intensity of pain, become uncooperative, or cling to a parent or other guardian and may be old enough to understand the secondary gains associated with pain. School-age children, without any cognitive impairment, should be able to not only verbalize pain but also use objective pain assessment scales. Self-reporting, which is the gold standard, would be the appropriate pain assessment scale in this age group. Adolescents possess the ability to localize and verbalize pain but may deny pain based on peer pressure and are more likely to be influenced by cultural and social issues.[12] Pain in this group may be expressed in behavioral changes, such as regressive or withdrawn behaviors and insomnia. In addition to self-reporting, there are scales based on observational and physiological (behavioral) data.

In newborns and infants, there are a variety of behavioral distress scales that are available based on facial expressions, crying and body movements. The most commonly used in newborns are the premature infant pain profile (PIPP) and the CRIES (crying, requires increased oxygen administration, increased vital signs, expression, sleeplessness) postoperative pain scales.[13] In children between the ages of two months and seven years, the FLACC (face, legs, activity, cry, and consolability) scale is often used to assessment postoperative pain. The child is observed by nursing staff for one to five minutes and a pain score is obtained, based on observed behaviors, which are matched to an assigned numeric score.[14]

In children between three and six years old, who are becoming more articulate in describing the location and sometimes intensity of pain, self-reporting scales which utilize drawings, pictures of faces, and graded changes are most appropriate. The poker chip scale, Wong-Baker Faces scale, Faces Pain Scale revised, and the Oucher scale are well-established self-reporting scales for this age group. The poker chip scale asks children to quantify the amount of pain by the "pieces of hurt," which are represented by each poker chip. The more poker chips, the greater the pain. The use of body outlines allows children to point to the location of their pain.[15] The Wong-Baker Faces Pain scale works by showing children images of faces and asking them to identify the face that best represents how they feel. Each face is associated with a numeric value, which is used to rate level of pain.[16] The Oucher scale uses actual photographs of other children depicting different levels of pain and is more realistic than drawings of the Wong-Baker scale. Children are asked to point out the face that best represents how they feel. Each face is assigned a pain score, which is used to determine the score of the patient using the scale[17]. It is important to emphasize that child must select the face that represents how he or she feels and not what the parents think the child is feeling. This allows children to rate their pain by matching their pain to the face of other children depicting the same pain level as their own. The Oucher scale has been well accepted in children over six years old.

In school-age children and adolescents, without developmental or cognitive impairments, verbal scales and visual analog pain scale (VAS) provide accurate pain assessment.[17,18] The VAS is usually reserved for children eight years or older who are able to comprehend the concept of assigning a numeric value, which is similar to their actual pain level. This scale has been well studied and validated in both sexes. The scale uses numbers from zero to 10 to denote level of pain, with zero corresponding to no pain and 10 corresponding to excruciating pain. The pain practitioner must utilize this scale and be careful with focusing on the exact numeric value as some children may assign higher numeric scores, which is not clinically accurate. One such example is the case of children with sickle cell disease, who may rate their pain with higher numbers, even when they are comfortable and have been observed playing games or enjoying activities. The practitioner must use all tools and observations when assessing pain in order to best guide treatment.[17–19]

In children with cognitive impairment, assessing pain is very difficult. In this population, it is important to understand expressions and behaviors that may indicate pain, as these patients do not express pain in the same way as other children of the same age. One such example would be children with Down's syndrome, who may express pain more slowly than other children.[20] Self-reporting scales will not be as useful in this population. Scales based on observational and behavioral data may be more useful

PHARMACOLOGICAL MANAGEMENT STRATEGIES

Opioid Pharmacologic Management

The term "opioid" describes any substance that acts on opioid receptors (mu, delta, and kappa) to produce morphine-like effects and includes several broad classes. Opiates are naturally occurring alkaloids derived from the opium poppy and include morphine, codeine, thebaine, and papaverine. Chemical modifications of opiates yielded semi-synthetic compounds with applications in clinical medicine, including dihydromorphone, buprenorphine, and oxycodone.[21] Synthetic opioids include fentanyl, methadone, alfentanil, remifentanil, and tapentadol.[21] Opioids can also be classified by their effect at opioid receptors as agonists, antagonists, or partial agonists.[21] An agonist binds to a receptor to produce a maximal effect. Antagonists produce no effect upon binding to a receptor but prevent agonists from binding and exerting effects on the receptor. Partial agonists yield only a partial functional response upon receptor binding, regardless of the amount of the drug that is administered.[22]

Opioids exert their pharmacologic effects through their interaction with opioid receptors in both pre- and postsynaptic sites in the brain, spinal cord, and peripheral nerve cells. Activation of mu, delta, and kappa opioid receptors within the CNS results in decreased release of excitatory neurotransmitters from presynaptic terminals.[22] Different effects are exerted at different receptor subclasses. For example, mu-1 activation mediates supraspinal analgesia and physical dependence whereas mu-2 activation results in respiratory depression, bradycardia, and gastrointestinal (GI) dysmotility.[23] The most common mu-agonist is morphine. Other mu-agonists include codeine, hydromorphone, fentanyl, meperidine, and methadone. In contrast, kappa activation yields analgesia without significant respiratory depression. Butorphanol, nalbuphine, buprenorphine, and nalorphine exert their effects at the kappa receptor.[23] Unique properties of different opioid compounds offer options for the clinician in selecting the appropriate agent for the desired analgesic effect while also considering potential side effects.

Opioids have an important role in the multimodal approach to pediatric postsurgical pain management where the goal is to provide adequate analgesia while also minimizing the side effects of individual drugs or techniques.[24] The clinician must be cautious with opioid administration in pediatric patients, particular in neonates and young infants. A quantitative imbalance in mu-1 and mu-2 receptors may result in an increased susceptibility to apnea, which is exacerbated by the fact that these patients already have a decreased ventilatory response to hypoxia and hypercapnia.[24] Furthermore, the combination of immature liver conjugation and renal filtration results in a markedly decreased metabolism and excretion of opioids.[24] The patient's respiratory rate must be monitored carefully, and drug dosages should be titrated slowly. There are different opioids available for pediatric postsurgical pain management, with varying routes of administration, and the agent and delivery mechanism must be tailored to the patient's individual needs, which is dependent on both the nature of the procedure as well as the patient's pain threshold.

For the treatment of mild to moderate pain in children, tramadol, a synthetic codeine analog, has medium potency and is useful due to its opioid-sparing effect.[24] In addition to its effects on the opioid receptors, tramadol inhibits serotonin and norepinephrine reuptake and results in less sedation and minimal effects on respiration when compared to morphine.[24] Tramadol is available as an oral agent in the United States and is administered 1 to 2 mg/kg every four to six hours.[25] In a study of postsurgical pediatric patients, tramadol showed a dose-ranging effect in which patients receiving the 2 mg/kg dose required 42% less rescue analgesics than those who received the 1 mg/kg dose.[25] A principal concern with tramadol is increased risk of postoperative nausea and vomiting, and treatment with ondansetron can result in inhibition of tramadol-induced analgesia.[26] Codeine is a naturally occurring opiate whose analgesic properties depend on its conversion to morphine, which binds to the mu-opioid receptor with an affinity 200 times that of codeine.[27] Although codeine can be useful in relieving mild to moderate pain (dose of 0.5–1 mg/kg, maximum of 60 mg/dose, with dosing interval of four to six hours), the hepatic CYP2D6 enzyme must first metabolize codeine to morphine, and up to 34% of pediatric patients are poor metabolizers, gaining no analgesic effect.[27] Conversely, ultra-rapid metabolizers can achieve dangerously high morphine levels. For these reasons, tramadol is preferred over codeine in treatment of mild to moderate pain. Codeine and acetaminophen combination products such as Tylenol #3 are not recommended for the same reasons as well as concern for liver toxicity at higher acetaminophen doses.[24] The clinician should be mindful of the maximum daily acetaminophen dose in children, which ranges from 800 mg in three-year-olds to 4000 mg in adolescents.[24]

Morphine is the most common opioid analgesic used for treatment of moderate to severe pain in pediatric patients due to its long duration of action and mild sedative effect.[24] The dose range is 0.05 to 0.1 mg/kg intravenous (IV) with a dosing interval of two to four hours.[24] Morphine undergoes extensive hepatic metabolism to morphine-6-glucuronide (M6G) and morphine-3-glucuronide (M3G), which then undergo renal excretion.[28] M6G is an active metabolite with half-potency of morphine at the mu-opioid receptor, and in the setting of renal failure, M6G accumulation can occur with subsequent oversedation and ventilatory depression.[28]

Fentanyl, with its shorter duration of clinically significant action, may be desirable in the immediate postsurgical recovery period due to more accurate titration. The dose range is 1 to 2 mcg/kg with dosing interval of 10 min to one hour.[24] Nasal fentanyl administration was also demonstrated to achieve a blood level which is comparable to that of IV administration.[29] Hydromorphone has a potency up to seven times that of morphine, has no active metabolites (and is therefore useful in patients with renal failure), and has been demonstrated to have fewer opioid-induced side effects.[28] The dose is 15 mcg/kg IV with a dosing interval of two to four hours.[24] Concerns associated with IV administration of opioids include breakthrough pain between peaks and troughs, as well as the concern for apnea with dose increases.[24] Morphine can also be administered by the intramuscular (IM) route, but due to pain with injection and concern for anxiety in the pediatric population, this method often results in ineffective analgesia due to avoidance of the IM injection.[24]

Meperidine is a synthetic alternative to morphine which is more lipid-soluble and has a faster onset of action and was initially thought to have fewer side effects and less risk of dependence.[24] It can be administered at the dose of 1 to 2 mg/kg by IV or IM route, with dosing interval of three to four hours. There is, however, a concern for development of seizures (even with normal renal function) and a risk of accumulation of the topic metabolite normeperidine with decreased renal function, which limit its use in the pediatric population.[30]

An alternative to IV bolus administration of opioids is IV patient-controlled analgesia (IV PCA). With IV PCA, the dose can be adjusted according to individual needs, the patient is given more autonomy in pain management decisions, and there are more consistent opioid blood levels.[24] Morphine is the most common agent used in IV PCA for pediatric patients, and the minimum PCA dose for satisfactory analgesia with minimal side effects is 0.015 to 0.02 mg/kg with a lockout period of 5 to 10 minutes.[24] A continuous opioid infusion can be added to the PCA dose to reduce the number of bolus doses needed, improve sleep quality, and improve overall analgesia. Basal infusion rate is commonly started at 0.015 mg/kg/hr.[24] In a study of postappendectomy pediatric patients given a PCA, the number of bolus doses administered was decreased by 50% and the total opioid consumption was lower in patients who were given a continuous infusion in addition to the PCA dose.[31] There was no statistical difference in pain scores, sedation, respiratory depression, or nausea.[31]

Although morphine is the most commonly used opioid for IV PCA, fentanyl and hydromorphone can also be used. Fentanyl IV PCA may be particularly useful in patients with intermittent, severe pain of short duration due to the more rapid onset and shorter duration of this agent.[24] Hydromorphone may offer an alternative to patients who are intolerant of morphine due to its lower side effect profile.[24] When a morphine IV PCA is initiated for moderate to severe pain, the clinician should consider a concurrent low-dose naloxone infusion at the rate of 0.25 mcg/kg/hr to decrease the incidence of opioid-induced side effects (e.g., pruritus) without reversing the analgesic effect.[32] Furthermore, when an IV PCA is initiated, it is prudent to consider concurrent administration of an nonsteroidal anti-inflammatory drug (NSAID) to reduce the overall opioid requirement.[33]

The IV PCA can be given to any child who understands that pushing the PCA button is indicated with worsening pain. An additional option is nurse-controlled analgesia wherein the nurse performs periodic pain assessments of the patient and administers doses through the PCA pump as necessary. Through this practice, young children and pediatric patients with cognitive impairment can reap the same benefits of IV PCA.[24] The nurse can immediately deliver the dose when needed, without leaving the bedside to obtain controlled substances.[34] For the process of weaning the IV PCA, the continuous infusion is routinely stopped first, at the time when a decrease in the number of demand doses is noted.[24] The total daily requirement of opioid is then used to determine an appropriate analgesic equivalent of oral analgesics.[24]

Oral oxycodone and hydromorphone are useful in the conversion from parenteral to enteral administration of opioids. With these agents, there is an approximately 60% bioavailability after oral ingestion.[24] Analgesia begins 20 minutes following administration, and the maximum effect is achieved in 60 to 120 minutes.[24] The dose for oxycodone is 0.1 to 0.2 mg/kg with a dosing interval of four to six hours and the dose for hydromorphone is 0.05 mg/kg with a dosing interval of three to four hours.[24] These agents are also available in sublingual form for young patients who are unable to swallow tablets.[35] Acetaminophen combinations with oxycodone or hydrocodone are also available (Percocet and Vicodin, respectively) but there is concern for liver toxicity with escalating doses required to provide adequate analgesia.[36]

An additional option for delivery of opioids is the transdermal route, particularly applicable to fentanyl. It is important to consider that, compared to adults, young children may require more time until a steady state is reached with transdermal delivery.[30] Furthermore, higher doses in reference to body mass may be required in young children compared with adolescents or adults. It is necessary to offer these patients sufficient medication for breakthrough pain in the initial period when transdermal therapy is started.[30] Due to poor patch adhesion, patients may need redosing at a 48-hour interval, rather than the traditional 72-hour interval.[30] However, when the dosing and administration changes are tailored to this population, these patients can achieve improved analgesia with potentially fewer side effects, particularly less GI dysmotility.[30]

Non-Opioid Pharmacologic Management

Non-opioid analgesics are often used conjunction with or in lieu of opioids whenever possible to minimize opioid side effects and tolerance. Studies have shown that the immediate preoperative administration of ketorolac and/or acetaminophen serves to decrease opioid requirements and postoperative nausea and vomiting in children undergoing tonsillectomy.[37] Common non-opioid analgesics which will be covered in this section include non-steroidal NSAIDs, acetaminophen, N-methyl-D-aspartic acid (NMDA) antagonists, α-agonists, muscle relaxants, antineuroleptics, and local anesthetics.

NSAIDs (ibuprofen, naproxen, diclofenac, celecoxib, ketorolac) are anti-inflammatories commonly used in children. Most NSAIDs inhibit both cyclooxygenase (COX)-1 and COX-2, leading to unwanted side effects and therapeutic effects, respectively.[38] Whereas COX-1 is constitutively produced, COX-2 production is induced by inflammation cytokines and cell damage.[38] Inhibition of COX-2 decreases prostaglandin formation associated with inflammation and pain. Inhibition of COX-1, which is produced by platelets, the kidneys, and gastric mucosa, is responsible for NSAID side effects such as bleeding, acute kidney injury, and gastritis.[38] These side effects are seen less commonly in children than in adults.[39] Potent NSAIDs such as indomethacin have been used to induce closure of the ductus arteriosus in premature infants before attempting surgical closure. These NSAIDS should be used with caution in infants with congenital heart defects, dependent on a patent ductus arteriosus for survival.[40] Ibuprofen is orally dosed 6 to 10 mg/kg every six hours with a maximum 24-hour dose of 400 to 600 mg.[41] Naproxen is orally dosed 5 to 6 mg/kg every 12 hours with a maximum 24-hour dose of 250 to 375 mg.[41] Diclofenac is available in IV (0.5 mg/kg), oral (2–3 mg/kg every 24 hours), and topical (1.3% DEPT Patch twice daily) formulations.[42-44] Celecoxib is a selective COX-2 inhibitor associated with a lower risk of gastric ulcers but an increased risk of cardiovascular events in adults.[45,46] Celecoxib can be used for children dosed at 3 to 6 mg/kg twice daily.[47]

Ketorolac is given intravenously and is dosed 0.5 mg/kg every six hours with a maximum single dose of 30 mg.[48] Two concerns that must be taken in mind when using ketorolac for postoperative pain control are the risk of postoperative bleeding (especially post-tonsillectomy) and non-union following orthopedic procedures. In a double-blinded trial comparing the use of intraoperative ketorolac versus rectal acetaminophen for tonsillectomy postoperative pain control, ketorolac provided better pain control but was associated with increased intraoperative blood loss.[49] Intraoperative ketorolac has also been shown to increase the risk of post-tonsillectomy hemorrhage and hospital admission.[50] However, there was no increased risk of post-tonsillectomy hemorrhage shown with postoperative use of ibuprofen.[51,52] In a retrospective study of patients undergoing spinal surgery, perioperative ketorolac was associated with an increased risk of bone non-union in comparison to celecoxib.[53] However, meta-analyses on the effect of normal-dose ketorolac on bone healing failed to reproduce this association. Further research is needed to determine the effects of ketorolac on bone healing and non-union.[54–56]

Acetaminophen (paracetamol, Ofirmev®) can be administered orally, rectally, or intravenously. The exact mechanism of analgesia is unknown; however, acetaminophen is believed to act predominantly through COX-2 inhibition, resulting in its antipyretic and anti-inflammatory effects.[57] Although acetaminophen can be used safely in children of all ages, it is important to note that supratherapeutic doses are known to cause acute liver failure and therefore liver function should be taken into account to ensure appropriate dosing. Supratherapeutic doses vary based on the age of the patient and are outlined as >40 mg/kg/day for preterm neonates less than 28-weeks postgestation; >60 mg/kg/day for preterm neonates 32 to 40 weeks postgestation; >75 mg/kg/day for term infants; >100 mg/kg/day for children, maximum of 4000 mg per day. The oral dose for children is 10 to 15 mg/kg every four hours with a maximum single dose of 650 to 1000 mg. The rectal dose for children is 35 to 45 mg/kg every six to eight hours with subsequent doses of 20 mg/kg due to delayed absorption.[41]

Ofirmev® (IV formulation of acetaminophen) is dosed 15 mg/kg every six hours for children older than two years and 10 mg/kg every six hours for children less than two years.[58] Pharmacokinetic studies of oral acetaminophen show increasing bioavailability of the drug with increasing doses with a maximum bioavailability of 87% at doses greater than 1000 mg. This bioavailability pattern is associated with first-pass metabolism by the liver and can be bypassed by using the IV preparation.[59] In a meta-analysis of single-dose IV acetaminophen for postoperative pain control, 1000 mg acetaminophen had the morphine equivalent of 1.3 mg and correlated with a 16% reduction in narcotic requirement.[60]

Ketamine is an NMDA receptor antagonist used for anesthesia, acute analgesia, chronic pain modulation, and the treatment of depression. In addition to NMDA receptors, ketamine also acts on mu, kappa, and delta opioid receptors, contributing to its analgesic effect. Unlike opioids, ketamine is not a respiratory depressant, and it can be used safely with opioids for synergistic pain control.[61] In high doses, ketamine can be associated with dysphoria; however, this rarely occurs in the dose range used for acute pain control.[61,62] Other side effects include nausea/vomiting, increased oral secretions, bronchodilation, nystagmus, and diplopia.[62] For treatment of postoperative pain, an IV dose of 0.5 mg/kg (0.25–1 mg/kg) is most commonly used. A meta-analysis of the intraoperative use of ketamine to treat postoperative pain in children showed that ketamine was associated with decreased pain in the early postoperative period compared to control.[63] In the trials included, doses varied widely from 0.25 to 6 mg/kg bolus ± 0.02 to 10 mg/kg/min infusion. Surgical procedures that were included in this analysis were tonsillectomy, adenoidectomy, inguinal hernia repair, circumcision, appendectomy, and scoliosis repair. Ketamine can also be given orally or intramuscularly for preoperative sedation.

Clonidine and dexmedetomidine are alpha-2 agonists used to treat pain. Although these medications were originally used as antihypertensive agents, their sedative, analgesic, and anxiolytic effects have made these medications useful in the operating room. Clonidine is peripherally acting and is proposed to decrease pain perception by direct blockade of nociceptive c-fibers and cross-reactivity with mu-opioid receptors.[64,65] Dexmedetomidine is a centrally acting alpha-2 agonist, which has been shown to downregulate nociceptive pathways at the level of the dorsal horn of the spinal cord.[64] It is proposed that dexmedetomidine may also have analgesic action at the level of the locus coeruleus.[66] One study showed that children 5 to 12 years old treated with oral clonidine 4 mcg/kg prior to surgery had lower postoperative pain scores in comparison to those who did not receive oral clonidine preoperatively.[67] Similar results have been shown with 1 mcg/kg transmucosal dexmedetomidine.[68] Alpha-2 agonists should be used with caution in children due to bradycardia, and some practitioners recommend co-administration with oral atropine. These medications are also useful as adjuvants for neuraxial analgesia, which is discussed later in this chapter.

Muscle relaxants such as baclofen, tizanidine, and diazepam are useful in treating pain due to muscle spasms. While baclofen and tizanidine are often used to manage chronic pain due to muscle spasms in cerebral palsy and severe scoliosis, diazepam has been shown to be useful in treating spasms following abdominal or spinal surgery. Additionally, there is some evidence to support that benzodiazepines treat pain by gabanergic modulation of nociceptive pathways independent of its antispasmodic properties.[69] It is important to note that diazepam is the only benzodiazepine with antispasmodic properties, and other benzodiazepines should not be prescribed to treat postoperative pain. Benzodiazepines should be used with caution in children especially in combination with opioids due to respiratory depression. Diazepam can be administered orally 0.1 to 0.2 mg/kg or intravenously 0.05 to 0.1 mg/kg every six hours.

Anti-neuroleptics such as gabapentin and pregabalin are well-established chronic neuropathic pain therapies, but they also can be useful in the treatment of acute postoperative pain. Pregabalin is a pro-drug with an identical backbone structure to gabapentin. The exact mechanism of action of gabapentin and pregabalin is unknown.[70] Both medications have sedating side effects, which are tolerated in the immediate postoperative period. A double-blinded randomized trial of pediatric patients undergoing spinal fusion showed that patients who were given 15 mg/kg gabapentin preoperatively required less total narcotics and had lower pain scores than controls.[71] One advantage of pregabalin over gabapentin is better bioavailability and a shorter dose interval to achieve steady state.[69]

Local anesthetics are useful in children; however, most children will not tolerate infiltration of soft tissue without sedation. Topical formulations also exist, such as EMLA cream (mixture of lidocaine and prilocaine).[41] Surgical incisions can be infiltrated with local anesthetic while the child is under general anesthesia to improve postoperative pain. Intraoperative lidocaine 2 mg/kg/hr infusions have been shown to decrease postoperative opioid requirements after laparoscopic abdominal surgery in adults, but data is limited in pediatrics.[72] It is important to note that safe local anesthetic dosing differs for neonates due to decreased clearance and higher drug availability in plasma due to lower levels of binding proteins.[73] For neonates, the maximum dose of lidocaine is 4 mg/kg and the maximum dose of lidocaine with epinephrine is 5 mg/kg. For neonates the maximum dose of bupivacaine (with or without epinephrine) is 2 mg/kg. Children follow similar dosing guidelines to adults (lidocaine 5 mg/kg maximum; lidocaine with epinephrine 7 mg/kg maximum; bupivacaine 2.5 mg/kg maximum).[41] The use of local anesthetic for regional and neuraxial blockade is addressed later in this chapter.

NONPHARMACOLOGIC MANAGEMENT STRATEGIES: REGIONAL ANESTHESIA

Introduction

Regional anesthesia has become an integral part of pain management for patients undergoing a variety of surgical procedures. While some peripheral nerve blocks (PNBs) such as brachial plexus blockade can be used for surgical anesthesia as well as postoperative analgesia in adults, regional anesthesia is generally used for postoperative pain control in children. One major difference between adults undergoing a PNB placement and children is the ability to cooperate with block placement due to different anxiety and developmental levels. As a result, PNBs are usually performed after the patient has been anesthetized. While there is concern for increased risk of undetected complications associated with placing PNBs under general anesthesia, there is a greater risk of complications if performed in an awake child who is uncooperative. Various studies have shown the benefits of an anesthetized patient who is not moving outweighs the risks of the risks of a moving and uncooperative patient.

Although there are no randomized controlled trials comparing complication rates of blocks placed under general anesthesia versus no sedation, a meta-analysis of case reports, observational studies, and experimental animal studies suggests no increased risk of seizure, cardiovascular toxicity, or nerve damage when ultrasound and appropriate test doses of epinephrine or isoproterenol are used to place a block under general anesthesia.[74] Taenzer et al. conducted a prospective observational multicenter study to determine the incidence of neurologic and cardiovascular complications and local anesthetic systemic toxicity (LAST) that occur in children having PNB placed under different forms of anesthesia. The patients were divided into four groups: general anesthesia with paralysis (GA + NMB), general anesthesia without paralysis (GA – NMB), sedation, or awake. Taenzer found that the complication rates were seven times higher in awake and sedated groups compared to those who had the blocks placed under general anesthesia. In fact, the postoperative neurological complications were noted in those who received sedation for PNB placement.[75]

Furthermore, based on animal studies, general anesthesia might decrease the risk of adverse outcome (seizure, cardiovascular collapse) in the event of local anesthetic intravascular injection.[76,77] Although paresthesias during block placement in the conscious patient would be considered a warning sign for nerve injury, the limited data neither supports nor refutes this conjecture.[78] The American Pain Society recommends the placement of continuous PNB catheters for postoperative pain control in children (strong recommendation, moderate evidence). But it is important to note that the failure rate is 20% to 25% depending on the block, and block failure should be discussed during informed consent.[1,79] This section discusses the use of interscalene, supraclavicular, infraclavicular, axillary, and digital blocks for pediatric upper extremity surgery.

Blocks for Upper Extremity Surgery

Interscalene Nerve Block

Of the blocks discussed in this section, the interscalene is the most proximal, targeting the trunks of the brachial plexus. A proper interscalene block covers the distal clavicle to the lateral elbow and is most commonly used for shoulder surgery.[80] For this block, the patient is positioned supine with the head of the bed at 45° with the head turned to the contralateral side. A rolled towel or blanket under the ipsilateral shoulder can optimize positioning.[81] The ultrasound probe is placed along the clavicle and is then traced up the neck toward the mandible until the trunks of the brachial plexus are seen between the anterior scalene muscle (medial) and middle scalene muscle (lateral). The brachial plexus appears as a classic "traffic light" at the level of the trunks. With the needle positioned lateral to and in plane with the ultrasound probe, advance the needle until the tip penetrates the nerve sheath between the upper and middle trunks. For children less than eight years old, it is recommended to use either 0.2% ropivacaine or 0.25% bupivacaine 0.5 cc/kg up to 20 cc. For children older than eight years, 0.5% ropivacaine or 0.5% bupivacaine 0.5 cc/kg up to 20 cc can be used.[81] Side effects of the procedure include ipsilateral phrenic nerve paralysis in 100% of patients; therefore, bilateral interscalene blocks should not be performed. Also, for this reason, interscalene blocks may not be suitable for children with respiratory compromise. Horner's syndrome and hoarseness can also be seen and disappear with block resolution. Other complications include intravascular injection and nerve injury.

Supraclavicular Nerve Block

A supraclavicular block targets the brachial plexus at the level of the divisions, and a successful block will cover the humerus to the hand, although distal coverage is incomplete.[80] Supraclavicular blocks can be used for surgery of the distal humerus and elbow. Positioning for a supraclavicular block is similar to that of the interscalene block, supine with the head of the bed at 45° and the head turned to the contralateral side. Again the ultrasound probe is placed flat to the clavicle. The divisions of the brachial plexus should be visible lateral to the subclavian artery and superficial to the first rib and pleura in a characteristic "bunch of grapes" appearance. Again with the needle positioned lateral to and in plane with the ultrasound probe, advance the needle until the tip of the needle is between the divisions. Proper needle placement should yield spread of local anesthetic between the divisions upon injection. Local anesthetic spread to the deep divisions will yield a more distal block. For children less than eight years old, it is recommended to use either 0.2% ropivacaine or 0.25% bupivacaine 0.5 mL/kg up to 20 mL. For children older than eight years, 0.5% ropivacaine or 0.5% bupivacaine 0.5 mL/kg up to 20 mL can be used.[81] Side effects are similar to that of an interscalene block. Ipsilateral phrenic nerve paralysis is not ubiquitous as in interscalene blocks; the rate is approximately 50%.[82] Transient Horner's syndrome and hoarseness may also occur.[80] Pneumothorax is a rare complication when the block is placed under ultrasound guidance in adults, but the risk is higher in children due to the anatomy of the superior thoracic aperture.[83,84]

Infraclavicular Nerve Block

An infraclavicular block targets the cords of the brachial plexus to provide anesthesia to the arm distal to the elbow. It is particularly useful for surgery of the elbow, forearm, and hand.[80] However, compared to the supraclavicular block, the infraclavicular block has less radial coverage.[85] For this block the patient is placed supine with the arm abducted 90°. The ultrasound probe is placed just caudate to the clavicle in the sagittal plane two-thirds from midline. The lateral, medial, and posterior cords will be seen surrounding the axillary artery, deep to the pectoris major and minor muscles and cephalad to the axillary vein. The needle is advanced in plane superior to the ultrasound probe approaching the lateral and posterior cords.[80] For children less than eight years old, it is recommended to use either 0.2% ropivacaine or 0.25% bupivacaine 0.5 mL/kg up to 20 mL. For children older than eight years, 0.5% ropivacaine or 0.5% bupivacaine 0.5 mL/kg up to 20 mL can be used.[81] Complications include intravascular injection, nerve injury, and pneumothorax; however, the rate of pneumothorax is less than with supraclavicular block.[86]

Axillary Nerve Block

The axillary block targets the brachial plexus at the levels of the branches. A proper axillary block should cover the forearm to the hand and is useful for distal radius, wrist, and hand surgery. For block placement, the arm is abducted 90° from the torso and the elbow is flexed 90° with the hand toward the head. The ultrasound probe is placed in the anterior third of the axilla along the lateral edge of the pectoris minor. The median, radial, and ulnar nerves will be surrounding the axillary artery with the musculocutaneous nerve cephalad and deep to the other structures. The needle should be advanced in plane with the ultrasound probe in the caudad direction. Injection of local anesthetic superficial and deep to the axillary artery and around the musculocutaneous nerve should yield a successful block.[80] The transarterial approach is not practiced in children due to an unacceptable risk of limb ischemia.[84] For children less than eight years old, it is recommended to use either 0.2% ropivacaine or 0.25% bupivacaine 0.3 cc/kg up to 20 cc. For children older than eight years, 0.5% ropivacaine or 0.5% bupivacaine 0.3 cc/kg up to 20 cc can be used.[81] A retrospective, nonrandomized study of nerve injury following axillary block showed an increased risk of nerve injury in children under age 14 compared to older children and adults. The study was not designed, however, to detect if this risk was increased in children who received an axillary block in comparison to children who did not receive a block.[74,87] The axillary block is considered very safe, and the most common complications include intravascular injection and infection especially if a catheter is placed.

Digital Blocks

Digital blocks or "ring blocks" target the four digital nerves, which innervate an individual finger or digit. This block is useful for minor surgery of the digit or other minor procedures including laceration repairs and nail injuries. Unlike the brachial plexus blocks previously mentioned, no imaging is used to increase the success of block placement or to decrease complication rates. For children less than eight years old, it is recommended to use either 0.2% ropivacaine or 0.25% bupivacaine 0.05 to 0.1 cc/kg up to 2 to 3 cc maximum at the lateral and medial base of the finger. For children older than eight years, 0.5% ropivacaine or 0.5% bupivacaine 0.05 to 0.1 cc/kg up to 2 to 3 cc can be used.[81,84] Complications are rare with digital blocks. Although it is generally recommended not to use local anesthetics with epinephrine due to theoretical risk of digit ischemia, this complication has not been reported.

Blocks for Lower Extremity Surgery

Lower extremity PNBs target the nerves of the lumbar plexus and sacral plexus. The lumbar plexus (L1–L4) provides innervation for most of the thigh and upper leg, giving branches to the femoral nerve, lateral femoral cutaneous nerve, and obturator nerve.[88] The sacral plexus (anterior rami of L4, L5, S1, S2, and S3) provides innervation to the lower leg, giving rise to the sciatic nerve.[88] A larger volume of local anesthetic is generally required for blocks of the lower extremity, compared to blocks of the upper extremity. For single-shot PNBs of the lower extremity in patients less than five to eight years old, the dose is 0.5 to 1 ml/kg of 0.25% bupivacaine or 0.2% ropivacaine.[88] In older children, the dose is commonly 0.5 ml/kg of 0.5% bupivacaine or 0.5% ropivacaine.[88] For continuous infusions through a catheter, suggested dosing for newborns and infants is 0.2 mg/kg/hr of 0.1% ropivacaine and for older children is 0.3 to 0.4 mg/kg/hr of 0.1% ropivacaine.[88] The clinician must make sure that the combined total dose of local anesthetic does not exceed the maximum for the patient's body mass. Dilute epinephrine can be added to the local anesthetic solution to quickly identify intravascular injection if ultrasound guidance is not employed during placement.

Femoral Nerve Block

The femoral nerve block is the most frequently performed lower extremity PNB in children and is useful in the setting of femoral fractures and for postoperative pain management following knee arthroscopy.[89]

The femoral nerve is blocked at the level of the crease at the groin, lateral to the femoral artery pulsation. The nerve stimulator needle should be inserted lateral to the palpable arterial pulsation, and quadriceps contraction should be observed.[89] An appropriate dose of local anesthetic is typically 0.2 to 0.3 ml/kg, distributed around the nerve sheath. A retrospective study was performed to evaluate the efficacy of femoral nerve blockade using different concentrations of local anesthetic. In 269 knee arthroscopy patients, femoral nerve block offered an opioid-sparing effect and a reduction in postoperative pain scores, and the higher concentrated local anesthetic (ropivacaine 0.5%) was superior to bupivacaine 0.25% or ropivacaine 0.2%.[90]

Adductor Canal Block

An alternative option for postoperative analgesia in pediatric patients undergoing knee surgery is the adductor canal block. In a case series report of pediatric patients (ages 7–15 years) undergoing surgery for habitual patellar dislocation requiring an open reduction and internal fixation, single-shot adductor canal blocks were administered with 0.2% ropivacaine. Pain scores were lower in patients who received the block, and systemic analgesic consumption was decreased compared to those patients who had not received the block.[91] Additionally, compared with patients receiving femoral nerve block, there was less motor blockade and decreased time to ambulation.[91]

Sciatic Nerve Block

The sciatic nerve, which innervates the posterior thigh and leg and most of the foot, is blocked at two anatomical areas: infragluteal and popliteal fossa. The preferred method for ease of access is the popliteal fossa block of the sciatic nerve. Approximately 5 to 8 cm above the popliteal crease, the sciatic nerve divides into the tibial and common peroneal nerves and a common epineural sheath covers both branches, resulting in blockade of both branches when local anesthetic is administered.[92] A lateral approach to the popliteal fossa is advantageous since anesthetized pediatric patients are usually supine. After the knee is flexed on the side of the block, the biceps femoris tendon is identified.[92] The needle is introduced between the vastus lateralis and the biceps femoris tendon approximately 5 to 6 cm above the popliteal crease.[92] Twitch responses of either the tibial or common peroneal nerve are adequate because the needle insertion is above the point of sciatic bifurcation.[92] A total volume of 0.5 ml/kg of local anesthetic is used.[89] With the infragluteal approach to sciatic block, the infragluteal (gluteal crease) line is marked.[92] A nerve stimulator needle is inserted at a point inferior to the gluteal crease and just medial to the biceps femoris tendon.[92] As with the popliteal approach, a total volume of 0.5 ml/kg of local anesthetic is used.[89]

Saphenous Nerve Block

Innervation of the knee and the medial leg distal to the knee is provided by the saphenous nerve, which is a branch of the femoral nerve. It courses within the adductor canal, adjacent to the sartorius muscle, and then continues to the medial aspect of the knee.[92] Saphenous nerve blockade is useful to provide sensory analgesia to the anterior aspect of the knee. While patient is supine, the leg is abducted and laterally rotated. The sartorius muscle is identified, and the needle is directed toward the saphenous nerve.[92] The saphenous nerve block can be performed in combination with a sciatic block to provide enhanced coverage for surgical procedures on the lower extremity.[93]

Lumbar Plexus Nerve Block

The lumbar plexus is composed of the T12 to L5 nerve roots, and branches include the femoral, lateral femoral cutaneous, and obturator nerves, which innervate the upper leg.[94] The lumbar plexus can be blocked along with the ipsilateral sciatic nerve for complete lower extremity analgesia.[94] The lumbar plexus block has been effectively performed in pediatric patients.[95] After the patient is placed in lateral decubitus position, the iliac crest and spinous processes are identified.[94] Erector spinae and quadratus lumborum muscles are deep to the transverse processes, and the lumbar plexus is deep to these muscles.[94] Nerve stimulation is often used with ultrasound imaging to position the needle adjacent to the plexus.[94]

Ankle Block

The ankle block is commonly performed for foot surgery in pediatric patients and provides effective pain relief in the postoperative period. The ankle block does not offer pain relief during tourniquet application, but this block is often performed in conjunction with general anesthesia.[89] Five nerves are blocked: posterior tibial, deep peroneal, superficial peroneal, saphenous, and sural. A low volume of local anesthetic is sufficient for blockade of these nerves since they are very superficial.[92] The tibial nerve, which supplies the plantar aspect of the foot, is located below the medial malleolus. The needle is advanced to the bone, withdrawn slightly, and a total volume of 5 to 8 ml of local anesthetic is injected.[89] The saphenous nerve (a branch of the femoral nerve) innervates the skin overlying the medial leg below the knee and ankle. A superficial ring along the medial malleolus is injected with a total of 5 ml of local anesthetic.[89] The deep peroneal nerve is blocked when 2 to 3 ml of local anesthetic solution is deposited just lateral to the extensor hallucis longus tendon.[89] Blockade of the superficial peroneal nerve, which supplies sensation on the dorsal aspect of the foot, is achieved through injection of a superficial ring of local anesthetic between the extensor hallucis longus tendon and the lateral malleolus.[89] The sural nerve supplies sensation to the lateral aspect of the foot, and injection of local anesthetic between the calcaneus and the lateral malleolus will achieve blockade.[89] The ankle block is relative facile and can be a useful adjunct to traditional modalities for postoperative pain control.

Another option for postoperative analgesia in pediatric patients undergoing lower extremity surgery is the placement of a lumbar epidural catheter. Clinical studies have shown a reduced incidence of hypoxemia, improved cardiovascular stability, faster return of GI function, and reduced intensive care stays for patients who received epidural analgesia as part of a multimodal postoperative pain management plan.[96] Lumbar epidural catheters can be safely placed while the patient is under general anesthesia.[97] Using a midline approach with a Touhy needle and loss of resistance syringe, the depth of the epidural space can be estimated to be 1 mm/kg, with a minimal distance of 10 mm.[97] The goal is to place the catheter tip close to the spinal level of nerves innervating the involved dermatomes in order to limit the dose of local anesthetic required and to reduce the incidence of local anesthetic toxicity.[97] Ropivacaine and levobupivacaine are the preferred local anesthetic agents.[98]

BLOCKS FOR ABDOMINAL SURGERY

Truncal Blocks

Truncal blocks are divided into two categories: anterior and posterior. The anterior truncal blocks include the rectus sheath block, transversus abdominis plane (TAP) block, and the ilioinguinal/iliohypogastric (IL/IH) block. The posterior truncal blocks include paravertebral nerve block (PVB), intercostal nerve block, and extra-pleural catheters, which are not commonly used in children and are not discussed in this chapter.

Rectus Sheath Block

The rectus sheath block, also known as paraumbilical block, is becoming increasingly popular in children undergoing abdominal surgeries due to the increased efficacy and safety achieved when performing the block under ultrasound guidance.[99] The rectus sheath block is ideal for providing sensory coverage for incisional pain involving the umbilicus such as umbilical hernia repair and umbilical port sites. The innervation of the umbilical area including the muscle is provided by the right and left thoracoabdominal intercostal nerves, which are derived from the anterior rami of spinal roots T8 to T12 and run just deep to the rectus abdominis. The anterior cutaneous branches of the thoracoabdominal intercostal nerves supply sensory innervation to the peri-umbilical dermis.[99] Local anesthetic deposited in a potential space between the rectus abdominis muscle and posterior rectus sheath is required for an effective block. When performed prior to surgical incision, rectus sheath blocks have been shown to reduce intraoperative opioid requirements as well as decrease the total dose of opioids required in the postanesthesia care unit (PACU).[99] Postoperative analgesia can last greater than six hours depending on the local anesthetic agent used, with bupivacaine providing the longest duration of analgesia. While non-opioid adjuvants such as NSAIDs and acetaminophen alone have been shown to provide effective analgesia for mild to moderate postoperative pain, the combination non-opioids with a PNB has been shown to provide effective analgesia superior to either modality alone.[99]

This synergistic analgesia has been shown to reduce and in some cases eliminate the need for postoperative opioids.[99] This block can be performed using either the landmark technique, otherwise known as the double pop technique, or more commonly using real-time ultrasonography due to concerns for increased risks of bowel perforation or damage to other important viscera such kidneys or spleen in smaller children. When performing this block using ultrasound guidance, the patient is placed in the supine position and a high-frequency linear probe (50 Hz) is placed lateral to the umbilicus locating the linea alba. Once the linea alba is found, the probe is then used to scan laterally until the rectus muscle is identified, and local anesthetics are deposited along the posterior sheath of the rectus muscle on both sides of the linea alba for the best coverage.[100] Intravascular injection or local anesthetic toxicity are other complications that have been associated with placement of a rectus sheath block.[101] Although surgical infiltration can also be used to decrease postoperative pain, ultrasound guided rectus sheath block has been associated with lower pain scores and less opiate requirements when compared to surgical site infiltration.[102]

Transversus Abdominis Plane Block

A TAP block provides the best pain control for any surgery involving the anterior abdominal wall—laparoscopic or open—including appendectomy, cholecystectomy, exploratory laparotomy, Nissan fundoplication, and some genitourinary procedures such as ureteral stent placement. The lateral abdominal wall is comprised of three muscle layers and their associated fascia: external oblique, internal oblique, and transversus abdominis. Sensory innervation to the anterolateral abdominal wall is provided by the branches of the anterior rami of T6 to L1: intercostal nerves (T7–T11), subcostal nerve (T12), and iliohypogastric/ ilioinguinal nerves (L1). In children, TAP blocks have been shown to provide superior pain control compared to wound infiltration for both inguinal hernia repair and open pyeloplasty.[103,104]

TAP blocks are now routinely performed using real time ultrasonography (US) as most of the children require general anesthesia in order to tolerate the procedure.

With the patient in the supine position, the US probe is placed superior to iliac crest in the midaxillary line. The external oblique (superficial), internal oblique (middle), and transversus abdominis (deep) muscles are then identified prior to insertion of the needle. A 22-gauge blunt stimuplex needle is inserted using the in-plane technique, and local anesthetic is injected between the internal oblique and transversus abdominis muscles. Although less commonly used in children, a blind landmark technique involving the triangle of petit has also been described. The triangle of petit is bordered by the iliac crest, the latissimus dorsi muscle, and the external oblique muscle.[105] Injection of local anesthetic into this space with the needle placed in the center of the triangle and perpendicular to the skin has been shown to result in consistent anatomic spread of local anesthetic.[106] Complications include bleeding, local infection, and (rarely) bowel perforation.

Ilioinguinal/Iliohypogastric Block

IL/IH blocks when used in combination provide pain control for surgeries of the inguinal area and groin—especially inguinal hernia repair, orchiopexy, and hydrocelectomy. In fact, IL block has been shown to provide superior pain relief to TAP blocks for surgeries of this region.[107] The IL and IH nerves stem from the L1 dorsal root and travel below the internal oblique muscle within the aponeurosis 1 to 3 cm medial to the anterior superior iliac spine. These nerves provide abdominal wall sensation to the inguinal area and the groin. Preoperative IL/IH nerve block has been shown to decrease PACU pain scores following open inguinal hernia repair.[108] Some studies show these blocks even have equivalent pain control to caudal block for unilateral groin surgery with fewer risks.[109]

This block is routinely placed under ultrasound guidance with the child under general anesthesia. With the probe placed over the anterior superior iliac spine, the external oblique, internal oblique, and transversus abdominis muscles should be seen, with the IL and IH nerves visible between the internal oblique and the transversus abdominis muscles. Advance the needle in plane with the probe and inject 0.1 to 0.2 mL/kg of 0.2% ropivacaine, fithydro-dissecting the internal oblique from the transversus abdominis muscle.[110] Landmark techniques are less reliable in children due to variations in anatomy based on age.[111] The use of US has not only increased the success rates for these procedures but is also associated with lower rates of complications. Risks are similar to other anterior truncal blocks and include colon perforation and pelvic hematoma.[110,112,113]

Caudal Blockade

Despite the increasing use of PNB such as the anterior truncal blocks, caudal blockade (CB) remains the gold standard for providing analgesia for most routine abdominal wall procedures. CB has been used with great success and efficacy in children undergoing a variety of procedures involving the groin (umbilical hernia repair), penile region (orchiopexy), and lower extremities such as heel cord releases.[114] Therefore, caudal anesthesia is one of the most important techniques that the pediatric anesthesiologist must master, as part of the arsenal against postoperative pain.[115] CB is typically performed using longer-acting local anesthetics such as bupivacaine with epinephrine or ropivacaine.[116] A variety of adjuncts such as clonidine have been used to successfully prolong CB.[117]

Clonidine 1 mcg/kg has been used to prolong the duration of anesthesia in children undergoing urologic procedures, and, in some institutions, this combination has eliminated the need for the placement of caudal catheters in procedures such as bilateral urethral reimplantations. Typically, the CB is performed after the induction of anesthesia and placement of the airway device, with the patient positioned in the lateral decubitus position. Landmarks for the CB are superior iliac spine and sacral hiatus, which forms an equilateral triangle. After sterile prepping of area, an angiocath needle is typically inserted below the S4 spinous process and is advanced at a 45° to 60° angle to the skin.[118]

The needle is advanced slowly using the loss of resistance technique. Once a slight loss is felt, the practitioner should drop the angle of the needle and advance the catheter while retracting the needle. After negative aspiration for blood or cerebrospinal fluid (CSF), a local anesthetic agent is then administered slowly, while palpating for any subcutaneous infiltration. Typically, a test dose is administered, while monitoring for changes in EKG tracing, specifically the ST-T segment changes such as inverted T waves and ST-T segment depressions or elevations. Tachycardia can also be seen but is a late finding, with a heart rate increase of 20% above baseline, as the indicator of intravascular injection of a local anesthetic agent.[119] Spinal anesthesia has been used successfully in premature infants for repair of inguinal hernia repair to avoid general anesthesia and the associated increased risks of apneic and bradycardiac episodes. Given the rapid production of CSF and increased CSF flow in infants, spinal anesthesia has a shorter duration than seen in adults. For this reason, tetracaine is an excellent choice as it provides surgical anesthesia 45 to 60 minutes. IL/IH blocks have been used to provide analgesia for children undergoing groin and urologic procedures such as inguinal hernia repair, orchiopexy, and hydrocelectomy. They have been shown to be equivalent or better than CB and are associated with minimal side effects and complications.[119]

Abualhassan et al. compared CB to US-guided IL/IH nerve block in a randomized prospective study and was able to show that the children who received the IL/IH nerve blocks had a longer time before they needed rescue analgesics in comparison to the children who received CB. He was also able to show that the children in the nerve block group received lower doses of local anesthesia in comparison to the CB group. This was attributed to the use of US, which allowed for visualization of nerves and a more precise allocation of local anesthesia.[109]

Blocks for Thoracic Surgery

Thoracic surgery in children is becoming increasingly more common due to the advances in surgical techniques that have significantly decreased the morbidities and mortalities associated with these high-risk procedures. Despite these advancements, postoperative pain continues to be of paramount importance, as thoracic surgeries are among the most painful operative procedures and poorly controlled postoperative pain can negatively influence patient outcomes. Effective management of acute postoperative pain can result in decreased morbidity by allowing for earlier ambulation, improved pulmonary toilet and improved patient satisfaction as well as reducing the incidence of developing chronic pain following the procedure.[120] Thoracic surgeries, particularly open procedures where there is removal of portion of the ribs or possibly the chest wall, have a high incidence of sympathetic mediated pain that can result in post-thoracotomy pain syndrome (PTPS) and neuropathic pain, which can be permanent if not managed early on in the perioperative period. This subsection focuses primarily on some of the more common blocks that are currently being performed for children undergoing a variety of thoracic procedures and the management of acute and chronic post-thoracotomy pain.

Posterior Truncal Blocks

Paravertebral Nerve Blocks

PVBs were first described in 1905 by Hugo Sellheim and have become increasingly more popular as a viable alternative to epidural blocks or CB in certain patient populations where placement of a neuraxial blockade is contraindicated (see Table 13.1). The paravertebral space is a potential space lateral to the spinous process, which contains the intercostal and sympathetic nerves. The borders of this space include the parietal pleura (anterior), the posterolateral aspect of the vertebra and the intervertebral foramen (medial), the parietal pleura (lateral), and the costotransverse ligament (posterior). This space has been estimated to be 1 cm caudad to the transverse process and 2.5 cm lateral to the spinous process in most adults.[99]

PVBs can be performed using loss of resistance, neurostimulation, or ultrasound guidance. The classic or landmark technique involves identifying the spinous process and marking the skin 2.5 cm laterally in adult patients or at the estimated location of the transverse process in children and using a Touhy needle to contact the posterior surface of the transverse process. Once the transverse process is contacted, the distance from the skin to the transverse process is measured and then the needle is withdrawn, angled at 15° to 60°, and advanced 1 cm caudally beyond the transverse process. Local anesthetics can be injected slowly following a negative drop technique. In the case of ultrasonography, the ultrasound probe, which is usually a high-frequency linear probe in smaller children, is placed parallel to the spine (sagittal approach) or perpendicular to the spine (longitudinal approach) and the spinous process is visualized along with the costotransverse ligament and the pleura. The needle is inserted 30° using the in-plane technique and the local anesthetic is deposited below the posterior aspect of the costo-transverse ligament pushing down the pleural line.

PVB is quickly becoming a new standard in regional anesthesia due to its versatility in providing analgesia for a variety of surgeries, including abdominal, thoracic, and urologic procedures. Lonnqvist et al. performed a landmark retrospective study

Table 13.1. Indications for Placement of Paravertebral Nerve Blocks

Difficult epidural placement due to severe kyphoscolosis or spinal surgery
Procedures where placement of a thoracic epidural has been associated with more complications as in the case of Nuss bar placement due to high blockade with profound hypotension and loss of cardio-accelerator fibers (T1–T4)
Coagulopathy (idiopathic due to hepatic dysfunction or renal failure)

comparing PVB to lumbar epidurals for children undergoing renal surgery, which showed that PVB are equal and/or superior to lumbar epidurals. Those patients in the PVB group required lower demand doses of supplemental morphine and there were a lower number of patients requiring supplemental morphine within 24 hours.[35] PVBs have also been shown to be superior in providing analgesia when compared to caudals for children undergoing inguinal hernia repair[121] or surgical infiltration.[122]

Epidurals

Epidural placement is the classic neuraxial approach to postoperative pain management, and although there are several other modalities currently being employed, epidural analgesia remains a useful and time-tested technique. An indwelling catheter in the epidural space allows for the continuous delivery of opioid or local anesthetic medications, or a combination of the two, and gives the clinician the opportunity to offer a patient-controlled approach to epidural analgesia in patients who are cooperative and demonstrate an understanding.

Post-Thoracotomy Pain Syndrome

Post-thoracotomy pain may be characterized as either acute or chronic. Pain in the acute phase is mediated by nociceptor stimulation from direct injury from the incision, and these afferent pain signals may be impacted and modulated by the duration of the stimulus, repeated stimuli, involvement of the sympathetic nervous system, and production of local inflammatory mediators.[123] When repeatedly stimulated, as in the setting of acute pain, alterations in central and peripheral neuronal physiology result in a different, enhanced response to a given stimulus, which can contribute to the development of chronic pain. This concept emphasizes the importance of effective management of acute pain in an effort to prevent development of chronic pain.[123] Thoracotomy is one of the surgical procedures most commonly associated with chronic pain and disability, so the topic of postoperative analgesia, particularly with a preemptive and proactive approach, is particularly relevant in patients undergoing thoracic surgery.[124]

The degree of pain a patient experiences following thoracic surgery is related to the extent of the surgical trauma, and therefore the smallest and least traumatic incision that can provide the surgeon with an appropriate level of exposure is preferred.[125] In the muscle-sparing approach to thoracotomy, the chest is accessed without division of the latissimus dorsi, and Hazelrigg et al. demonstrated in a prospective randomized trial that postoperative pain scores and narcotic requirements were lower as compared to traditional thoracotomy.[126] Ochroch et al. compared axillary, vertical, muscle-sparing thoracotomy with posterolateral thoracotomy and found no differences in post-operative pain.[127] There is a lack of conclusive data revealing which incisional approach has a better outcome from the standpoint of postoperative pain. Video-assisted thoracoscopic surgery (VATS) is the minimally invasive approach to thoracic surgery which evolved from a biopsy modality into a therapeutic technique. Multiple studies have revealed that VATS patients experience significantly less postoperative pain in the acute setting but long-term results in relation to chronic pain have been mixed.[120]

Effective control of acute pain following thoracic surgery results in decreased risk for atelectasis and pneumonia as well as a decreased neurohumoral stress response.[128] IV opioids have an important role in the treatment of acute pain because of their rapid onset and predictable clinical course.[123] Although the side effects (including respiratory depression, sedation, nausea/vomiting, ileus, and urinary retention) can be limiting, opioids are particularly useful for management of breakthrough pain in the postoperative period.[123] PCA (commonly used with fentanyl, morphine, or hydromorphone) can offer an individualized approach to pain control but alone is inferior to epidural analgesia and is most effectively used as an adjunct to thoracic analgesia in a multimodal approach.[129]

Epidural analgesia is the gold standard for control of acute postoperative pain after thoracic surgery.[130] Using a combination of opioids and local anesthesia, the epidural approach offers effective segmental block of pain with adequate coverage of incision and chest tube sites.[129] Paravertebral block offers an alternative to epidural analgesia with its effect directed at the sympathetic chain, dorsal rami of spinal nerves, and intercostal nerves.[131] Numerous studies have demonstrated that, with a continuous infusion of local anesthetic through a paravertebral catheter, the efficacy is similar to epidural analgesia.[131] Furthermore, continuous PVBs have demonstrated improved lung function on spirometry testing as compared with epidural blockade.[132] Adjuvant medications include NSAIDs (such as ketorolac) and NMDA antagonists (such as ketamine).[123]

In its chronic form, PTPS usually presents as pain that recurs or persists along a thoracotomy scar >2 months following surgery.[133] The reported incidence of PTPS is 30% to 55%, and a large retrospective study indicated a 52% overall incidence.[134] Patients typically experience localized aching or tenderness at the area of the incision.[135] This chronic pain is a type of neuropathic pain syndrome which is thought to be caused by injury to the intercostal nerves, through which pain is transmitted from the chest wall and costal pleura, and the injury may occur during surgical incision, rib retraction, placement of trocars, or suturing.[136] There has been considerable research done to determine if the incidence of PTPS can be decreased by factors such as the type of surgical incision, which was inconclusive.[137] Furthermore, the notion that VATS have a lower incidence of PTPS when compared to open procedure has not been yielded conclusive results. A retrospective study found that VATS led to reduced PTPS when compared with muscle-sparing thoracotomy.[138] A prospective study demonstrated no difference in PTPS incidence when comparing VATS with the classic posterolateral approach.[139] Prospective studies designed to compare the various incision approaches to the development of chronic PTPS are lacking, and thus no conclusion can be drawn regarding one approach versus another.[137]

Several different anesthetic approaches have been attempted with the goal of reducing PTPS, mainly focusing around the concept of preventive analgesia, which involves blocking afferent pain signals from the surgical wound from incision time and through the healing process, thereby preventing central sensitization.[140] Thoracic epidural placement still remains one of the most common techniques employed for managing acute postoperative pain in patients undergoing VATS or thoracotomy. In a randomized controlled trial, Senturk et al. compared three different approaches to analgesia: preoperative initiation of thoracic epidural analgesia (TEA), postoperative initiation of TEA, and IV PCA. Preoperative initiation of TEA resulted in diminished incidence and severity of PTPS, but there was no difference between postoperative initiation of TEA and IV PCA, emphasizing the importance of preemptive analgesia.[141] In contrast, Ochroch et al. conducted a randomized controlled trial involving 157 patients presenting for open thoracotomy who received TEA either at incision time or at time of rib approximation. They concluded that TEA initiation prior to incision did not significantly reduce pain, and although TEA may effectively reduce PTPS, timing of initiation did not have a significant clinical impact.[142]

PVBs offer an alternative to TEA for pain control in the postoperative period in patients undergoing thoracotomy and VATS. Compared to TEA, PVBs provide adequate pain control, are associated with improved respiratory function, have fewer adverse effects on hemodynamic status, and are useful in patients in whom TEA is contraindicated (e.g., coagulopathy).[143] To date, no studies have investigated the role of PVBs in preventing development of PTPS. The use of intercostal nerve blocks has been limited due to concern for high levels of vascular uptake of local anesthetic, and this technique has been shown to be ineffective in reducing the incidence of PTPS.[137]

Following the development of PTPS, antineuroleptic medications have been shown to play a significant role in the treatment of the neuropathic component of the pain, for which systemic opioids may be ineffective.[144] Solak et al. compared gabapentin with naproxen in the treatment of PTPS and concluded that gabapentin is a safe and effective option, with high patient compliance.[145] Other treatment options include medications which have been generally shown to be useful in treatment of neuropathic pain, including pregabalin, tricyclic antidepressants, serotonin-norepinephrine reuptake inhibitors, transdermal lidocaine, and tramadol.[146]

CONCLUSION

The management of postoperative pain in pediatric surgical patients is now receiving the much-needed attention that has allowed for advancements in the different modalities that are now available for use in this patient population. Providers are becoming more attentive and concerned not only with the treatment of postoperative pain but also with its prevention. This new focus has increased the number of regional and neuraxial procedures that are being performed for surgeries. Even routine ambulatory procedures are now being managed not just through IV and oral opioids but also with this multimodal approach, using single-shot PNBs for better optimization of postoperative pain immediately following surgery as well as facilitating expedient discharge home.

REFERENCES

1. Chou R, Gordon DB, de Leon-Casasola OA, et al. Management of postoperative pain: a clinical practice guideline from the American Pain Society, the American Society of Regional Anesthesia and Pain Medicine, and the American Society of Anesthesiologists' Committee on Regional Anesthesia, Executive Committee, and Administrative Council. *J Pain.* 2016;17(2):131–157.

2. Apfelbaum JL, Chen C, Mehta SS, Gan TJ. Postoperative pain experience: results from a national survey suggest postoperative pain continues to be undermanaged. *Anesth Analg.* 2003;97(2):534–540.

3. Merskey H. Pain terms. In: Merskey H, Bogduk N, eds. *Classification of Chronic Pain.* Seattle: IASP Press; 1994; 209–214.

4. Fitzgerald M, Walker SM. Infant pain management: a developmental neurobiological approach. *Nat Clin Pract Neurol.* 2009;5(1):35–50.

5. Grichnik K, Ferrante F. The difference between acute and chronic pain. *Mount Sinai J Med.* 1991;58(3):217–220.

6. Gregory GA, Andropoulos DB. *Gregory's Pediatric Anesthesia.* New York: John Wiley; 2012.

7. Taddio A, Katz J, Ilersich AL, Koren G. Effect of neonatal circumcision on pain response during subsequent routine vaccination. *Lancet.* 1997;349(9052):599–603.

8. Pattinson D, Fitzgerald M. The neurobiology of infant pain: development of excitatory and inhibitory neurotransmission in the spinal dorsal horn. *Reg Anesthes Pain Med.* 2004;29(1):36–44.

9. Walker SM. Pain in children: recent advances and ongoing challenges. *Br J Anaesth.* 2008;101(1):101–110.

10. Zeltzer L, Krell H, Kliegman R, Behrman R, Jenson H, Stanton B. Pediatric pain management. In: *Nelson Textbook of Pediatrics*, 18th ed. Philadelphia: Saunders Elsevier; 2007:479.

11. Pawar D, Garten L. Pain management in children. In: Kopf A, Patel NB, eds. *Guide to Pain Management in Low-Resource Settings.* 2010:255.

12. Perquin CW, Hazebroek-Kampschreur AA, Hunfeld JA, et al. Pain in children and adolescents: a common experience. *Pain.* 2000;87(1):51–58.

13. Stevens B, Johnston C, Petryshen P, Taddio A. Premature infant pain profile: development and initial validation. *Clin J Pain.* 1996;12(1):13–22.

14. Voepel-Lewis T, Shayevitz JR, Malviya S. The FLACC: a behavioral scale for scoring postoperative pain in young children. *Pediatr Nurs.* 1997;23:293–297.

15. Hester N, Foster R, Kristensen K. Measurement of pain in children—generalizability and validity of the pain ladder and the poker chip tool. *Adv Pain Res Ther.* 1990;15:79–84.

16. Hicks CL, von Baeyer CL, Spafford PA, van Korlaar I, Goodenough B. The Faces Pain Scale–Revised: toward a common metric in pediatric pain measurement. *Pain.* 2001;93(2):173–183.

17. Beyer JE, Denyes MJ, Villarruel AM. The creation, validation, and continuing development of the Oucher: a measure of pain intensity in children. *J Pediatr Nurs.* 1992;7:335.

18. Cohen LL, Lemanek K, Blount RL, et al. Evidence-based assessment of pediatric pain. *J Pediatr Psychol.* 2008;33(9):939–955.

19. von Baeyer CL. Children's self-report of pain intensity: what we know, where we are headed. *Pain Res Manage.* 2009;14(1):39–45.

20. Hennequin M, Morin C, Feine J. Pain expression and stimulus localisation in individuals with Down's syndrome. *Lancet.* 2000;356(9245):1882–1887.

21. Pathan H, Williams J. Basic opioid pharmacology: an update. *Br J Pain.* 2012;6(1):11–16.

22. McDonald J, Lambert D. Opioid receptors. *Cont Educ Anaesth Crit Care Pain.* 2005;5(1):22–25.

23. Dhawan B, Cesselin F, Raghubir R, et al. International Union of Pharmacology. XII. Classification of opioid receptors. *Pharmacolog Rev.* 1996;48(4):567–592.

24. Verghese ST, Hannallah RS. Acute pain management in children. *J Pain Res.* 2010;3(2):105–123.

25. Finkel JC, Rose JB, Schmitz ML, et al. An evaluation of the efficacy and tolerability of oral tramadol hydrochloride tablets for the treatment of postsurgical pain in children. *Anesth Analg.* 2002;94(6):1469–1473.

26. Arcioni R, della Rocca M, Romanò S, Romano R, Pietropaoli P, Gasparetto A. Ondansetron inhibits the analgesic effects of tramadol: a possible 5-HT3 spinal receptor involvement in acute pain in humans. *Anesth Analg.* 2002;94(6):1553–1557.

27. Dean L. Codeine therapy and CYP2D6 genotype. *Med Genet Summary.* 2016 Mar 16.

28. Felden L, Walter C, Harder S, et al. Comparative clinical effects of hydromorphone and morphine: a meta-analysis. *Br J Anaesth.* 2011;107(3):319–328.

29. Galinkin JL, Fazi LM, Cuy RM, et al. Use of intranasal fentanyl in children undergoing myringotomy and tube placement during halothane and sevoflurane anesthesia. *J Am Soc Anesthesiologists.* 2000;93(6):1378–1383.

30. Zernikow B, Michel E, Anderson B. Transdermal fentanyl in childhood and adolescence: a comprehensive literature review. *J Pain.* 2007;8(3):187–207.

31. Yildiz K, Tercan E, Dogru K, Ozkan U, Boyaci A. Comparison of patient-controlled analgesia with and without a background infusion after appendicectomy in children. *Pediatr Anesth.* 2003;13(5):427–431.

32. Maxwell LG, Kaufmann SC, Bitzer S, et al. The effects of a small-dose naloxone infusion on opioid-induced side effects and analgesia in children and adolescents treated with intravenous patient-controlled analgesia: a double-blind, prospective, randomized, controlled study. *Anesth Analg.* 2005;100(4):953–958.

33. Sutters K, Shaw B, Gerardi J, Hebert D. Comparison of morphine patient-controlled analgesia with and without ketorolac for postoperative analgesia in pediatric orthopedic surgery. *Am J Orthoped.* 1999;28(6):351–358.

34. Monitto CL, Greenberg RS, Kost-Byerly S, et al. The safety and efficacy of parent-/nurse-controlled analgesia in patients less than six years of age. *Anesth Analg.* 2000;91(3):573–579.

35. Lönnqvist P-A, Morton N. Postoperative analgesia in infants and children. *Br J Anaesth.* 2005;95(1):59–68.

36. Heubi JE, Barbacci MB, Zimmerman HJ. Therapeutic misadventures with acetaminophen: hepatoxicity after multiple doses in children. *J Pediatr.* 1998;132(1):22–27.

37. Mather SJ, Peutrell JM. Postoperative morphine requirements, nausea and vomiting following anaesthesia for tonsillectomy: comparison of intravenous morphine and non-opioid analgesic techniques. *Paediatr Anaesthes.* 1995;5(3):185–188.

38. Vane JR, Botting RM. Mechanism of action of nonsteroidal anti-inflammatory drugs. *Am J Med.* 1998;104(3a):2S–8S; discussion 21S–22S.

39. Lesko SM, Mitchell AA. The safety of acetaminophen and ibuprofen among children younger than two years old. *Pediatrics.* 1999;104(4):e39.

40. Heymann MA, Rudolph AM, Silverman NH. Closure of the ductus arteriosus in premature infants by inhibition of prostaglandin synthesis. *N Engl J Med.* 1976;295(10):530–533.

41. Berde CB, Sethna NF. Analgesics for the treatment of pain in children. *N Engl J Med.* 2002;347(14):1094–1103.

42. Rømsing J, Østergaard D, Drozdziewicz D, Schultz P, Ravn G. Diclofenac or acetaminophen for analgesia in paediatric tonsillectomy outpatients. *Acta Anaesthesiol Scand.* 2000;44(3):291–295.

43. Korpela R, Olkkola K. Pharmacokinetics of intravenous diclofenac sodium in children. *Eur J Clin Pharmacol.* 1990;38(3):293–295.

44. McCarberg B, Argoff C. Topical diclofenac epolamine patch 1.3% for treatment of acute pain caused by soft tissue injury. *Int J Clin Pract.* 2010;64(11):1546–1553.

45. Deeks JJ, Smith LA, Bradley MD. Efficacy, tolerability, and upper gastrointestinal safety of celecoxib for treatment of osteoarthritis and rheumatoid arthritis: systematic review of randomised controlled trials. *BMJ.* 2002;325(7365):619.

46. Caldwell B, Aldington S, Weatherall M, Shirtcliffe P, Beasley R. Risk of cardiovascular events and celecoxib: a systematic review and meta-analysis. *J Royal Soc Med.* 2006;99(3):132–140.

47. Foeldvari I, Szer IS, Zemel LS, et al. A prospective study comparing celecoxib with naproxen in children with juvenile rheumatoid arthritis. *J Rheumatol.* 2009;36(1):174–182.

48. Forrest JB, Heitlinger EL, Revell S. Ketorolac for postoperative pain management in children. *Drug Saf.* 1997;16(5):309–329.

49. Rusy LM, Houck CS, Sullivan LJ, et al. A double-blind evaluation of ketorolac tromethamine versus acetaminophen in pediatric tonsillectomy: analgesia and bleeding. *Anesth Analg.* 1995;80(2):226–229.

50. Splinter WM, Rhine EJ, Roberts DW, Reid CW, MacNeill HB. Preoperative ketorolac increases bleeding after tonsillectomy in children. *Can J Anaesth.* 1996;43(6):560–563.

51. Pickering A, Bridge H, Nolan J, Stoddart P. Double-blind, placebo-controlled analgesic study of ibuprofen or rofecoxib in combination with paracetamol for tonsillectomy in children. *Br J Anaesth.* 2002;88(1):72–77.

52. Krishna S, Hughes LF, Lin SY. Postoperative hemorrhage with nonsteroidal anti-inflammatory drug use after tonsillectomy: a meta-analysis. *Arch Otolaryngol Head Neck Surg.* 2003;129(10):1086–1089.

53. Reuben SS, Ablett D, Kaye R. High dose nonsteroidal anti-inflammatory drugs compromise spinal fusion. *Can J Anaesth.* 2005;52(5):506–512.

54. Dodwell ER, Latorre JG, Parisini E, et al. NSAID exposure and risk of nonunion: a meta-analysis of case–control and cohort studies. *Calcif Tissue Int.* 2010;87(3):193–202.

55. Li Q, Zhang Z, Cai Z. High-dose ketorolac affects adult spinal fusion: a meta-analysis of the effect of perioperative nonsteroidal anti-inflammatory drugs on spinal fusion. *Spine.* 2011;36(7):E461–E468.

56. Jirarattanaphochai K, Jung S. Nonsteroidal antiinflammatory drugs for postoperative pain management after lumbar spine surgery: a meta-analysis of randomized controlled trials. *J Neurosurg Spine.* 2008;9(1):22–31.

57. Graham GG, Scott KF. Mechanism of action of paracetamol. *Am J Ther.* 2005;12(1):46–55.

58. Fusco NM, Parbuoni K, Morgan JA. Drug utilization, dosing, and costs after implementation of intravenous acetaminophen guidelines for pediatric patients. *J Pediatr Pharmacol Ther.* 2014;19(1):35–41.

59. Rawlins M, Henderson D, Hijab A. Pharmacokinetics of paracetamol (acetaminophen) after intravenous and oral administration. *Eur J Clin Pharmacol.* 1977;11(4):283–286.

60. McNicol E, Tzortzopoulou A, Cepeda M, Francia M, Farhat T, Schumann R. Single-dose intravenous paracetamol or propacetamol for prevention or treatment of postoperative pain: a systematic review and meta-analysis. *Br J Anaesth.* 2011;106(6):764–775.

61. Schmid RL, Sandler AN, Katz J. Use and efficacy of low-dose ketamine in the management of acute postoperative pain: a review of current techniques and outcomes. *Pain.* 1999;82(2):111–125.

62. Hollister G, Burn J. Side effects of ketamine in pediatric anesthesia. *Anesth Analg.* 1974;53(2):264–267.

63. Dahmani S, Michelet D, Abback PS, et al. Ketamine for perioperative pain management in children: a meta-analysis of published studies. *Paediatr Anaesth.* 2011;21(6):636–652.

64. Chan AKM, Cheung CW, Chong YK. Alpha-2 agonists in acute pain management. *Expert Opin Pharmacother.* 2010;11(17):2849–2868.

65. Calvillo O, Ghignone M. Presynaptic effect of clonidine on unmyelinated afferent fibers in the spinal cord of the cat. *Neurosci Lett*. 1986;64(3):335–339.

66. Correa-Sales C, Rabin BC, Maze M. A hypnotic response to dexmedetomidine, an alpha 2 agonist, is mediated in the locus coeruleus in rats. *Anesthesiology*. 1992;76(6):948–952.

67. Mikawa K, Nishina K, Maekawa N, Asano M, Obara H. Oral clonidine premedication reduces vomiting in children after strabismus surgery. *Can J Anaesth*. 1995;42(11):977–981.

68. Schmidt AP, Valinetti EA, Bandeira D, Bertacchi MF, Simoes CM, Auler JO Jr. Effects of preanesthetic administration of midazolam, clonidine, or dexmedetomidine on postoperative pain and anxiety in children. *Paediatr Anaesth*. 2007;17(7):667–674.

69. Kraemer FW, Rose JB. Pharmacologic management of acute pediatric pain. *Anesthesiol Clin*. 2009;27(2):241–268.

70. Taylor CP, Angelotti T, Fauman E. Pharmacology and mechanism of action of pregabalin: the calcium channel α 2–δ (alpha 2–delta) subunit as a target for antiepileptic drug discovery. *Epilepsy Res*. 2007;73(2):137–150.

71. Rusy LM, Hainsworth KR, Nelson TJ, et al. Gabapentin use in pediatric spinal fusion patients: a randomized, double-blind, controlled trial. *Anesth Analg*. 2010;110(5):1393–1398.

72. Lauwick S, Kim DJ, Michelagnoli G, et al. Intraoperative infusion of lidocaine reduces postoperative fentanyl requirements in patients undergoing laparoscopic cholecystectomy. *Can J Anesth*. 2008;55(11):754.

73. Mazoit JX, Denson DD, Samii K. Pharmacokinetics of bupivacaine following caudal anesthesia in infants. *Anesthesiology*. 1988;68(3):387–391.

74. Bernards CM, Hadzic A, Suresh S, Neal JM. Regional anesthesia in anesthetized or heavily sedated patients. *Reg Anesth Pain Med*. 2008;33(5):449–460.

75. Taenzer AH, Walker BJ, Bosenberg AT, et al. Asleep versus awake: does it matter? Pediatric regional block complications by patient state: a report from the Pediatric Regional Anesthesia Network. *Reg Anesth Pain Med*. 2014;39(4):279–283.

76. Lee VC, Moscicki JC, DiFazio CA. Propofol sedation produces dose-dependent suppression of lidocaine-induced seizures in rats. *Anesth Analg*. 1998;86(3):652–657.

77. Ohmura S, Ohta T, Yamamoto K, Kobayashi T. A comparison of the effects of propofol and sevoflurane on the systemic toxicity of intravenous bupivacaine in rats. *Anesth Analg*. 1999;88(1):155–159.

78. Faryniarz D, Morelli C, Coleman S, et al. Interscalene block anesthesia at an ambulatory surgery center performing predominantly regional anesthesia: a prospective study of one hundred thirty-three patients undergoing shoulder surgery. *J Shoulder Elbow Surg*. 2006;15(6):686–690.

79. Ahsan ZS, Carvalho B, Yao J. Incidence of failure of continuous peripheral nerve catheters for postoperative analgesia in upper extremity surgery. *J Hand Surg*. 2014;39(2):324–329.

80. Kwofie K, Shastri U, Vandepitte C. Standard approaches for upper extremity nerve blocks with an emphasis on outpatient surgery. *Curr Opin Anaesthesiol*. 2013;26(4):501–508.

81. Buckenmaier C. *Military Advanced Regional Anesthesia and Analgesia Handbook*. Washington, DC: Government Printing Office; 2009.

82. Mak P, Irwin M, Ooi C, Chow B. Incidence of diaphragmatic paralysis following supraclavicular brachial plexus block and its effect on pulmonary function. *Anaesthesia*. 2001;56(4):352–356.

83. Kapral S, Krafft P, Eibenberger K, Fitzgerald R, Gosch M, Weinstabl C. Ultrasound-guided supraclavicular approach for regional anesthesia of the brachial plexus. *Anesth Analg*. 1994;78(3):507–513.

84. Miller RD, Eriksson LI, Fleisher LA, Wiener-Kronish JP, Young WL. *Anesthesia.* Philadelphia: Elsevier Health Sciences; 2009.

85. Arcand G, Williams SR, Chouinard P, et al. Ultrasound-guided infraclavicular versus supraclavicular block. *Anesth Analg.* 2005;101(3):886–890.

86. Fleischmann E, Marhofer P, Greher M, Waltl B, Sitzwohl C, Kapral S. Brachial plexus anaesthesia in children: lateral infraclavicular vs axillary approach. *Pediatr Anesth.* 2003;13(2):103–108.

87. Ben-David B, Barak M, Katz Y, Stahl S. A retrospective study of the incidence of neurological injury after axillary brachial plexus block. *Pain Pract.* 2006;6(2):119–123.

88. Hadzic A. *Textbook of Regional Anesthesia and Acute Pain Management.* New York: McGraw-Hill Professional; 2007.

89. Ivani G, Mazzarello G, Lampugnani E, DeNegri P, Torre M, Lonnqvist P. Ropivacaine for central blocks in children. *Anaesthesia.* 1998;53(Suppl 2):74–76.

90. Veneziano G, Tripi J, Tumin D, et al. Femoral nerve blockade using various concentrations of local anesthetic for knee arthroscopy in the pediatric population. *J Pain Res.* 2016;9:1073.

91. Chen J-Y, Li N, Xu Y-Q. Single shot adductor canal block for postoperative analgesia of pediatric patellar dislocation surgery: a case-series report. *Medicine.* 2015;94(48).

92. Suresh S, Wheeler M. Practical pediatric regional anesthesia. *Anesthesiol Clin North Am.* 2002;20(1):83–113.

93. Miller BR. Ultrasound-guided proximal tibial paravenous saphenous nerve block in pediatric patients. *Pediatr Anesth.* 2010;20(11):1059–1060.

94. Shah R, Suresh S. Applications of regional anaesthesia in paediatrics. *Br J Anaesth.* 2013;111(Suppl 1):i114–i124.

95. Jöhr M. The right thing in the right place: lumbar plexus block in children. *J Am Soc Anesthesiologists.* 2005;102(4):865–866.

96. Giaufre E, Dalens B, Gombert A. Epidemiology and morbidity of regional anesthesia in children: a one-year prospective survey of the French-Language Society of Pediatric Anesthesiologists. *Anesth Analg.* 1996;83(5):904–912.

97. Patel D. Epidural analgesia for children. *Cont Educ Anaesth Crit Care Pain.* 2006;6(2):63–66.

98. Lerman J, Nolan J, Eyres R, et al. Efficacy, safety, and pharmacokinetics of levobupivacaine with and without fentanyl after continuous epidural infusion in children: a multicenter trial. *J Am Soc Anesthesiologists.* 2003;99(5):1166–1174.

99. Oliver J-A, Oliver L-A. Beyond the caudal: truncal blocks an alternative option for analgesia in pediatric surgical patients. *Curr Opin Anaesthesiol.* 2013;26(6):644–651.

100. Orebaugh SL, Bigeleisen PE. *Ultrasound-Guided Regional Anesthesia and Pain Medicine.* New York: Lippincott Williams & Wilkins; 2009.

101. Yuen PM, Ng PS. Retroperitoneal hematoma after a rectus sheath block. *J Am Assoc Gynecol Laparoscopists.* 2004;11(4):448.

102. Dingeman RS, Barus LM, Chung HK, et al. Ultrasonography-guided bilateral rectus sheath block vs local anesthetic infiltration after pediatric umbilical hernia repair: a prospective randomized clinical trial. *JAMA Surg.* 2013;148(8):707–713.

103. Kendigelen P, Tutuncu AC, Erbabacan E, et al. Ultrasound-assisted transversus abdominis plane block vs wound infiltration in pediatric patient with inguinal hernia: randomized controlled trial. *J Clin Anesth.* 2016;30:9–14.

104. Lorenzo AJ, Lynch J, Matava C, El-Beheiry H, Hayes J. Ultrasound guided transversus abdominis plane vs surgeon administered intraoperative regional field infiltration with bupivacaine for early postoperative pain control in children undergoing open pyeloplasty. *J Urol.* 2014;192(1):207–213.

105. Suresh S, Chan VW. Ultrasound guided transversus abdominis plane block in infants, children and adolescents: a simple procedural guidance for their performance. *Pediatr Anesth*. 2009;19(4):296–299.

106. Jankovic ZB, du Feu FM, McConnell P. An anatomical study of the transversus abdominis plane block: location of the lumbar triangle of Petit and adjacent nerves. *Anesth Analg*. 2009;109(3):981–985.

107. Fredrickson MJ, Paine C, Hamill J. Improved analgesia with the ilioinguinal block compared to the transversus abdominis plane block after pediatric inguinal surgery: a prospective randomized trial. *Pediatr Anesth*. 2010;20(11):1022–1027.

108. Bærentzen F, Maschmann C, Jensen K, Belhage B, Hensler M, Børglum J. Ultrasound-guided nerve block for inguinal hernia repair: a randomized, controlled, double-blind study. *Reg Anesth Pain Med*. 2012;37(5):502–507.

109. Abdellatif AA. Ultrasound-guided ilioinguinal/iliohypogastric nerve blocks versus caudal block for postoperative analgesia in children undergoing unilateral groin surgery. *Saudi J Anaesth*. 2012;6(4):367–372.

110. Tsui BC, Suresh S. Ultrasound imaging for regional anesthesia in infants, children, and adolescents: a review of current literature and its application in the practice of extremity and trunk blocks. *J Am Soc Anesthesiologists*. 2010;112(2):473–492.

111. HONG JY, Kim W, Koo B, Kim Y, Jo Y, Kil H. The relative position of ilioinguinal and iliohypogastric nerves in different age groups of pediatric patients. *Acta Anaesthesiol Scand*. 2010;54(5):566–570.

112. Vaisman J. Pelvic hematoma after an ilioinguinal nerve block for orchialgia. *Anesth Analg*. 2001;92(4):1048–1049.

113. Johr M, Sossai R. Colonic puncture during ilioinguinal nerve block in a child. *Anesth Analg*. 1999;88(5):1051–1052.

114. Dalens B, Hasnaoui A. Caudal anesthesia in pediatric surgery: success rate and adverse effects in 750 consecutive patients. *Anesth Analg*. 1989;68(2):83–89.

115. Ansermino M, Basu R, Vandebeek C, Montgomery C. Nonopioid additives to local anaesthetics for caudal blockade in children: a systematic review. *Paediatr Anaesth*. 2003;13(7):561–573.

116. Wulf H, Peters C, Behnke H. The pharmacokinetics of caudal ropivacaine 0.2% in children. *Anaesthesia*. 2000;55(8):757–760.

117. Lee JJ, Rubin AP. Comparison of a bupivacaine-clonidine mixture with plain bupivacaine for caudal analgesia in children. *Br J Anaesth*. 1994;72(3):258–262.

118. Rowney DA, Doyle E. Epidural and subarachnoid blockade in children. *Anaesthesia*. 1998;53(10):980–1001.

119. Goeller JK, Bhalla T, Tobias JD. Combined use of neuraxial and general anesthesia during major abdominal procedures in neonates and infants. *Paediatr Anaesth*. 2014;24(6):553–560.

120. Karmakar MK, Ho AM. Postthoracotomy pain syndrome. *Thorac Surg Clin*. 2004;14(3):345–352.

121. Tug R, Ozcengiz D, Günes Y. Single level paravertebral versus caudal block in paediatric inguinal surgery. *Anaesthes Intensive Care*. 2011;39(5):909.

122. Visoiu M, Cassara A, Yang CI. Bilateral paravertebral blockade (T7-10) versus incisional local anesthetic administration for pediatric laparoscopic cholecystectomy: a prospective, randomized clinical study. *Anesth Analg*. 2015;120(5):1106–1113.

123. Koehler RP, Keenan RJ. Management of postthoracotomy pain: acute and chronic. *Thorac Surg Clin*. 2006;16(3):287–297.

124. Khelemsky Y, Noto CJ. Preventing post-thoracotomy pain syndrome. *Mt Sinai J Med*. 2012;79(1):133–139.

125. d'Amours RH, Riegler FX, Little AG. Pathogenesis and management of persistent postthoracotomy pain. *Chest Surg Clin North Am.* 1998;8(3):703–722.

126. Hazelrigg S, Landreneau R, Boley T, et al. The effect of muscle-sparing versus standard posterolateral thoracotomy on pulmonary function, muscle strength, and postoperative pain. *J Thorac Cardiovasc Surg.* 1991;101(3):394–400; discussion 400–391.

127. Ochroch EA, Gottschalk A, Augoustides JG, Aukburg SJ, Kaiser LR, Shrager JB. Pain and physical function are similar following axillary, muscle-sparing vs posterolateral thoracotomy. *Chest J.* 2005;128(4):2664–2670.

128. Kruger M, McRae K. Pain management in cardiothoracic practice. *Surg Clin North Am.* 1999;79(2):387–400.

129. Block BM, Liu SS, Rowlingson AJ, Cowan AR, Cowan JA Jr, Wu CL. Efficacy of postoperative epidural analgesia: a meta-analysis. *JAMA.* 2003;290(18):2455–2463.

130. Soto RG, Fu ES. Acute pain management for patients undergoing thoracotomy. *Ann Thorac Surg.* 2003;75(4):1349–1357.

131. Ochroch EA, Gottschalk A. Impact of acute pain and its management for thoracic surgical patients. *Thorac Surg Clin.* 2005;15(1):105–121.

132. Berrisford RG, Sabanathan SS. Direct access to the paravertebral space at thoracotomy. *Ann Thorac Surg.* 1990;49(5):854.

133. Merskey H. International Association for the Study of Pain. Subcommittee on Taxonomy. Classification of chronic pain: descriptions of chronic pain syndromes and definitions of pain terms. *Pain Suppl.* 1986;3:S1–26.

134. Pluijms W, Steegers M, Verhagen A, Scheffer G, Wilder-Smith O. Chronic post-thoracotomy pain: a retrospective study. *Acta Anaesthesiol Scand.* 2006;50(7):804–808.

135. Kalso E, Perttunen K, Kaasinen S. Pain after thoracic surgery. *Acta Anaesthesiol Scand.* 1992;36(1):96–100.

136. Conacher I. Pain relief after thoracotomy. *Br J Anaesth.* 1990;65(6):806–812.

137. Wildgaard K, Ravn J, Kehlet H. Chronic post-thoracotomy pain: a critical review of pathogenic mechanisms and strategies for prevention. *Eur J Cardiothorac Surg.* 2009;36(1):170–180.

138. Landreneau RJ, Mack MJ, Hazelrigg SR, et al. Prevalence of chronic pain after pulmonary resection by thoracotomy or video-assisted thoracic surgery. *J Thorac and Cardiovasc Surg.* 1994;107(4):1079–1086.

139. Furrer M, Rechsteiner R, Eigenmann V, Signer C, Althaus U, Ris H. Thoracotomy and thoracoscopy: postoperative pulmonary function, pain and chest wall complaints. *Eur J Cardiothorac Surg.* 1997;12(1):82–87.

140. Dahl JB, Kehlet H. Preventive analgesia. *Curr Opin Anesthesiol.* 2011;24(3):331–338.

141. Sentürk M, Özcan PE, Talu GK, et al. The effects of three different analgesia techniques on long-term postthoracotomy pain. *Anesth Analg.* 2002;94(1):11–15.

142. Ochroch EA, Gottschalk A, Augostides J, et al. Long-term pain and activity during recovery from major thoracotomy using thoracic epidural analgesia. *J Am Soc Anesthesiologists.* 2002;97(5):1234–1244.

143. Vila Jr H, Liu J, Kavasmaneck D. Paravertebral block: new benefits from an old procedure. *Curr Opin Anesthesiol.* 2007;20(4):316–318.

144. Przewlocki R, Przewlocka B. Opioids in neuropathic pain. *Curr Pharmaceut Design.* 2005;11(23):3013–3025.

145. Solak O, Metin M, Esme H, et al. Effectiveness of gabapentin in the treatment of chronic post-thoracotomy pain. *Eur J Cardiothorac Surg.* 2007;32(1):9–12.

146. Dworkin RH, O'connor AB, Audette J, et al. Recommendations for the pharmacological management of neuropathic pain: an overview and literature update. Paper presented at: Mayo Clinic Proceedings, 2010.

14 Nonpharmacologic Management of Postsurgical Pain

Jessica Carter and Srinivas Pyati

INTRODUCTION

Multimodal Therapy

As a component of a multimodal analgesic approach, psychological and behavioral interventions are gaining popularity and importance with a goal to reduce the doses of the analgesics consumed during the perioperative period.[1] In this chapter, we review the use of neurostimulation, including transcutaneous electrical stimulation (TENS), in the postoperative period. While TENS therapy has quickly become a mainstay for the treatment of chronic pain, several alternative therapies have been trialed in postoperative patients.

The concomitant use of allopathic and alternative therapies is frequently referred to as complementary medicine, defined by the National Center for Complementary and Integrative Health.[2] The evidence supporting and challenging the use of music therapy, acupuncture, aromatherapy, and mind-body techniques as postoperative pain therapy adjuncts is also presented. Ultimately, the goal of this chapter is to broaden perspectives on possible components of a multimodal, patient-centered regimen that includes pharmacologic and nonpharmacologic therapies to improve the postoperative experience.

Brief History of Complementary Medicine

Alternative medicine strategies have existed for thousands of years. They often coexisted with what is now referred to as allopathic medicine until the Flexner report was published in 1910. This report promoted a focus on biomedical sciences and hands-on clinical training[3] and helped to catalyze the marginalization of alternative medical strategies. However, in the early 2000s, after the Institute of Medicine published a report that nearly one-third of Americans had used alternative medical therapies in their lifetime, academic medical institutions again began to develop an interest in integrative medicine.[4] Between 1991 and 2008, 30 academic integrative health centers were established.[5] This trend has been closely followed by increased clinical trials and observational studies to investigate the role of complementary therapies for the treatment of a variety of medical conditions. In this chapter we review the application of these complementary therapies in the postsurgical patient population with the ultimate goal of creating practical applications.

INTERVENTIONS

Neurostimulation

Transcutaneous Electrical Nerve Stimulation

Perhaps one of the most widely trialed nonpharmacologic pain management strategies for chronic pain is TENS therapy. TENS therapy is the application of low-voltage electrical current to the skin at various frequencies and intensity.[6] Common TENS therapy frequency patterns include continuous, burst, high-frequency, and low-rate frequency, and proposed mechanisms include central activation of opioid, muscarinic, and serotonergic receptors.[7-9] The success of TENS therapy in treating neuropathic and myofascial pain syndromes is a natural segue into acute pain therapy.[10]

One of the earliest studies of TENS therapy after abdominal surgery was conducted by Cuschieri et al. in 1985. In a study including 106 patients randomized to either TENS therapy or sham after open abdominal surgery, a modified rectangular fixed pulse width and rate was used twice daily for the first three postoperative days. This study excluded any patients with a comorbid psychiatric diagnosis or previous history of opioid use. The outcomes assessed were pain score, oxygen and carbon dioxide tension, and intramuscular morphine requirement over first three postoperative days. Additionally, the authors assessed the rate of chest infection after surgery. Interestingly, no difference between the treatment and sham groups was shown.[11] Because of their limited exclusion criteria, it is possible that this study failed to identify the specific patient subpopulations that would most benefit from TENS therapy. A specific example of this contrast was reported in a study by Ali et al., which excluded smokers and obese patients, that reported decreased analgesic doses in the TENS versus control group in the first 72 hours.[12]

A more recent randomized study in open living-donor kidney surgery compared TENS therapy to placebo as well. With a total of 74 patients, a significant reduction in pain intensity, increase in respiratory muscle strength, and increase in vital capacity were reported in the TENS group. This study excluded patients with a history chronic lung disease, surgical reintervention within the data collection period, and death within six hours of surgery. The results were promising: the interventional group had significantly better outcomes.[13] Similar positive results were reported in a post-thoracotomy pain population observed from postoperative day zero to two.[14] Additionally, in a meta-analysis of TENS therapy after thoracic surgery that included nine studies, seven studies supported TENS as an excellent pain therapy in combination with narcotics. While TENS therapy alone was ineffective in treating severe post-thoracotomy pain, the use of TENS after thoracoscopic surgeries may be appropriate. TENS therapy along with narcotics decreased total narcotic dose, improved tolerance of chest physiotherapy, and improved forced vital capacity.[15]

Though large, multicenter, prospective randomized trials are still lacking, as well as investigations into the best frequency, duration, and interval of TENS therapy, the reduced opioid consumption in postoperative patients is a promising outcome. TENS therapies is also a feasible long-term intervention with a low side-effect profile. However, important relative contraindications to TENS therapy are implantable cardiodefibrillator device and pacemakers, as TENS machines can interact unfavorably with these devices.[16] Lastly, TENS units are portable patient-administered therapies that can be used in a variety of settings, including after patients return to work, without similar increase risk in the workplace that is more commonly associated with more sedating pharmacological pain therapies.

Acupuncture

Acupuncture is a form of Eastern medicine that stimulates certain anatomical points using a variety of stimuli. Generally, needles are inserted and manipulated manually or connected to electrical stimulation.[17] Acupuncture needles, as postulated by Pomeranz and Stux, stimulate A-delta thereby interrupting ascending pain transmission in the spinal cord, trigger midbrain structures to send descending inhibitory signals within the spinothalamic tract, and stimulate the pituitary-hypothalamic complex to release beta endorphins and adrenocortical hormone (Figure 14.1).[18]

Acupuncture in the postoperative period has shown promising results when performed by experienced practitioners.[19] It has been shown to be a relatively cost-effective therapy compared to other interventions in the chronic pain setting.[20,21] Acupuncture not only can treat postoperative pain but can also help prevent and treat postoperative nausea and vomiting and postoperative ileus.[19,22,23] In a meta-analysis by Asher et al., acupuncture was shown to decrease postoperative analgesic use and pain intensity.[24]

Specifically, breast surgery patients who had access to acupuncture therapy throughout the duration of their hospital stay had significantly lower anxiety, muscular discomfort, and pain. In a study by Mallory and colleagues, acupuncture was offered from postoperative day 1 throughout the duration of the hospital stay. The participants reported pain using the visual analog scale and a satisfaction survey before and after each visit. This group also was able to integrate acupuncture into a busy clinical setting; in fact, the only two patients who dropped out of this study did so due to scheduling difficulties. Additionally, all of the patients in this study reported high patient satisfaction scores.[25]

Another common general surgical procedure is inguinal hernia repair. Taghavi et al. performed a prospective, randomized trial including 90 male patients. Their postoperative pain was assessed by a blinded observer. They compared acupuncture needle placement alone at LI4 and SD36 versus electroacupuncture offered at 0.5 hours preoperatively and at 1 and 2 hours postoperatively. Not only did the electroacupuncture group have decreased opioid requirements and decreased pain intensity, but they also reported decreased opioid-related dizziness and nausea.[26]

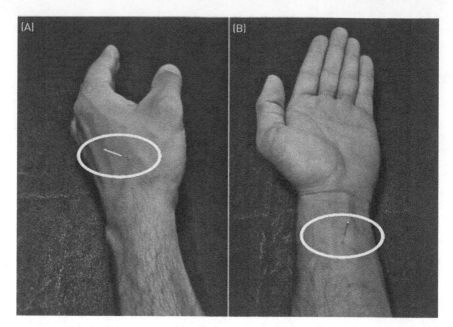

FIGURE 14.1. (A) Hegu-LI4. Stimulation of this point has antinociceptive effects for head and neck. (B) Neiguan-Pc6. Stimulation of this point can decrease postoperative nausea and vomiting and decrease myocardial ischemia in patients with CAD.[66] Reprinted with permission from Elsevier.

A third study, comparing manual versus electroacupuncture, has also been performed during the postoperative period after thyroid surgery for benign lesions. Iacabone et al. randomized 121 patients to three groups, excluding those with severe OA (osteoarthritis), myofascial pain syndromes, and previous head or neck trauma: no acupuncture or manual or electrical acupuncture point stimulations were employed. The only co-analgesics offered to these patients were acetaminophen and ketorolac. The pain intensity was only significantly decreased inpatients in the electroacupuncture group when compared to the control. Both manual and electroacupuncture patients used significantly less acetaminophen on postoperative days 2 and 3. This study, while excluding malignancy, is unique in comparing manual versus electroacupuncture.[27]

A systematic review by Sun et al. identified 126 studies published from 1966 to 2007, of which 15 fit the inclusion criteria, on the use of acupuncture for postoperative pain. They reported that acupuncture not only decreased pain intensity but also attenuated opioid-related side effects, such as nausea, pruritis, and sedation.[28] Similarly, a larger and more recent meta-analysis by Liu and colleagues ultimately included 59 randomized controlled trials conducted from 1986 to 2014 using acupuncture-point stimulation for postoperative pain control after any type of surgery. While insufficient evidence was found to support that acupuncture-point stimulation can decrease pain intensity, it was consistently linked to decreased analgesic requirements. No serious adverse events were reported; however, discomfort and pain at the insertion site, minor bruising, and constitutional symptoms were reported. Some of the limitations highlighted in this meta-analysis include short follow-up periods, participant and interventions variability, and overall lack of rigorous methodological quality.[29] One large barrier to methodological rigor is the challenge of performing double-blinded trials. While, sham needles do exist, nearly 70% of patients and 85% of practitioners were able distinguish treatment versus sham acupuncture stimulation.[30] Finally, though rare, acupuncture is not without risk; infection, hemothorax, and pneumothorax have been documented.[31-34]

While acupuncture requires access to a trained practitioner in the postoperative period, clinical nurses, pain management physicians, and physical therapists can be trained to perform basic acupuncture-point stimulation. Acupuncture has also been repeatedly shown to be a relatively cost-effective intervention compared to some conventional therapies. Acupuncture carries a low side-effect profile and has been used for thousands of years in Eastern medicine. It can be integrated into a postsurgical ward and could likely also be integrated into a rehabilitation process after surgery.

Music Therapy

The American Music Therapy Association defines music therapy as the clinical and evidence-based use of music interventions to accomplish individualized goals within a therapeutic relationship by a credentialed professional who has completed an approved music therapy program to address physical, emotional, cognitive, and social needs of individuals.[35] Across all human cultures, music is an integral part of various ritual activities, social organization, and caregiving and influences group cohesion.[36] There is evidence that music therapy can reduce postoperative anxiety, analgesic use, and pain scores.[37-39] While some studies say music selected by the patients is preferred, others highlight the importance of a music therapist in choosing the most effective musical rhythms.[40-42]

Akin to dosing long-acting oral analgesics prior to surgery, using music therapy preoperatively to influence the postoperative period has been studied. In a study that randomized 54 healthy patients to two groups, self-selected music versus none, the patients who listened to music in the preoperative setting had lower bispectral index values after midazolam dosing.[43] Preoperative music therapy has also been correlated to less postoperative pain intensity, anxiety, and analgesic demands after colorectal surgery.[44]

Music therapy in same-day surgery pediatric patients is also correlated to attenuated pain scores and stress response. In a 42-patient study, children were randomized to either no music as a control or classical music as an intervention in the recovery period. Those children exposed to the intervention had an attenuated blood glucose rise, lower blood pressure, and lower FLACC (face, legs, activity, cry, consolability) scores.[45]

Music therapy has been studied in adult ambulatory postoperative laparoscopic cholecystectomy patients. One researcher-chosen musical selection was used for all patients in a music pillow placed behind the head from the preoperative area until discharge. Interesting, music therapy showed a significant influence on pain intensity on postoperative day 7, not 1.[46] Lastly, Matsota et al. suggested that music therapy in the perioperative setting depends on the patient's severity of pain stimulus and disposition.[47] Similar results were reported for a study including 151 patients having variceal surgery or herniotomy, in which those patients who were randomized to listen to music intraoperatively and postoperatively had lower pain intensity and decreased morphine requirements.[48]

A meta-analysis by Hole et al. examined 73 randomized controlled trials that used music as therapy in the perioperative period. This group reported that timing and choice of delivery mode had little effect on outcomes. The most important outcomes were that music decreased pain scores, decreased analgesic use, and improved patient satisfaction but did not affect length of stay. Music was also found to improve outcomes when used intraoperatively for patients under a general anesthetic.[39]

Finally, given the increasing knowledge about the phenomenon of immuno-suppression after surgical stress, there is evidence that music therapy may have immunomodulation properties.[49] In a small study that measured salivary cortisol in patients randomized to either one hour of postoperative music or standard care, those patients in the music group had significantly less salivary cortisol. This may indicate an attenuated stress response. However, the long-term implication of this change was not investigated due to a short follow-up period.[50] These findings are supported by a study that included 75 patients scheduled for open hernia repair. The patients were randomized to receive silence, intraoperative music, or postoperative music. There was a significant difference in pain intensity and serum cortisol levels two hours after surgery in those patients who received postoperative music therapy as compared to controls.[51]

Ultimately, music therapy is a helpful tool that can be low cost, improve patient satisfaction, decrease pain intensity, and decrease postoperative opioid requirements. Still, there are still no specific indications or contraindications to music therapy. Additionally, further studies to identify the neurological action of music therapy would be helpful to develop standardized patient protocols for its use in the postoperative period.

Aromatherapy

There is very little data on aromatherapy as an adjunct therapy for postoperative pain. Most studies involving aromatherapy in the postoperative period focus on its role to prevent and treat postoperative nausea and vomiting and decrease perceived stress.[52-54] After coronary artery bypass surgery, lavender essential oil inhalation had no effect on postoperative pain reduction.[52,55] Similarly, after breast biopsy lavender oil did not affect analgesic use or time to discharge but was associated with higher patient satisfaction scores.[56] Certainly, the data do not yet support a role for aromatherapy as a pain therapy adjunct, but this modality could still be considered for addressing other common postoperative patient complaints, such as postoperative nausea and vomiting.

Mind-Body Interventions

Mind-body therapies are defined as "interactions among the brain, the rest of the body, the mind, and behavior, and examination of the ways in which emotional, mental, social, spiritual, experiential, and behavioral factors can directly affect health."[57] Mind-body interventions have been investigated in a variety of chronic pain states: chronic low back pain, fibromyalgia, failed back surgery syndrome, chronic pain, musculo-skeletal pain, and diabetic neuropathy.[58,59] These interventions, including hypnosis, imagery, biofeedback, and mirror feedback, have also been reported sparingly in the postoperative setting for abdominal surgery, phantom limb pain, and breast surgery. However, mind-body interventions in the postoperative period are sparse and poorly powered.

Hypnosis, or the "set of techniques designed to enhance concentration, minimize one's usual distractions, and heighten responsiveness to suggestions to alter one's thoughts, feelings, behavior, or physiological state," has also been reported sparingly in the postoperative period.[60] Some research into the neurophysiology of the post-hypnotic state indicates an important role of the anterior cingulate cortex. This area of the brain is involved in executive attention, error detection, and mediating conflict between competing cognitive processes.[61] In an experimental pain study, posthypnosis patients failed to activate the anterior cingulate cortex and associated somatosensory cortical brain tissue when exposed to a painful stimulus, unlike their control counterparts.[62] In a clinical hypnosis therapy, a group of patients undergoing breast biopsy underwent hypnosis prior to surgery. Ninety patients were randomized to either a 15-minute presurgical hypnosis suggestion or a 15-minute attention control session. While excisional biopsies are not considered extremely painful surgeries, the anxiety of the patient due to the threat of cancer can complicate postoperative pain management. Those patients who received presurgical hypnosis had both reduced pain and anxiety.[63]

Lastly, one of the most interesting studies into mind-body therapies is the delivery of complimentary therapies via mobile devices. A novel study in Iceland randomized 105 same-day surgery patients to one of five groups: standard therapy, audio relaxation, music therapy, nature videos plus music therapy, or nature videos without music therapy. They were exposed to each intervention for 15 minutes twice daily during the first four postoperative days. Compared to controls, the findings were not significant in terms of pain intensity or anxiety; however, this study highlights the feasibility of offering these therapies to patients remotely. Mobile delivery, after more research into optimal use and patient populations, may increase the number of patients who can receive therapy with a limited supply of trained practitioners.[64]

The limitations to hypnosis research are that it is difficult to perform a double-blinded trial. Further, mind-body interventions, like biofeedback and guided imagery, require trained professionals as facilitators. Still, based on the currently available literature, no recommendations on the use of these therapies can be made. Among all of the interventions discussed in this chapter, mind-body interventions in the postoperative period have the greatest need for further large-scale trials with adequate follow-up.

CONCLUSION AND RECOMMENDATIONS

Postsurgical pain control improves comfort and patient satisfaction, facilitates return to normal activities, results in reduced morbidity, and can decrease the likelihood of developing chronic pain conditions.[65] Ultimately, multimodal analgesia allows decreased patient exposure to opioids, which have many unwanted side effects. Optimal postsurgical pain management will continue to rely on multimodal, patient-centered regimens focused on setting expectations preoperatively and pharmacologic and patient-selected nonpharmacologic solutions. The evidence for nonpharmacological therapies in the postoperative period varies in strength and generalizability. More well-powered, randomized, controlled trials are needed, especially in acupuncture, aromatherapy, music therapy, and mind-body interventions, in order to create indications, contraindications, and dosing and administration recommendations for their use in the postoperative period. Additionally, many of the therapies discussed in this chapter are unfamiliar to Western providers, and bias toward evidence-based medicine is often a barrier to their incorporation into practice. Conversely, patient bias toward conventional medical therapies, especially in the age of advertising medication on television, may also be a barrier to using integrative medicine strategies. The solution, however, relies on consistent patient education. Finally, to improve patient-centered outcomes and Hospital Consumer Assessment of Healthcare Providers and Systems scores, adequate acute pain management involves a collaborative effort and a multidisciplinary and integrative approach.

Some recommendations to practically integrate TENS and alternative therapeutic interventions into the postoperative period include the following.

1. Coordination of multimodal pain management plans that incorporate pharmacological and nonpharmacological interventions is best accomplished in a multidisciplinary team model led by a dedicated acute pain management consult service.
2. In the preoperative period, patients should receive teaching on TENS therapy from physical therapists.
3. TENS therapy, acupuncture, music therapy, and mind-body interventions are safe and cost-effective interventions with minimal adverse effects.
4. Patient and provider bias favoring conventional medical therapies can be mediated by novel education programs.
5. Partnership development with local integrative medicine centers can maximize the ability to provide acupuncture, aromatherapy, and other alternative therapies in the postoperative inpatient and postanesthesia recovery contexts.
6. Integrative medicine strategies and improved pain control are correlated to improved patient satisfaction even when they do not decrease opioid requirements.

REFERENCES

1. Kumar M, Kumar J, Saxena I. The role of mental distraction on the pain response in healthy young Indian adults. *J Clin Diagn Res.* 2012;6:1648–1652.
2. Complementary, alternative, or integrative health: what's in a name? In: *National Center for Complementary and Integrative Health*, Vol. 2016. Washington, DC: U.S. Department of Health & Human Services, National Institutes of Health; 2008. https://nccih.nih.gov/sites/nccam.nih.gov/files/Whats_In_A_Name_08-11-2015.pdf
3. Flexner A. Medical education in the United States and Canada: A report to the Carnegie Foundation for the Advancement of Teaching. In: *The Carnegie Foundation for the Advancement of Teaching*, Bulletin No. 4 346. New York; 1910.
4. Barnes PM, Bloom B, Nahin RL. Complementary and alternative medicine use among adults and children: United States, 2007. *Natl Health Stat Rep.* 2008:1–23.

5. Ehrlich G, Callender T, Gaster B. Integrative medicine at academic health centers: a survey of clinicians' educational backgrounds and practices. *Fam Med.* 2013;45:330–334.

6. DeSantana JM, Walsh DM, Vance C, Rakel BA, Sluka KA. Effectiveness of transcutaneous electrical nerve stimulation for treatment of hyperalgesia and pain. *Curr Rheumatol Rep.* 2008;10:492–499.

7. Sluka KA, Lisi TL, Westlund KN. Increased release of serotonin in the spinal cord during low, but not high, frequency transcutaneous electric nerve stimulation in rats with joint inflammation. *Arch Phys Med Rehab.* 2006;87:1137–1140.

8. Sluka KA, Deacon M, Stibal A, Strissel S, Terpstra A. Spinal blockade of opioid receptors prevents the analgesia produced by TENS in arthritic rats. *J Pharmacol Exp Ther.* 1999;289:840–846.

9. Tulgar M, McGlone F, Bowsher D, Miles JB. Comparative effectiveness of different stimulation modes in relieving pain. Part II. A double-blind controlled long-term clinical trial. *Pain.* 1991;47:157–162.

10. Johnson M, Martinson M. Efficacy of electrical nerve stimulation for chronic musculoskeletal pain: a meta-analysis of randomized controlled trials. *Pain.* 2007;130:157–165.

11. Cuschieri RJ, Morran CG, McArdle CS. Transcutaneous electrical stimulation for postoperative pain. *Ann Royal Coll Surgeons Engl.* 1985;67:127–129.

12. Ali J, Yaffe CS, Serrette C. The effect of transcutaneous electric nerve stimulation on postoperative pain and pulmonary function. *Surgery.* 1981;89:507–512.

13. Galli TT, Chiavegato LD, Liebano RE. Effects of TENS in living kidney donors submitted to open nephrectomy: a randomized placebo-controlled trial. *Eur J Pain.* 2015;19:67–76.

14. Fiorelli A, Milione R, Laperuta P, et al. Control of post-thoracotomy pain by transcutaneous electrical nerve stimulation: effect on serum cytokine levels, visual analogue scale, pulmonary function and medication. *Eur J Cardiothorac Surg.* 2012;41:861–868; discussion 868.

15. Freynet A, Falcoz PE. Is transcutaneous electrical nerve stimulation effective in relieving postoperative pain after thoracotomy? *Interact Cardiovasc Thorac Surg.* 2010;10:283–288.

16. Holmgren C, Carlsson T, Mannheimer C, Edvardsson N. Risk of interference from transcutaneous electrical nerve stimulation on the sensing function of implantable defibrillators. *Pacing Clin Electrophysiol.* 2008;31:151–158.

17. Traditional Chinese medicine: in depth. In: *National Center for Complementary and Integrative Health*, Vol. 2016. Bethesda, MD: National Institutes of Health; 2009. https://nccih.nih.gov/health/whatiscam/chinesemed.htm

18. Chernyak GV, Sessler DI. Perioperative acupuncture and related techniques. *Anesthesiology.* 2005;102:1031–1049; quiz 1077–1038.

19. Gliedt JA, Daniels CJ, Wuollet A. Narrative review of perioperative acupuncture for clinicians. *J Acupunct Meridian Stud.* 2015;8:264–269.

20. Witt CM, Jena S, Selim D, et al. Pragmatic randomized trial evaluating the clinical and economic effectiveness of acupuncture for chronic low back pain. *Am J Epidemiol.* 2006;164:487–496.

21. Reinhold T, Witt CM, Jena S, Brinkhaus B, Willich SN. Quality of life and cost-effectiveness of acupuncture treatment in patients with osteoarthritis pain. *Eur J Health Econ.* 2008;9:209–219.

22. Frey UH, Funk M, Lohlein C, Peters J. Effect of P6 acustimulation on post-operative nausea and vomiting in patients undergoing a laparoscopic cholecystectomy. *Acta Anaesthesiol Scand.* 2009;53:1341–1347.

23. You XM, Mo X-S, Ma L, et al. Randomized clinical trial comparing efficacy of simo decoction and acupuncture or chewing gum alone on postoperative ileus in patients with hepatocellular carcinoma after hepatectomy. *Medicine.* 2015;94:e1968.

24. Asher GN, et al. Auriculotherapy for pain management: a systematic review and meta-analysis of randomized controlled trials. *J Altern Complement Med.* 2010;16:1097–1108.

25. Mallory MJ, et al. Acupuncture in the postoperative setting for breast cancer patients: a feasibility study. *Am J Chinese Med.* 2015;43:45–56.

26. Taghavi R, et al. The effect of acupuncture on relieving pain after inguinal surgeries. *Korean J Pain.* 2013;26:46–50.

27. Iacobone M, et al. The effects of acupuncture after thyroid surgery: a randomized, controlled trial. *Surgery.* 2014;156:1605-1612; discussion 1612–1603.

28. Sun Y, Gan TJ, Dubose JW, Habib AS. Acupuncture and related techniques for postoperative pain: a systematic review of randomized controlled trials. *Br J Anaesth.* 2008;101:151–160.

29. Liu XL, Tan JY, Molassiotis A, Suen LK, Shi Y. Acupuncture-point stimulation for postoperative pain control: a systematic review and meta-analysis of randomized controlled trials. *Evid Based Complement Altern Med.* 2015:657809.

30. Vase L, et al. Can acupuncture treatment be double-blinded? An evaluation of double-blind acupuncture treatment of postoperative pain. *PloS One.* 2015;10:e0119612.

31. He C, et al. Unusual case of pyogenic spondylodiscitis, vertebral osteomyelitis and bilateral psoas abscesses after acupuncture: diagnosis and treatment with interventional management. *Acupunct Med.* 2015;33:154–157.

32. Singh Lubana S, Alfishawy M, Singh N, Brennessel DJ. First reported case of methicillin-resistant staphylococcus aureus vertebral osteomyelitis with multiple spinal and paraspinal abscesses associated with acupuncture. *Case Rep Med.* 2015:524241.

33. Karavis MY, et al. Acupuncture-induced haemothorax: a rare iatrogenic complication of acupuncture. *Acupunct Med.* 2015;33:237–241.

34. Brogan RJ, Mushtaq F. Acupuncture-induced pneumothorax: the hidden complication. *Scott Med J.* 2015;60:e11–e13.

35. What is music therapy? In: *What Is Music Therapy,* Vol. 2016. Silver Spring MD: American Music Therapy Association; 2018. http://www.musictherapy.org/about/musictherapy/

36. Trehub SE, Becker J, Morley I. Cross-cultural perspectives on music and musicality. *Philos Trans R Soc Lond B Biol Sci.* 2015;370:20140096.

37. Kumar TS, Muthuraman M, Krishnakumar R. Effect of the raga ananda bhairavi in post operative pain relief management. *Indian J Surg.* 2014;76:363–370.

38. Liu Y, Petrini MA. Effects of music therapy on pain, anxiety, and vital signs in patients after thoracic surgery. *Complement Ther Med.* 2015;23:714–718.

39. Hole J, Hirsch M, Ball E, Meads C. Music as an aid for postoperative recovery in adults: a systematic review and meta-analysis. *Lancet.* 2015;386:1659–1671.

40. Vetter D., et al. Effects of art on surgical patients: a systematic review and meta-analysis. *Ann Surg.* 2015;262:704–713.

41. Bernatzky G, Presch M, Anderson M, Panksepp J. Emotional foundations of music as a non-pharmacological pain management tool in modern medicine. *Neurosci Biobehav Rev.* 2011;35:1989–1999.

42. Gooding L, Swezey S, Zwischenberger JB. Using music interventions in perioperative care. *South Med J.* 2012;105:486–490.

43. Ganidagli S, Cengiz M, Yanik M, Becerik C, Unal B. The effect of music on preoperative sedation and the bispectral index. *Anesth Analg.* 2005;101:103–106.

44. Tusek DL, Church JM, Strong SA, Grass JA, Fazio VW. Guided imagery: a significant advance in the care of patients undergoing elective colorectal surgery. *Dis Colon Rectum.* 1997;40:172–178.

45. Calcaterra V, et al. Music benefits on postoperative distress and pain in pediatric day care surgery. *Pediatr Rep.* 2014;6:5534.

46. Graversen M, Sommer T. Perioperative music may reduce pain and fatigue in patients undergoing laparoscopic cholecystectomy. *Acta Anaesthesiol Scand.* 2013;57:1010–1016.

47. Matsota P., et al. Music's use for anesthesia and analgesia. *J Altern Complement Med.* 2013;19:298–307.

48. Nilsson U, Rawal N, Unosson, MA. Comparison of intra-operative or postoperative exposure to music—a controlled trial of the effects on postoperative pain. *Anaesthesia.* 2003;58:699–703.

49. Kehlet H. The surgical stress response: should it be prevented? *Can J Surg.* 1991;34:565–567.

50. Miluk-Kolasa B, Obminski Z, Stupnicki R, Golec L. Effects of music treatment on salivary cortisol in patients exposed to pre-surgical stress. *Exp Clin Endocrinol.* 1994;102:118–120.

51. Nilsson U, Unosson M, Rawal N. Stress reduction and analgesia in patients exposed to calming music postoperatively: a randomized controlled trial. *Eur J Anaesthesiol.* 2005;22:96–102.

52. Bikmoradi A., et al. Effect of inhalation aromatherapy with lavender essential oil on stress and vital signs in patients undergoing coronary artery bypass surgery: a single-blinded randomized clinical trial. *Complement Ther Med.* 2015;23:331–338.

53. Braden R, Reichow S, Halm MA. The use of the essential oil lavandin to reduce preoperative anxiety in surgical patients. *J Perianesth Nurs.* 2009;24:348–355.

54. McIlvoy L., et al. The efficacy of aromatherapy in the treatment of postdischarge nausea in patients undergoing outpatient abdominal surgery. *J Perianesth Nurs.* 2015;30:383–388.

55. Salamati A, Mashouf S, Sahbaei F, Mojab F. Effects of inhalation of lavender essential oil on open-heart surgery pain. *Iran J Pharmaceutic Res.* 2014;13:1257–1261.

56. Kim JT, et al. Evaluation of aromatherapy in treating postoperative pain: pilot study. *Pain Pract.* 2006;6:273–277.

57. Mind-body medicine practices in complementary and alternative medicine. NIH Fact Sheets, Vol. 2016. Bethesda, MD: National Center for Complementary and Alternative Medicine. https://report.nih.gov/nihfactsheets/viewfactsheet.aspx?csid=102, 2010

58. Lee C, Crawford C, Hickey A. Mind-body therapies for the self-management of chronic pain symptoms. *Pain Med.* 2014;15(Suppl 1):S21–S39.

59. Jensen MP, Patterson DR. Hypnotic approaches for chronic pain management: clinical implications of recent research findings. *Am Psychologist.* 2014;69:167–177.

60. Hypnosis for the relief and control of pain. Research in Action Vol. 2016. Washington, DC: American Psychological Association; 2004. http://www.apa.org/research/action/hypnosis.aspx, 2004

61. Vanhaudenhuyse A, Laureys S, Faymonville ME. Neurophysiology of hypnosis. *Neurophysiol Clin.* 2014;44:343–353.

62. Vanhaudenhuyse A, et al. Pain and non-pain processing during hypnosis: a thulium-YAG event-related fMRI study. *Neuroimage.* 2009;47:1047–1054.

63. Montgomery GH, Weltz CR, Seltz M, Bovbjerg DH. Brief presurgery hypnosis reduces distress and pain in excisional breast biopsy patients. *Int J Clin Exp Hypn.* 50, 17–32 (2002).

64. Hansen MM. A feasibility pilot study on the use of complementary therapies delivered via mobile technologies on Icelandic surgical patients' reports of anxiety, pain, and self-efficacy in healing. *BMC Complement Altern Med.* 2015;15:92.

65. Kumar K, Wilson JR. Factors affecting spinal cord stimulation outcome in chronic benign pain with suggestions to improve success rate. *Acta Neurochirurg Suppl.* 2007;97:91–99.

66. Mayor D. An exploratory review of the electroacupuncture literature: clinical applications and endorphin mechanisms. *Acupunct Med.* 2013;31:409–415.

15 Pain Management in the Patient with Substance Use Disorder

Thomas Hickey and Jessica Feinleib

INTRODUCTION

Substance use disorders are prevalent and present unique challenges to the perioperative team. There are a wide range of abused substances, all presenting different perioperative concerns. National Institute on Drug Abuse 2015 data on adults show that 55% drink alcohol regularly, 20% smoke cigarettes, 6.5% use marijuana, 8% use illicit drugs, and approximately 1% use cocaine (https://www.drugabuse.gov/national-survey-drug-use-health). In a given year, approximately 1% of adults have been prescribed long-term opioids, and the care of these patients is often further complicated by coexisting chronic pain syndromes.[1] This chapter describes a basic team-based approach and then describes each substance in detail.

Communication

As is typical of any perioperative challenge, aggressive communication between patient, surgeon, anesthesiologist, and other clinicians (i.e. addiction medicine, primary care) is of the utmost importance. Discussions in advance of surgery should weigh risk and benefit, establish reasonable expectations about pain management, and develop a mutually agreed-upon plan. This plan should be included in the multiple nursing hand-offs that accompany the perioperative period. Surgeons and anesthesiologists should take advantage of this opportunity to provide resources to help their patients overcome their addiction.

Key Dangers

Perioperative providers should know the risks of *overdose* and *withdrawal* associated with their patient's drug addiction.

Key Benefits

A multimodal analgesia plan that delivers well-controlled postoperative analgesia reduces the likelihood of chronic postoperative pain, pulmonary and cardiovascular complications, unexpected admissions in ambulatory patients, and increased length of stay for inpatients.

SUBSTANCES

Alcohol

Caring for an alcoholic around the time of surgery is an extremely common event.

In any suspected alcoholic it is important to gather what information is known about liver function. It is helpful to remember the Model for End-Stage Liver Disease (MELD) score, which consists of serum bilirubin, serum creatinine, and INR to estimate hepatic function. Hyponatremia is another useful prognosticator. Medications metabolized by the liver (which include most analgesic medication) should be used cautiously in alcoholics suspected to have impaired hepatic function or with known cirrhosis. Acetaminophen and nonsteroidal anti-inflammatory drugs (NSAIDs) in particular should be used cautiously in cirrhosis given the increased risk of acute liver injury. An initial approach of "titration to effect," particularly with opioid medications, is reasonable.

In considering analgesics, it is worth remembering that alcoholism causes disease in multiple organ systems. Alcoholics are more likely to have cardiovascular disease, pulmonary disease, hepatic disease, anemia and coagulopathy, psychiatric disease, neurological disease, renal disease, and gastrointestinal disease including esophagitis, gastritis, and pancreatitis.

Moreover, withdrawal from chronic alcohol may confound our interpretation of a patient's postoperative pain. Withdrawal can range from mild irritability to seizure and life-threatening delirium tremens; the latter typically occurs 48 to 96 hours after the last drink. If there is concern for withdrawal, patients should recover in a setting where they are aggressively monitored for signs and symptoms of withdrawal (agitation, hyperthermia, tachycardia, arrhythmia, hypo- and hypertension, seizure). Scales including the Clinical Institute Withdrawal Assessment may assist with assessment and management. Treatment ranges from benzodiazepines and beta blockers for mild symptoms to supportive intensive care unit care for severe cases.

Benzodiazepine

Keep in mind that some benzodiazepines are used for analgesic purposes. For example, diazepam is often prescribed for its muscle relaxant properties. Patients on benzodiazepines chronically should be continued on their home doses or tapered off perioperatively. The reversal agent flumazenil can be given when an acute intoxication is suspected. On the other hand, postoperative withdrawal is characterized by anxiety, insomnia, tremors, and seizure. Be aware that the combination of a patient's home benzodiazepines and postoperative opioids, especially in the opioid-naïve patient, can result in profound respiratory depression. Such patients should not suffer from a lack of monitoring.

Tobacco

While the risks of cigarette smoking are beyond the scope of this book and chapter, it is among the most common addictions. It is well established that smoking increases the risk of nearly all postoperative complications (including wound infection, sepsis, hernia, stroke, myocardial infarction, mechanical ventilation, reintubation, pneumonia, and overall mortality), which in turn may complicate postoperative pain management. However, the main consideration in postoperative pain management is to minimize the risk of exacerbating baseline pulmonary disease. As described earlier, a multimodal analgesia technique minimizing opioid-induced respiratory depression is optimal.

Marijuana

Generally, concerns with marijuana users are two-fold. For one, there are the respiratory concerns associated with cigarette smoking. Second, patients may be using marijuana medicinally for chronic pain, which may make perioperative pain management more challenging. Medical marijuana is increasingly common in clinical practice, and its use is well supported in chronic pain, neuropathic pain, and spasticity associated with multiple sclerosis.[2] In these patients, if practical, it may be beneficial to begin, continue, or increase baseline cannabinoid use. In the future there may be a role within a multimodal analgesia strategy for cannabinoids, but strong perioperative data is not yet available. Withdrawal symptoms are mild.

Opioids/Heroin

Side effects of acute and chronic use include sedation, respiratory depression, constipation, nausea, and pruritis. Chronic users develop tolerance, which can increase overall analgesia requirements and predispose them to poorly controlled postoperative pain. Note that opioid-tolerant patients may need over twice the opioid required by the opioid-naïve patient postoperatively. A multimodal analgesia regimen such as the one suggested later should be employed.

These patients should be maintained on equianalgesic doses of their usual home opioid regimen at a minimum. An equianalgesic dosing table is included as Table 15.1, and a conversion example is provided in the next section.

Patients on chronic opioids not receiving postoperative opioids should be monitored for withdrawal. Symptoms of withdrawal include anxiety, craving, mydriasis, diaphoresis, fever, irritability, nausea, vomiting, pain, tachycardia, and hypertension. Withdrawal is rarely life-threatening.

Table 15.1. Opioid Equianalgesic Dose Chart

Opioid	PO (mg)	IV (mg)
Morphine	30	10
Oxycodone	20	NA
Hydrocodone	20	NA
Hydromorphone	7.5	1.5
Fentanyl	n/a	0.1

PO = by mouth; IV = intravenous; NA = not applicable.

Equianalgesic Conversion Example

Your patient takes 20 mg TID Oxycontin (sustained-release oxycodone) and 10 mg Q3H oxycodone PRN pain. He estimates he takes the PRN dose six times a day. You would like to convert him to a morphine infusion in recovery. First, the total daily dose of oxycodone is 60 mg (basal) + 60 mg (breakthrough) = 120 mg. From the table, we know that 20 mg oral (PO) oxycodone is equivalent to 10 mg intravenous (IV) morphine. Therefore the equianalgesic dose of morphine is 60 mg. We typically reduce that dose by 25% to account for incomplete cross-tolerance, which leaves us with 45 mg morphine. Over 24 hours that would give us an infusion rate of approximately 1.9 mg/hour. (Note that this would not be a common prescription for postoperative analgesia; it is provided here only as an example of converting between one opioid and another.)

Management of Opioid-Related Side Effects

An opioid-sparing, multimodal analgesia plan such as the one described earlier is the most effective overall way to reduce side effects. A bowel regimen including a mild laxative and stool softener should be initiated along with opioids. Ondansetron (4 mg IV Q6H), scopolamine patch (Q72H), metoclopramide (10 mg IV Q6H), prochlorperazine (25 mg PR Q12H), or haloperidol (1 mg IV Q6H) may be useful for nausea and vomiting. Pruritis should be treated with a partial opioid antagonist such as nalbuphine (5 mg IV Q6H) rather than an antihistamine. True allergies to opioids are a rare, but in these cases an opioid of another class can be chosen. Sedation and delirium are best treated by reducing opioids and other sedatives as tolerated.

Management of Opioid-Induced Respiratory Depression

Management should start with an assessment at the bedside and discontinuation of opioid-containing medications. A patient who is somnolent with SaO2 < 90% and a respiratory rate <5 despite stimulation deserves the attention of an emergency response team. The arousable patient should be monitored in-person until stable for at least 30 minutes. For the arousable patient who becomes unstable, an emergency response is indicated. Emergency responders in any case should assist the patient's ventilation, administer supplemental oxygen as needed, and administer naloxone. An ampule of naloxone (0.4 mg) should be diluted in 9 cc of normal saline for a final 40 mcg/cc concentration; 1 to 2 cc boluses should be given every few minutes until an appropriate clinical response is seen. Note that naloxone's half-life is less than most opioids, requiring that the patient be monitored closely for subsequent respiratory depression with additional naloxone at the ready.

Buprenorphine

Patients with opioid addiction are increasingly prescribed opioid partial agonists such as buprenorphine and naltrexone. Buprenorphine, the ingredient of interest in suboxone, has a modest analgesic effect, but its major relevance in perioperative pain management is that it binds the opioid receptor so tightly that the typical opioid medications (fentanyl, oxycodone, hydromorphone) have very little effect unless huge doses are used. Thus, if more than mild postoperative pain is expected, buprenorphine should ideally be discontinued for 72 hours so that its effect can "wear off." Note that the prescriber will be rightly concerned with relapse and withdrawal, necessitating a carefully coordinated interdisciplinary plan around each patient, weighing the risk of relapse and withdrawal against the benefit of better postoperative analgesia. If there is concern for withdrawal, the prescriber may give the patient another opioid to take over the 72-hour abstinence period as needed. Patients who present for surgery still on buprenorphine may require *very* high doses of opioids to achieve any effect. A patient receiving those high doses while the effect of the buprenorphine is dissipating are a set-up for opioid-induced respiratory depression. Thus, these patients' respiratory status should be monitored closely postoperatively.

For the patient in whom minimal postoperative pain is expected, buprenorphine can be continued perioperatively with acute pain managed with a multimodal strategy. The buprenorphine dosing can be increased for additional analgesia; however, note that a ceiling for analgesia is reached at a dose of 32 mg/day.[3]

Naltrexone

This is a full opioid antagonist used in opioid and alcohol use disorders. A similar approach to buprenorphine should be employed. That is, patients should hold their once-daily dosing for at least 48 hours, ideally 72 hours, prior to surgery to allow sufficient time to elapse to allow opioids to be used effectively. Note that the effect of intramuscular naltrexone is clinically significant for 30 days. Elective surgery expected to cause more than mild postoperative pain should be delayed for 30 days from the last dose if possible.

Methadone

Methadone is an opioid commonly used to treat both opioid addiction and chronic pain. It is especially effective for the latter in that it acts not only at the opioid receptor but via a number of other mechanisms, including at the N-methyl-D-aspartate receptor. Patients on methadone for pain are typically on a Q8H dosing schedule, whereas once-daily dosing in the opioid-dependent patient is sufficient to prevent withdrawal. Clinicians should be aware of the stigma historically associated with methadone.

Patients on home methadone should be continued perioperatively and acute pain supplemented by a multimodal strategy including other opioids. If patients are unable to take oral methadone postoperatively, they can be given it via IV; the most common initial ratio for conversion from oral to IV is 2:1. Some patients may require gradual dose escalation after conversion.

High doses of methadone may cause QT prolongation. It is reasonable to record a baseline EKG on initiation of therapy and begin monitoring the QT interval if patients are increased to greater than 200 mg/day. Methadone can be lethal in patients predisposed to Torsade de Pointe, a type of arrhythmia. Also, given its long half-life, methadone takes three to five days to achieve a steady state. Escalation of doses can cause their individual effects to "stack," potentially causing sedation and respiratory depression. Initiating or adjusting methadone doses should be done in consultation with an acute pain service.

Stimulants

Cocaine increases circulating catecholamines, potentially leading to hypertension, tachycardia, arrhythmia, myocardial infarction, paranoia, psychosis, seizure, stroke, aortic dissection, QTc prolongation, and respiratory depression. Cocaine withdrawal is typically mild, and the immediate symptoms range widely from anxiety and irritability to dysphoria and exhaustion, followed by lethargy. Cocaine and other stimulants, such as amphetamines, do not appear to have much direct relevance in pain management, but they can confound assessments for the deleterious effects of pain management.

MULTIMODAL STRATEGY

Most patients deserve some elements of multimodal analgesia. The chronic pain, chronic opioid patient may deserve a more "kitchen sink" approach. First, a careful medical reconciliation should be completed preoperatively. Patients should take their regular home analgesic regimen (including muscle relaxants, opioids, alpha agonists, benzodiazepines, anticonvulsants, antidepressants, etc.). Regional and neuraxial techniques should be employed if possible, but at a minimum the skin should be infiltrated prior to incision. More discussion on regional and neuraxial techniques appears later in this chapter.

Consider premedication with NSAIDs (i.e., celecoxib 200-400 mg PO), acetaminophen (1 g PO), clonidine (3mcg/kg PO), and/or gabapentin (300 or greater mg PO). Intraoperatively consider dexamethasone 0.1 mg/kg IV; ketamine 0.5 mg/kg IV bolus preincision, which can be continued at 0.2 mg/kg/hr intra- and postoperatively if required; or ketorolac 30 mg IV (15 mg IV if the patient is more than 65 years old, and use caution if NSAIDs are given preoperatively). Also, IV lidocaine 1.5 mg/kg bolus followed by a 2 mg/kg/h infusion intraoperatively may be especially useful for laparotomies where epidurals are contraindicated. Some centers continue the lidocaine infusion for 24 hours postoperatively at that rate.

Postoperatively, most patients benefit from a continuation of the multimodal approach initiated in the preoperative and intraoperative period. Examples follow, with dosing for the healthy adult unless otherwise indicated. In our experience, the combination of standing acetaminophen and standing NSAID, with an opioid for breakthrough, will typically be sufficient. The other medications can be employed if the initial strategy is inadequate.

- Acetaminophen, 3–4 g/day, 2 g/day maximum in cirrhosis.
- NSAIDs.
  - Ibuprofen PO to 2,400 mg/day, < 1,500 mg/day minimizes gastrointestinal complications, or
  - Naproxen PO to 1,500 mg/day, or
  - Ketorolac IV to 120 mg/day
- Lidoderm patch to affected area 12 hours/day.
- Gabapentin, typically initiated in the naïve patient at 100 mg PO TID and increased by 100 mg Q2–3 days, up to 1,200 mg TID. Gabapentin may be particularly useful for major orthopedic procedures and can be continued for two to four weeks postoperatively.
- Clonidine patch (0.2 mg/day). A patch lasts one week; if used for a longer period, the patient must be monitored for rebound hypertension.
- Postoperative abdominal pain due to flatus can be treated safely with simethicone, an orally administered nonabsorbable antifoaming agent, 125 mg PO.
- Muscle relaxant (if muscle spasm is contributing).
  - Baclofen 5mg PO TID, or
  - Tizanidine 4 mg PO TID, or
  - Diazepam 5 mg PO BID
- For discomfort due to bladder spasm, belladonna (16.2 mg) and opium (30 mg) suppository is effective if NSAIDs have been ineffective.
- If anxiety is a significant contributor to pain, small amounts of benzodiazepine can be considered (i.e., lorazepam 0.5–1 mg PO TID PRN anxiety)
- Ketamine infusion (initiate at 0.1–0.2 mg/kg/hr) may require management by an acute pain service.

Regional/Neuraxial Anesthesia

Peripheral nerve blocks are well-established methods to increase patient satisfaction, decrease postoperative pain scores, and reduce postoperative opioid consumption. The widespread use of ultrasound has made these techniques highly safe, reliable, and effective for a wide range of surgeries. Most practicing anesthesiologists are adept at ultrasound-guided regional techniques for the upper and lower extremity, and a growing number can perform regional techniques for abdominal and chest surgery (i.e., transversus abdominus plane and paravertebral blocks, respectively). Many peripheral nerve blocks can be maintained for several days using a catheter-based technique. Some centers routinely use catheter-based techniques in ambulatory patients, often using elastomeric pumps to deliver local anesthetic safely and predictably.

Neuraxial techniques (i.e., epidural catheters) provide similar analgesic benefit and in a meta-analysis actually reduced mortality, likely due to the multitude of reduced vascular, respiratory, and gastrointestinal morbidity when compared to systemic analgesia.[4]

Regardless of the regional technique used, patients on chronic opioids should be maintained on or gradually weaned down from their chronic opioids perioperatively.

Also, a functioning regional technique does not obviate the need for multimodal analgesia, especially in the ambulatory patient. These patients in particular need an established plan in place for multimodal analgesia prior to the resolution of the sensory block.

REFERENCES

1. Volkow ND, McLellan AT. Opioid abuse in chronic pain—misconceptions and mitigation strategies. *N Engl J Med*. 2016;374:1253–1263
2. Hill KP. Medical marijuana for treatment of chronic pain and other medical and psychiatric problems: a clinical review. *JAMA*. 2015 Jun 23-30;313(24):2474–2483.
3. Bryson EO. The perioperative management of patients maintained on medications used to manage opioid addiction. *Curr Opin Anesthesiol*. 2014;27:359–364.
4. Pöpping DM, Elia N, Van Aken HG, et al. Impact of epidural analgesia on mortality and morbidity after surgery. *Ann Surg*. 2014;259:1056–1067.

FURTHER READING

Blaudszun G, Lysakowski C, Elia N, Tramèr MR. Effect of perioperative systemic α2 agonists on postoperative morphine consumption and pain intensity. *Anesthesiology*. 2012 Jun;116(6):1312–1322.

Brill S, Ginosar Y, Davidson EM. Perioperative management of chronic pain patients with opioid dependency. *Curr Opin Anaesthesiol*. 2006 Jun;19(3):325–331.

Buvandendran A, Kroin J. Multimodal analgesia for controlling acute postoperative pain. *Curr Opin Anaesthesiol*. 2009 Oct;22(5):588–593.

Carroll IR, Angst MS, Clark JD. Management of perioperative pain in patients chronically consuming opioids. *Reg Anesth Pain Med*. 2004 Nov-Dec;29(6):576–591.

De Oliveira GS Jr, Almeida MD, Benzon HT, McCarthy RJ. Perioperative single dose systemic dexamethasone for postoperative pain: a meta-analysis of randomized controlled trials. *Anesthesiology*. 2011 Sep;115(3):575–588.

De Oliveira GS Jr, Fitzgerald P, Streicher LF, Marcus RJ, McCarthy RJ. Systemic lidocaine to improve postoperative quality of recovery after ambulatory laparoscopic surgery. *Anesth Analg*. 2012 Aug;115(2):262–267.

Devin CJ, Lee DS, Armaghani SJ, et al. Approach to pain management in chronic opioid users undergoing orthopaedic surgery. *J Am Acad Orthop Surg*. 2014 Oct;22(10):614–622.

Farrell C, Mcconaghy P. Perioperative management of patients taking treatment for chronic pain. *BMJ*. 2012 Jul 3;345:e4148.

Garrison RN, Cryer HM, Howard DA, Polk HC Jr. Clarification of risk factors for abdominal operations inpatients with hepatic cirrhosis. *Ann Surg*. 1984;199:648–655.

Kiamanesh D, Rumley J, Moitra VK. Monitoring and managing hepatic disease in anaesthesia. *Br J Anaesth*. 2013;111(Suppl 1):i50–i61.

Kopf A, Banzhaf A, Stein C. Perioperative management of the chronic pain patient. *Best Pract Res Clin Anaesthesiol*. 2005 Mar;19(1):59–76.

Kopf A. Managing a chronic pain patient in the perioperative period. *J Pain Palliat Care Pharmacother*. 2013 Dec;27(4):394–396.

Memtsoudis SG. Perioperative comparative effectiveness of anesthetic technique in orthopedic patients. *Anesthesiology*. 2013 May;118(5):1046–1058.

Moran S, Isa J, Steinemann S. Perioperative management in the patient with substance abuse. *Surg Clin North Am*. 95 (2015) 417–428.

Pulley DD. Preoperative evaluation of the patient with substance use disorder and perioperative considerations. *Anesthesiology Clin.* 2016;34:201–211.

Recart A, Issioui T, White PF, et al. The efficacy of celecoxib premedication on postoperative pain and recovery times after ambulatory surgery: a dose-ranging study. *Anesth Analg.* 2003 Jun;96(6):1631–1635.

Segal IS, Jarvis DJ, Duncan SR, White PF, Maze M. Clinical efficacy of oral-transdermal clonidine combinations during the perioperative period. *Anesthesiology.* 1991 Feb;74(2):220–225.

Waldron NH, Jones CA, Gan TJ, Allen TK, Habib AS. Impact of perioperative dexamethasone on postoperative analgesia and side-effects: systematic review and meta-analysis. *Br J Anaesth.* 2013 Feb;110(2):191–200.

16 Postoperative Pain Management

Q. Cece Chen and Shengping Zou

PREOPERATIVE PAIN ASSESSMENT

It would be ideal to establish a plan for postoperative pain management preoperatively, in the surgeon's office and/or preadmission testing center, prior to any intervention, and communicated to all care team members. This helps to form a common goal among the care teams, alleviates patient anxiety, and sets appropriate expectations. Establishing an early pain management plan is especially important for patients with chronic pain who are dependent on long-term opioid regimens resulting in increased opioid requirement, who often are medically challenging due to underlying psychosocial and behavioral issues. A comprehensive pain management plan should be established preoperatively and communicated effectively to the care teams including nurses, surgeons, anesthesiologists, and postanesthesia care unit teams with the goal to provide smooth transition between each phase of care from the operating room to the recovery room then to the ward.

Preoperative evaluation of patients for postoperative pain management should begin with a proper history and physical exam. Patients should be assessed for not only medical but also psychiatric comorbidities, medication history, history of chronic pain, substance abuse, previous pain regimen, and, if available, previous postoperative treatment regimen and response.[1] A history of opioid abuse may affect the pain medications used and may indicate a need for a weaning protocol, monitoring, and follow-up. Several states have implemented prescription monitoring programs which should always be utilized as part of the initial pain assessment. In addition to opioid abuse, history of alcohol abuse, psychoactive substance, and benzodiazepine abuse may also affect pain management. While obtaining the medication history, practitioners should also assess the patient for compliance issues which may affect the choices for

- History of chronic pain and chronic opioid use which is equal to daily consumption of at least 30 mg equivalent of morphine for more than six months
- History of chronic benzodiazepine use
- History of or active substance abuse
- Chronic pain patients with history of psychiatric comorbidity
- History of allergic reaction to opioids
- Complex medical comorbidities that place patients at increased risk for opioid-related complications. These comorbidities include obstructive sleep apnea liver and renal disease, heart disease, morbid obesity.
- Presence of intrathecal pump or spinal cord stimulator

discharge medication and the discharge plan. Table 16.1 lists the risk factors that may be associated with challenging pain management patients.

PREOPERATIVE PAIN MANAGEMENT PLAN

Pain management plans should be tailored to each patient. They should be specific to the surgery the patient will be undergoing, modified by the patient's history and assessment. Considerations should be given to the potential benefit of preoperative pain intervention such as regional blocks and/or catheters placement, epidural catheters placement, or administration of pain medications preoperatively such as gabapentin, acetaminophen, and pregabalin, which studies have shown reduce opioid requirements both intraoperatively and postoperatively.[2] Chronic pain patients especially may benefit from the administration of adjuvant analgesics to help reduce perioperative opioid requirements. Continuation or discontinuation of a patient's home pain medications should also be addressed preoperatively in order to either avoid withdrawal or optimize pain control. However, per the American Pain Society guideline, there is insufficient evidence regarding recommendation for preoperative opioid use.[1]

PREOPERATIVE COMMUNICATION

In addition to forming a preoperative pain management plan, it is also important to establish communication with the patient, the family, and all care teams. The conversation should begin in the surgeon's office. Communication should involve setting realistic short-term, intermediate, and long-term expectations for the patient's pain management goals. Each patient and family should be provided with education, a pain management plan, and expectations that are appropriately tailored to the patient and type of surgery. Education should include a discussion of the different treatment options available such as interventional, integrative, and pharmacological treatment methods. Patients should be encouraged to participate in the decision-making process and given the opportunity to have any concerns or questions addressed prior to undergoing surgery. This process may help to lessen perioperative anxiety and identify patient needs and preferences, which may be especially important for those with psychosocial comorbidities or different cultural backgrounds.

POSTOPERATIVE PAIN MANAGEMENT

The important aspects of postoperative pain management are to apply ongoing assessment of the patient to determine efficacy of pain control, identify side effects and complications, and promote ambulation and return of function. The American Pain Society recently published guidelines that recommend the use of validated pain assessment tools as part of the postoperative pain evaluation.[1] Based on the pain assessment, changes in the pain management modalities, whether pharmacological or interventional, should then be determined. For patients with cognitive deficits, developmental delay, or other factors that may prevent them from being able to report their pain, behavioral assessment tools should be used, and, in addition, input from the caregivers should also be included in the assessment. Because pain is largely a subjective matter, in its guidelines the American Pain Society recommends that "clinicians should not rely solely on objective measures such as pain related behaviors or vital signs in lieu of patient self report to determine the presence of or intensity of pain because such measures are neither valid or reliable."[1] Examples of various pain assessment tools are numeric rating scales, verbal rating scales, visual analogue scales, pain thermometers, and FACES rating scales.

In general, postoperative pain assessment should include questions asking for the onset, pattern, location, intensity, and quality of pain. In addition, aggravating and relieving factors should be identified. Commonly, a numerical pain scale system is an accepted scale used to determine the intensity of pain. Practically, pain reduction by 30% to 50% of baseline may be considered sufficient. Adequacy of pain control can also be assessed based on patient's functionality, pain with deep breathing, coughs, getting out of bed, and ambulation. Improvement in a patient's functionality and mobility is the ultimate goal of pain management. Quality of sleep is another important aspect of pain control outcome. With each assessment, proper documentation should be written to not only record the patient's progress but also to communicate with the other care teams regarding the efficacy of pain management and the patient's recovery status.

As with forming a preoperative pain management plan, communication is also important for the postoperative period. With each patient, an appropriate postoperative expectation and goal for pain control should be established early on. The patient should be aware that a pain level of zero may not be achievable during the early recovery period, but a pain score at which the patient can be functional may be a more appropriate expectation and goal. Beginning from the preoperative period, communication with surgeons and nurses should also be maintained to involve all the care team members in the patient's recovery process.

In addition to improving pain control, practitioners should monitored the patient closely to minimize side effects from the pain regimen. Potential side effects from opioids can include sedation, respiratory depression, pruritus, nausea, vomiting, and opioid-associated constipation. Side effects from nonsteroidal anti-inflammatory drugs (NSAIDs) can include abdominal pain, gastrointestinal (GI) bleed, GI ulcer, and renal injury. Concomitant use of opioids with benzodiazepines can place the patients at even greater risk for oversedation and overdose. According to the Centers for Disease Control and Prevention (CDC), 31% to 61% of fatal overdoses were associated with concurrent use of benzodiazepines.[4]

In general, patient populations that are at the greatest risk for opioid-related complications include those with sleep apnea, hepatic, or renal disease; pregnant women; patients older than 65 years of age; patients with a history of depression, suicidal behavior, or other mental health disorders; and patients with a history of or ongoing substance abuse and alcohol abuse.

Sleep apnea. Opioids are known to cause respiratory depression which in patients who have underlying sleep apnea can lead to worsened central sleep apnea. In general, studies have also found that a large percentage of patients on chronic opioid therapy have abnormal apnea-hypopnea index.[4]

Hepatic/renal disease. Given that opioids depend on the liver and kidneys for metabolism and elimination, reduced function in these organ systems can led to increased peak effect, longer duration, respiratory depression, sedation, and overdose at lower doses.

Pregnant women. In addition to the opioid-related side effects that may affect the mother, opioid use during pregnancy may also place the fetus at risk for congenital defects, reduced fetal growth, premature delivery, still birth, and neonatal opioid withdrawal syndrome.[4]

Postpartum. Neonatal toxicity and death have been reported in breast-feeding infants whose mothers are taking codeine. If used, they should be limited to the lowest possible dose and to a four-day supply.[4]

Elderly population. Patients who are older than 65 years of age may have age-related decreased liver and renal function that can place them at increased risk for opioid-related complications even at lower dose of opioids.

Mental health disorders/history of substance and alcohol abuse. Pain management is often complicated by underlying behavior issues and high opioid requirements due to opioid dependency and tolerance. A psychiatry specialist may be consulted for these types of challenging patients.

PAIN MANAGEMENT OPTIONS AND POSTOPERATIVE ISSUES FOR SPECIAL CASES

Thoracotomy

Pain management options for thoracotomy include thoracic epidural, paravertebral block, and patient-controlled-analgesia initially, especially for patients with chest tubes, then transition to an oral pain regimen.

Thoracic epidurals are currently part of the standard of care for thoracic surgeries. Epidural catheters are commonly placed preoperatively unless there are contraindications for catheter placement such as requirement for therapeutic anticoagulation or patient refusal. Epidural catheters are particularly useful for patients who are at high risk for perioperative complications such as those with poor pulmonary functions at baseline. Intraoperative administration of local anesthetics +/– opioids via the epidural catheter serves as an adjunct for pain management, which may then be utilized to assist in transitioning into the recovery phase. To optimize the benefit of having an epidural catheter, the catheter should be continued until chest tube removal.[6]

A paravertebral block/catheter may be performed as a single injection or through a catheter. A paravertebral catheter may be either placed percutaneously by a trained anesthesiologist or intraoperatively by a surgeon. The paravertebral catheter may be used when an epidural is contraindicated due to anticoagulation use or coagulopathy.[6]

Postoperative issues include hypotension, referred shoulder pain, chest tube pain, and pulmonary splinting.

Possible causes of hypotension include iatrogenic fluid restriction and vasodilation due to sympathetic block from epidural local anesthetics. Management includes fluid administration if appropriate and use of epidural opioid solutions +/– a lower concentration of local anesthetics with epinephrine.

Studies have shown that greater than 75% of post-thoracotomy patients report ipsilateral shoulder pain.[5] Possible etiologies include overstretching of the shoulder during surgical positioning and referred pain transmitted through the phrenic nerve due to diaphragmatic irritation. Post-thoracotomy shoulder pain is often difficult to treat even with intravenous opioids. In addition, shoulder pain only responds partially to NSAID treatments. Various studies have attempted to search for more effective methods for pain treatment. Overall, superficial cervical plexus and interscalene blocks were effective in some patients while suprascapular nerve blocks were not helpful. Given that the phrenic nerve is believed to be responsible for the transmission of the referred pain, for some patients, intraoperative phrenic nerve block was found to help reduce overall pain by 33% to 85%.[5] Currently there is no single modality that can completely treat this pain. Therefore, the most effective method is to utilize a multimodal approach involving nonopioid and interventional techniques.

Cesarean Section

The patient population that undergoes cesarean sections are typically young, healthy females who present to the hospital solely for delivery of their babies. Consequently, their expectation of the hospital experience is positive and pleasant. Therefore the treatment goal for managing these post-Cesarean section patients is to promote and enhance this expected experience.

This may be achieved through epidural patient-controlled analgesia (PCA). The "walking" epidural catheter is an effective pain management modality that at a concentration of 0.15% bupivacaine with 3 mcg/ml fentanyl with 1:2000,000 epinephrine allows for adequate pain control and ambulation to improve patient satisfaction. However, the side effects of such a technique include pruritus, numbness, and anxiety. For pruritus, patients can be placed on a naloxone PCA at a low dose, which helps to relieve the pruritus without affecting any pain relief. However, this can be cumbersome for the patients.[7,9]

Duramorph is less effective than epidural PCA for pain control with a risk for respiratory depression in addition to pruritus.[8,10]

Gastric Bypass

Patients undergoing gastric bypass are an unique population in that they tend to have a high opioid requirement and have multiple comorbidities that may complicate their pain management, including obesity and obstructive sleep apnea. In such cases, an epidural catheter may provide effective pain control while minimizing the potential side effects such as sedation and respiratory depression.

Postoperative issues include nausea, vomiting, nothing by mouth status, respiratory depression, obstructed airway, abdominal splinting, delayed ambulation, ileus, opioid-induced constipation, and chronic opioid use.

Various studies have investigated the increase in opioid use despite weight reduction surgery. Given that obesity is considered one contributing factor to pain, it was assumed that, after weight reduction, the requirement for opioids would also be reduced. However, studies have shown that, on the contrary, postoperatively these patients not only have an ongoing requirement for opioids but some had increased opioid requirements. Factors contributing to the increased opioid use may be multifactorial. Obese patients may in general have increased pain sensitivity and lower pain tolerance, and this baseline-altered pain perception may be responsible for persistent opioid requirements even after weight reduction surgery.[11]

Spine Surgery

The patient population undergoing spine surgeries typically has underlying chronic pain that may be complicated by behavior, dependency, and tolerance issues. Additionally, due to the extensiveness of the surgical procedure, the restriction on postoperative mobility, and the limitations on the types of pain modalities that can be used, pain management for these patients often can be challenging. In these patients, in addition to a PCA, patients may benefit from long-acting opioid medications, optimization of non-opioid regimens such as muscle relaxants, acetaminophen and gabapentin. Ketorolac however is usually prohibited from use in spinal fusion patients.

Postoperatively, pain is particularly severe and difficult to control during the initial one to three days. Patients may benefit from a long-acting opioid medication for consistent baseline pain control combined with a PCA for breakthrough pain. The goal is to help manage pain in the acute postoperative period, after which the patient can be taken off or weaned off the opioid regimen as appropriate.

Due to concerns regarding effects on bone healing and bleeding, NSAIDs are commonly avoided during the postoperative period for spine surgery.

For patients who fail conventional pain management methods, administration of low-dose ketamine infusion may be more beneficial and effective. In addition, ketamine is believed to either reduce or reverse opioid tolerance via its inhibition of N-methyl-D-aspartate receptor. In general, however, utilization of a ketamine infusion would require placing patients in a monitored setting.

Postoperative issues in spine surgery patients include sedation, respiratory depression, anxiety, hypotension, high opioid requirements, muscle spasms, delayed ambulation, and oversedation from valium/benzodiazepines that are commonly ordered by surgeons for muscle spasms.

PAIN MANAGEMENT MULTIMODALITIES

- Regional nerve blocks and nerve catheters
- Intraoperative local anesthetic administration by surgeon
- PCA

When transitioning from intravenous (IV) to oral pain regimens, consider the following.

- For optimal transition, calculate the patient's 24-hour requirement of the IV opioid then convert to an oral regimen using the equianalgesic table. Due to concern for cross-tolerance, when converting to an oral regimen, consider decreasing the dosage by 25% to 50%.
- Consider providing options for breakthrough pain medication during the transition period.
- Monitor the patient closely and frequently assess him or her during the transition period, as too much opioid medication can increase the chance for side effects during this period and inadequate pain medications can lead to increased pain and poor patient satisfaction.

DISCHARGE PLAN

Prior to discharge, the patient should be assessed to ensure that he or she will be able to tolerate routine daily activities while on the pain regimen that will be prescribed at the time of discharge. The patient should be encouraged to try the pain regimen while in the hospital setting to assess for side effects and potential complications and determine whether additional adjustments are needed. Patients, caregivers, and family members should also be provided with education regarding each of the medications in the pain regimen and should be made aware of the symptoms of the side effects, how to manage them, and how to seek medical help. The overall goal is to ensure optimal comfort and safety while the patient is recovering at home.

Prior to leaving the hospital, patients should schedule a follow-up appointment at a pain management clinic, especially those on high-dose opioids who underwent complicated surgery and had a difficult recovery process. While in the outpatient setting, the pain physician should continue to assist the patient through the recovery process and rehabilitation, identify any issues that may be delaying recovery, and adjust the pain regimen accordingly. In addition, the pain physician should provide further education and support to the patient, caregivers, and family as needed. For certain patients, the pain physician may provide an opioid wean protocol when opioids are no longer indicated or the benefits no longer outweigh the risks. This may also help to reduce the risk for opioid abuse. Establishing such postoperative care not only provides continuation of care from the hospital but may also increases patient comfort, satisfaction, and HCAHPS pain score.

According to the CDC guidelines for prescribing opioids, there is evidence that treating acute pain with opioids may increase the risk for long-term opioid use. The CDC recommends that, in most cases, opioids prescribed should be limited to less than three to seven days during which the lowest effective dose should be used.[2] The lowest effective dose can be determined by using titration. The CDC recommends that opioids be prescribed for only the period during which pain is expected to be severe enough to indicate opioid use. More specifically for postsurgical patients, the CDC guideline makes reference to the Washington State Agency Medical Directors' guideline for prescribing opioids. This guideline suggests that for the acute pain phase that is between zero to six weeks after surgery, opioids may be indicated; however, beyond this phase, opioids should rarely be needed. For minor surgeries, it recommends a limited supply of opioids for two to three days. For chronic pain patients who were on opioids prior to surgery, the guideline recommends that opioids be tapered to at least the preoperative dose within the initial six-week period. For patients who require opioids beyond six weeks postoperatively, opioids should not be continued unless there is evidence of clinical improvement in regards to function and pain. In addition, patients should be evaluated for mental health issues and signs of opioid misuse with a urine drug test and checking the opioid prescription registry. Opioids should be discontinued when the benefit no longer outweighs the risks, there is no longer an evidence of clinical improvement, or aberrant behaviors are identified. When discontinuing opioids, considerations should be made in tapering the dosages to minimize potential withdrawal symptoms.[3]

SPECIAL CASES: OPIOID ALLERGY DESENSITIZATION PROTOCOL FOR PATIENTS WITH AN ALLERGY TO FENTANYL

New York University Langone Medical Center protocol:

1. The patient should be preadmitted to a monitored setting.
2. The desensitization protocol should be followed without gaps in between administration of the medications. A 48-hour gap between administration of the medications will place the patient at risk for redeveloping allergy to fentanyl.
3. Vital signs should be rechecked between each dose.
4. For desensitization, three types of solutions with different concentrations of fentanyl should be used.

Solution:	Total Volume	Concentration	Dose
Solution 1	250 mL	0.008 mcg/mL	2 mcg
Solution 2	250 mL	0.06 mcg/mL	15 mcg
Solution 3	250 mL	0.60 mcg/mL	150 mcg

5. The following steps should be followed while using these solutions at different stages of the protocol.

Step	Solution#	Rate (mL/hr)	Time (minutes)	Volume infused per step (mL)	Dose administered with this step (mcg)	Cumulative dose (mcg)
1	1	2	30	0.5	0.004	0.004
2	1	5	30	1.25	0.01	0.014
3	1	10	30	2.5	0.02	0.034
4	1	20	30	5	0.04	0.074
5	2	5	30	1.25	0.075	0.149
6	2	10	30	2.5	0.15	0.299
7	2	20	30	5	0.3	0.599

Step	Solution#	Rate (mL/hr)	Time (minutes)	Volume infused per step (mL)	Dose administered with this step (mcg)	Cumulative dose (mcg)
8	2	40	30	10	0.6	1.199
9	3	10	30	2.5	1.5	2.699
10	3	20	30	5	3	5.699
11	3	40	30	10	6	11.699
12	3	80	30	230.50	138.301	150

6. The patient should be monitored closely for any signs of allergic reactions. The infusion should be stopped immediately if there is evidence of hypotension, changes in mental status, dyspnea, skin changes, sensation of swelling or itching in the throat, changes in voice, wheezing, or any symptoms that may be concerning for airway involvement or anaphylaxis.

7. Medications for anaphylaxis or airway obstruction should be readily available, including epinephrine, diphenhydramine, albuterol, and steroids, as well as nebulizer equipment, oxygen, and an airway cart.

8. Mild allergic symptoms such as rashes or hives that develop at high infusion rates generally do not require cessation of infusion. The infusion rate may be reduced to the last tolerated rate, and patients may be treated with diphenhydramine and/or prednisone until the symptoms subside. The infusion rate can then be increased back to the initial rate.

9. After completion of desensitization treatment, allergic reactions can still occur; however, major allergic reactions are unusual. The patient should receive treatment as clinically indicated.

REFERENCES

1. Chou R, Gordon DB, de Leon-Casasola OA, et al. Management of postoperative pain: a clinical practice guideline from the American Pain Society, the American Society of Regional Anesthesia and Pain Medicine, and the American Society of Anesthesiologists' Committee on Regional Anesthesia, Executive Committee, and Administrative Council. *J Pain.* 2016;17(2):131–147.

2. Pulos N, Sheth D. Perioperative pain management following total joint arthroplasty. *Ann Orthoped Rheumatol.* 2014;2(3):1029.

3. Washington State Agency Medical Directors' Group. AMDG 2015 interagency guideline on prescribing opioids for pain. Olympia, WA: Washington State Agency Medical Directors' Group; 2015. http://www.agencymeddirectors.wa.gov/guidelines.asp

4. Dowell D, Haegerich TM, Chou R. CDC guideline for prescribing opioids for chronic pain—United States, 2016. Atlanta: Centers for Disease Control and Prevention; March 18, 2016. https://www.cdc.gov/mmwr/volumes/65/rr/rr6501e1.htm

5. Gerner P. Post-thoracotomy pain management problems. *Anesthesiol Clin.* 2008 Jun; 26(2):355–vii.

6. Gottschalk A, Cohen SP, Yang S, Ochroch EA. Preventing and treating pain after thoracic surgery. *Anesthesiology.* 2006;104(3):594–600.

7. Harrison DM, Sinatra R, Morgese L, Chung JH. Epidural narcotic and patient-controlled analgesia for post-cesarean section pain relief. *Anesthesiology.* 1988;68(3):454–456.

8. Donchin Y, Davidson JT, Magora F. Epidural morphine for the control of pain after cesarean section. *Survey Anesthesiol.* 1982;26(4):238–239.

9. Cohen S, Amar D, Pantuck DB, et al. Postcesarean delivery epidural patient-controlled analgesia. *Anesthesiology.* 1993;78(3):486–491.

10. Singh SI, Rehou S, Marmai KL, Jones PM. The efficacy of 2 doses of epidural morphine for postcesarean delivery analgesia. *Anesth Analg.* 2013;117(3):677–685.

11. Raebel MA, Newcomer SR, Reifler LM, et al. Chronic use of opioid medications before and after bariatric surgery. *JAMA.* 2013;310(13):1369.

12. Bajwa SJ, Haldar R. Pain management following spinal surgeries: an appraisal of the available options. *J Craniovert Junct Spine.* 2015;6(3):105.

17 Clinical Consequences of Inadequate Pain Management and Barriers to Optimal Pain Management

Evan Goodman, Magdalena Anitescu, and Tariq M. Malik

INTRODUCTION

Treating pain is a challenge faced by physicians across all specialties and disciplines. Attempts at achieving adequate analgesia are often met with failure because of a physician's misunderstanding of the human experience of pain. According to the International Association for the Study of Pain (IASP), pain is "an unpleasant sensory and emotional experience associated with actual or potential tissue damage, or described in terms of such damage." Pain, therefore, does not have a single target. Treatment must consider the subjective psychological and emotional experience with the objective physiology of pain perception. The perception of pain varies between individuals. Biospsychosocial treatment, which accounts for the individual experience of pain, is all too commonly left out of treatment plans. As a result of its complexity, pain is often left undertreated, producing clinical, social, and economic consequences.

The unmet need for pain control is apparent when patients return to an emergency department with pain scores unchanged, when postoperative patients have pain weeks after surgery, when geriatric patients with chronic degenerative conditions suffer as they age, and when cancer patients experience excruciating pain during their final moments of life. In a study of 842 patients who presented to an emergency department, pain intensity score stayed the same or increased for 41% of the patients by the time of discharge.[1] In another study of the effectiveness of postoperative pain management with multiple analgesic techniques, 30% of patients reported moderate to severe postoperative pain and 11% reported severe postoperative pain.[2]

As our population advances in age, we are seeing the morbidity of diseases such as cancer increase while mortality decreases. The prevalence of acute and chronic pain in newly diagnosed cancer patients is 30%, 50% to 70% in those undergoing treatment, and 60% to 80% in individuals with advanced disease.[3] In a study of 573 cancer patients, 11% were not receiving any analgesic medications and 50% of the participants felt that their health care providers did not consider their quality of life in their treatment plans.[4] Twelve percent of these individuals also felt that their health care providers did not understand that pain is a problem.[4] With such astonishing numbers, the need for better pain management will only continue to grow.

Control of pain is inadequate despite our most advanced practices of medicine. In 2001 the U.S. Congress named the beginning decade as the decade of pain control and research.[5] Initiatives were set in motion by the Joint Commission, a nonprofit organization that acts to accredit hospital systems and holds them to the highest standards for providing safe, effective, and quality care, and by the World Health Organization (WHO), which acts to promote the highest level of health care for the people of the world. These organizations established guidelines and standards for the assessment and treatment of pain and have developed evidence-based tools, such as the analgesic ladder, to assist physicians in effectively managing pain.

With this relatively contemporary focus on pain management, research into new treatment modalities is showing promise in mitigating the epidemic of undertreated pain.

CLASSIFICATION OF PAIN

Pain can be classified as acute, chronic, or cancer-related. Acute pain is the body's physiologic response to noxious stimuli (nociception), which aids in the awareness and prevention of injury. Acute pain manifests as intense sensations with both neuroendocrine and autonomic responses. The causes of acute pain can be somatic or visceral. Somatic pain is the result of destruction or injury to skin, subcutaneous tissue, joints, or bones. Pain of a somatic origin is often easily localized. Visceral pain, which is the result of destruction or damage to or malfunction of organs and their coverings, is less easily localized. Somatic and visceral pain are types of acute pain. If an inflamed appendix (visceral) is removed, or if a laceration of the skin (somatic) heals, the symptoms of pain resolve. If the experience of pain persists well beyond the end of tissue injury or destruction, the pain is considered chronic.

According to the IASP, chronic pain is "pain without apparent biological value that has persisted beyond the normal tissue healing time usually taken to be 3 months." Like acute pain, chronic pain can be the result of persistent nociceptive pain. Injuries to the central nervous system or inherent structural or functional abnormalities result in the neuropathic etiology of chronic pain. Chronic pain comes from persistent injury or destruction to musculoskeletal, visceral, or neural tissues as in osteoarthritis, sickle cell anemia, and diabetic neuropathy, respectively. One of the most profound features of chronic pain is how it is influenced by a patient's psychosocial well-being. A patient's outlook, understanding of the condition, and coping mechanisms affect pain control. The experience of pain varies by gender, race, and genetic predisposition.

Unfortunately this is often overlooked. What was once thought of as a balancing act between titrating opioid dosages to pain scores and side effect profiles, managing chronic pain is now the art of incorporating patient emotion, cognition, and coping abilities into intricate treatment plans.

PHYSIOLOGY OF PAIN

The perception of pain starts at the peripheral nociceptors. Nociception is the conversion of chemical, mechanical, or thermal energy into neural impulses. The neural impulses travel via primary afferent nerve fibers that can be categorized based on their physiologic properties and capabilities. A∂ fibers, which are small and thinly myelinated, carry fast, sharp, well-localized pain. C fibers, which are larger and unmyelinated, carry slow, dull achy pain. Both fibers travel in conjunction with even larger and myelinated Aß fibers, which carry non-noxious stimuli such as touch and vibration. The cell bodies of the primary afferent neurons are located in the dorsal root. Their endings synapse with second-order neurons in the dorsal horn of the spinal cord. The dorsal horn of the spinal cord is additionally the area where modulation of pain signals take place via interneurons which exhibit their excitatory and/or inhibitory effects and where higher centers of the brain (the periaqueductal grey and nucleus raphe magnus) send their descending inhibitory tracts.[6] The dorsal horn can be subdivided into laminae, which are specific to the termination points of A∂ (lamina I and V), and C fibers (lamina II). Aß fibers do not synapse in the dorsal horn. They travel lateral to the dorsal horn and course through to the medial columns, while giving off projections that end in lamina III, IV, and V and also synapse with C fibers in laminae II. When Aß fibers are activated, via non-noxious stimuli in the periphery (rubbing a thumb after it is stuck by a hammer), they can influence inhibitory interneurons located in laminae II to modulate the slow, achy pain signals being transmitted by C fibers in this region.

Second-order neurons leave the dorsal column, decussate, and travel toward the brain via the spinothalamic and spinoreticular tracts. Second-order neurons then synapse in the thalamus where somatosensory information is processed. From the thalamus, third-order neurons synapse with second-order neurons and project to the cortices of the brain were the perception of pain occurs.

Neuropathic pain is the result of abnormalities arising from injury or acquired defects in the physiologic pathways that lead to the perception of pain. In neuropathic pain, the patient perceives pain but no apparent injury or noxious stimulus is present. Neuropathic pain is characterized by numbness, tingling, and burning sensations in constant or random patterns. It can be pain in response to non-noxious stimuli (allodynia) or pain out of proportion to a noxious stimulus (hyperalgesia). Additionally, injury and acquired defects of the nervous system can cause pain resulting from abnormal sympathetic discharges. The prototypical example is complex regional pain syndrome. In this syndrome the patient experiences not only symptoms of neurogenic abnormalities such as allodynia but also components of sympathetically mediated vasogenic, motor, and pseudomotor changes like alterations in temperature and skin color, decreased range of motion, and sweating, respectively. Because of the plasticity of the central nervous system, with repetitive painful stimulation, the threshold for pain can be altered: patients become more sensitive to similar stimuli and their threshold for response is decreased.

CLINICAL CONSEQUENCES OF INADEQUATE PAIN MANAGEMENT

What happens when pain goes untreated? In the acute phases patients experience increases in heart rate, blood pressure, systemic vascular resistance, respiratory rate, and stress on the endocrine system. Typically, the patient populations that are more commonly prone to experiencing severe acute pain are postsurgical patients, the elderly with chronic disease, and cancer patients. The physiologic stress of acute pain puts them at risk for myocardial infarction, cerebral vascular accidents, poor wound healing, or immunosuppression. Severe pain can manipulate the body's circulating hormones. Stress on the endocrine system stimulates the hypothalamic-pituitary-adrenal-thyroid-gonadal system, to increase an array of stress hormones: cortisol, pregnenolone, dehydroepiandrosterone, progesterone, testosterone, estrogen, and thyroid hormone. The hormones are essential to the stages of healing, metabolic activity, and immunologic response to injury, and even for the control of pain.[7] When acute pain continues for prolonged periods of time, the hormones can become exhausted, which delays tissue and nerve healing, as well as deranges metabolic activity.

What happens if pain continues without intervention? The severity of postoperative pain is a strong predictor of the development of chronic pain.[8] The central nervous system has a neuroplastic response to repetitive stimuli from acute pain. The neurons that transmit the sensation of pain are remodeled to become more sensitive to stimuli and ultimately result in the processes of "wind up" and "central sensitization."[8] This process is one of the most significant driving factors behind the development of chronic pain.

Inadequately treated postoperative pain also affects recovery. Patients may suffer from hypoxemia and hypoventilation as a result of the inability to take sufficient breaths from poorly controlled pain (splinting). Additionally pain prohibits a patient's ability to ambulate and participate in physical therapy, which has a multitude of adverse effects such as decreases in bowel functioning (paralytic ileus), urinary retention, and the development of deep venous thrombosis.[9]

Equally as profound are the psychological, social, and economic consequences. Patients who suffer from chronic pain decline in health and well-being because of impaired sleep, depression, and reduced mobility and physical activity. The vicious cycle of symptoms intensifies the patient's physical and emotional experience of pain. Ultimately, the morbid nature of chronic pain prevents many patients from productive participation in society. The economic impact includes lost workdays, hospital readmission, and utilization of health care and government resources. Lost production because of common pain conditions in actively working individuals costs the United States approximately $61.2 billion per year.[10]

The overwhelming influence that pain has at the individual and societal level has brought significant attention to the field of pain medicine. What has not changed, however, are the barriers that stand in the way of implementing new strategies for treating pain.

The consequences of undertreated pain have become so significant over the years that the Joint Commission for the Accreditation of Health Care Organizations, the IASP, the World Health Organization, and the U.S. Congress have made efforts to create guidelines and standards of practice for the evaluation and treatment of pain.[11] However, many barriers still exist that prevent effective pain management. By dividing the barriers to managing pain into physician, nursing, patient, hospital, and societal factors, the complexities in treating pain quickly reveal themselves.

In today's health care system, hospitals are incentivized to reduce the duration of a patient's length of stay. This incentive has created a significant hospital-driven barrier to pain management as patients are being discharged from emergency departments and postoperatively well before their pain is adequately controlled. When patients leave the hospital with untreated pain, their risk of developing chronic pain, and the morbidity associated with it, dramatically increases.

Many of the patient-focused barriers to pain management are driven by the fears of the adverse effects associated with treatment strategies. In a national survey of 250 patients, 94% believed that pain medications prescribed after surgery caused adverse effects, and, if given a choice, 72% of these patients would choose nonnarcotic medications as they are less addictive (49%) and have fewer side effects (18%).[12] More often than not, patients are not educated about the side effects of the treatments and the physician's ability to manage and prevent them. As a result, many patients prefer to suffer from pain than be potentially exposed to constipation, nausea, vomiting, addiction, and hyperalgesia.[12] Patients not educated about the effects of treatment strategies may be noncompliant with treatment. Nurses too are affected by similar fears and lapses in education. As the gatekeepers of analgesic regimens, nurses administer them as needed. With nurses' fears of side effects and subjective decisions about a patient's need for medication, pain control often falls short.[13] Another contributor to noncompliance by a patient is the fear of the stigma because of reliance on opioids. Patients may think that others may view them as drug addicts. Their chronic reliance on medications to function (pseudoaddiction) may affect their social relationships or careers.

Another profound patient-centered barrier that contributes to noncompliance is the belief that treatments such as opioids should be reserved for the end of the course of a disease. Patients may think the need for pain medication is an indicator of worsening disease progression. In these situations, noncompliance results from denial or not wanting to be viewed negatively by a physician for having poor outcomes.

The key to removing these patient barriers to pain control is communication between the physician and patient. The successful treatment of pain relies on the physician and patient working together to titrate regimens for analgesia that are tolerable. Physicians must offer realistic expectations about the management of pain, possible adverse effects, and solutions when adverse effects arise. The physician must either possess the ability, or provide resources, to support the patient's emotional component of pain to remove the barriers to successful treatment.

Overcoming patient-specific barriers is still not sufficient to adequately treat pain. Physicians must overcome barriers of their own. The most prominent barrier that currently plagues the United States is the lack of training in pain management in the medical school curriculum. In a study of 879 oncologists, 12% reported excellent training in the treatment of cancer pain during medical school while 36% reported their training to be fair and 52% reported theirs to be poor.[14] Of this same group, only 27% of the physicians reported their training in pain management during residency to be excellent or good.[14] This lack of education produces physician discomfort in treating pain and which ultimately leads to inadequate management. With this deficiency in education, physicians often fear subjecting their patients to the potential for addiction or adverse effects from treatment regimens. To tailor a treatment regimen specific to a patient's experience of pain, the physician has to develop an accurate assessment of the type and quality of that pain. Unfortunately, many physicians who have not been trained in pain management lack the skills necessary to generate a useful assessment. As a result, tools such as the visual analog scale, verbal rating scales, the McGill pain questionnaire, and pain inventories have been developed to assist physicians in their attempts.[3]

Another overwhelming barrier to the management of pain from the physician perspective is the fear of litigation. In attempts to provide adequate pain management and limit illicit substance abuse, there are often lines that are blurred between what is deemed appropriate management and excessive prescribing. Ultimately this fear of litigation is another result of a lack of physician education about appropriate pain management regimens.

With the recognition that many of the physician-related barriers to adequate pain management stem from a lack of education, clinical practice guidelines and national education programs have been instituted. For example, the WHO's "analgesic ladder" offers a framework to treat patients with persistent pain in a stepwise fashion without the fears of legal scrutiny. Programs like Topics on Pain Medicine, a virtual textbook sponsored by the American Academy of Pain Physicians, attempts to fill the void in the US medical education curriculum.[11] Once physicians are adequately educated in the assessment and management of pain, the barriers to pain management can be removed, and the modern strategies for mitigating pain can be applied.

MODERN STRATEGIES IN PAIN MANAGEMENT

The recent attention in the field of medicine to addressing the world need for adequate pain control has brought forward many new treatment modalities and techniques which have improved patient satisfactions scores and have spared the use of significant amounts of opioids. For instance, the advent of the patient-controlled analgesic pump has removed the nursing barrier to pain management. With this device, patients decide when an opioid is needed rather than relying on a nurse's subjective evaluation of their pain or even their availability. This allows patients to stay on top of their requirements rather than catching up later (requiring additional opioids) when pain is no longer tolerable. One of the most promising strategies is "multimodal analgesia." Multimodal analgesia is "the administration of two or more drugs that act by different mechanisms for providing analgesia."[15] This approach to treating pain targets multiple contributors to the perception of pain at the same time rather than specifically targeting opioid receptors. The goal of multimodal analgesia is to provide analgesia while limiting the amount of opioid necessary. Typical non-opioid analgesics and adjuvants used in multimodal therapies include nonsteroidal anti-inflammatory drugs, COX inhibitors, acetaminophen, tricyclic antidepressants, and anticonvulsants such as gabapentin. Infusions of local anesthetics such as lidocaine and subanesthetic doses of ketamine have been used to treat intraoperative, postoperative, and chronic pain. These adjuvants modulate pain pathways and opioid receptors so that opioid requirements are reduced for analgesia in patients with a high tolerance for opioids. The effectiveness of multimodal analgesia has been proven through multiple meta-analyses. As a result, the American Society of Anesthesiologists recommends this method to treat acute pain in the perioperative setting.[15]

Another aspect of multimodal analgesia with promise for reducing opioid requirements in treating pain is regional anesthesia. The minimally invasive techniques of regional anesthesia have become so advanced with the increased utilization of ultrasound that they can now be applied to acute postoperative, traumatic, chronic, or cancer pain. Regional anesthesia directly targets the area of pain sensation continuously with epidural and peripheral nerve catheters or intermittently with single-shot nerve blocks and epidural injections. With these techniques, the acute phases of pain are blunted at a time when opioid requirements would otherwise be at their highest.

While these methods for managing pain are promising, their utilization requires the skill set of individuals trained in the specialty of pain management. To make these treatment modalities more accessible in the inpatient setting, hospitals systems are starting to create acute pain services for consultation about methods to reduce pain and limit the use of opioids or to suggest and coordinate treatment beyond the capabilities of the primary service.

Recognizing the importance of the biopsychosocial component of the perception of pain, hospitals and ambulatory pain management centers focus on a multidisciplinary team model for the treatment of pain. On the teams are anesthesiologists, nurses, psychiatrists or psychologists, physiotherapists, and occupational therapists. The treating physicians lead the multidisciplinary team. Nurses are patient liaisons, who educate patients and coordinate their care. Because depression is found to be 15% to 56% more prevalent in patients who suffer chronic pain[16] and, along with anxiety, acts to exacerbate the pain experience, psychiatrists and psychologists play an integral role. They use cognitive-behavioral therapy and relaxation techniques such as biofeedback to develop coping mechanisms and insight to help facilitate the patient's ability to live with a chronic pain condition. Physiatrists and occupational therapists, on the other hand, assist in the restoration of patient mobility and function through exercise and education. The aim is to improve a patient's quality of life and functioning even if the chronic pain never fully resolves.[17]

The recent surge in research in the field of pain management has deepened our understating of the complex pathways of pain perception and its interconnection with emotions. As barriers to adequate pain management are removed by patient and physician education and communication, and as strategies in pain management that encompass the biopsychosocial component of pain are applied, we come closer to fulfilling our society's unmet need of adequate pain control.

REFERENCES

1. Todd KH, Ducharme J, Choiniere M, et al. Pain in the emergency department: results of the pain and emergency medicine initiative (PEMI) multicenter study. *J Pain.* 2007;8(6):460–466.

2. Dolin SJ, Cashman JN, Bland JM. Effectiveness of acute postoperative pain management: I. Evidence from published data. *Br J Anaesth.* 2002;89(3):409–423.

3. Jacobsen R, Liubarskiene Z, Moldrup C, et al. Barriers to cancer pain management: a review of empirical research. *Medicina.* 2009;45(6):427–433.

4. Breivik H, Cherny N, Collett B, et al. Cancer-related pain: a pan-European survey of prevalence, treatment, and patient attitudes. *Ann Oncol.* 2009;20(8):1420–1433.

5. Brennan F. The US Congressional decade on pain control and research 2001–2011: a review. *J Pain Palliat Care Pharmacother.* 2015;29(3):212–227.

6. Steeds CE. The anatomy and physiology of pain. *Surgery.* 2009;27(12):507–511.

7. Tennant F. The physiologic effects of pain on the endocrine system. *Pain Ther.* 2013;2(2):75–86.

8. Voscopoulos C, Lema M. When does acute pain become chronic? *Br J Anaesth.* 2010;105(Suppl 1):I69–185.

9. Joshi GP, Ogunnaike BO. Consequences of inadequate postoperative pain relief and chronic persistent postoperative pain. *Anesthesiol Clin North Am.* 2005;23(1):21–36. HERE

10. Stewart, WF, Ricci JA, Chee E, Morganstein D, Lipton R. Lost productive time and cost due to common pain conditions in the US workforce. *JAMA* 2003;290(18):2443–2454.

11. Brennan F, Carr DB, Cousins M. Pain management: a fundamental human right. *Anesth Analg.* 2007;105(1):205–221.

12. Apfelbaum JL, Chen C, Mehta SS, Gan TJ. Postoperative pain experience: results from a national survey suggest postoperative pain continues to be undermanaged. *Anesth Analg.* 2003;97(2):534–540.

13. Taylor A, Stanbury L. A review of postoperative pain management and the challenges. *Curr Anaesth Crit Care.* 2009;20(4):188–194.

14. Von Roenn A, Cleeland C, Gonin R, Hatfield A, Kishan P. Physician attitudes and practice in cancer pain management: a survey from the Eastern Cooperative Oncology Group. *Ann Intern Med.* 1993:119(2):121.

15. American Society of Anesthesiologists Task Force on Acute Pain Management. Practice guidelines for acute pain management in the perioperative setting: an updated report by the American Society of Anesthesiologists Task Force on Acute Pain Management. *Anesthesiology.* 2012;116(2):248–273.

16. Trescot AM, Helm S, Hansen H, et al. Opioids in the management of chronic non-cancer pain: an update of American Society of the Interventional Pain Physicians' (ASIPP) guidelines. *Pain Physician.* 2008;11(Suppl 2):S5–S62.

17. Holdcroft A, Jaggar S, eds. *Core Topics in Pain.* Cambridge, UK: Cambridge University Press; 2005.

18 Prevention of Adverse Effects in Perioperative Pain Management for General and Plastic Surgeons

Daniel Krashin, Natalia Murinova, and Alan D. Kaye

INTRODUCTION

Pain is a feared complication of surgery which may result in worse outcomes and prolonged hospitalization. As the populations of developed countries grow older, the number of patients suffering chronic pain prior to surgery increases as well. In the United States, large numbers of patients are currently or have previously been treated with high dose opioids for chronic pain and will require alterations in their care. Treatments for pain, particularly opioid analgesics, can have many adverse effects and even lead to serious complications. In addition, research suggests that treatment strategies around the time of surgery can influence the rate of persistent postoperative pain. Therefore, it is worthwhile to consider pain management in every patient who may be undergoing surgical treatment.

PREOPERATIVE ASSESSMENT

The preoperative assessment should include both general questioning and a focused pain history. A patient may present with intense anxiety about postoperative pain based on past experiences with pain, from reading on the Internet, or from a family member. The pain portion of the preoperative evaluation should review the patient's previous pain experience, including specific diagnoses if possible.

The interviewer should elicit past and current use of medications for pain, as well the duration and dosage of treatment if possible. This list should be reviewed with the patient to identify medications which were not tolerated due to adverse effects and which were particularly effective. For controlled substances, it may also be helpful to review a prescription database, which is available in most of the United States and will usually provide a list of controlled substance prescriptions over the past year along with the names of prescribers. It is worth noting that, depending on the region, not all health care systems will report their prescriptions to this database; for example, Veterans Administration clinics, methadone maintenance clinics, and some Indian health care clinics will not report controlled substance prescriptions. The importance of this detailed history cannot be overstated, and it is often worthwhile to bring in family members or caregivers if the patient is a poor historian. Many medications relevant to pain, such as long-acting opioids, psychiatric medications, and neuropathic pain medications should be continued perioperatively. Sudden discontinuation will predictably cause a pain crisis which will distress the patient and may trigger a fruitless search for surgical complications.

The specifics to address pre-existing conditions and medication regimens are discussed in greater detail later in this chapter. However, notifying the patient during the interview of its purpose and that this information will be used to ensure a good postoperative pain course will often reassure patients and make them more forthcoming with relevant details.

The patient's concerns regarding pain may also be assessed at this time to help guide patient education. Patients who understand their surgical care plan are better able to manage postoperative pain.[1] Some psychological factors have been noted to interfere with postoperative recovery. Anxiety before surgery impairs recovery and prolongs hospital stays.[2] High anxiety levels are also associated with higher rates of complications in joint replacements and cardiac surgery.[3,4] Behavioral interventions prior to surgery have been shown to improve these outcomes.[5] Catastrophization, the tendency to describe one's pain in terms such as "terrible" or "unbearable," is strongly associated with postoperative pain.[6] It is unclear whether this behavior pattern can be modified, although small studies have shown improvements with a behavioral intervention for catastrophization.[7]

Patient with substance use disorders, particularly opioid use disorders, may also pose a special challenge to perioperative pain care. Several of the medications used in medication-assisted treatment of addiction are also relevant to perioperative management.

This type of preoperative behavioral screening and intervention goes well beyond the standard of care in most surgical settings; however, even more modest interventions can help improve a patient's pain coping.

Setting expectations for surgery is essential. No one on the surgical and anesthesia teams can or should promise painless surgery. Providers should explain that some postoperative pain is normal and to be expected at the same time that pain treatment plans are discussed. Since health care literacy varies widely, education should not assume prior knowledge and should explain pain plans in simple, patient-focused terms. Since many patients are nervous and do not retain information well at these visits, consider also providing handouts or links to educational videos, which can also be provided in multiple languages.[8] If the patient is not familiar with patient-controlled analgesia (PCA), this may be discussed as well.

Pain relief should be discussed in functional terms at these visits; for example, saying "we will help you with your pain so that you can work with physical therapy and get some rest" rather than specifying a particular value on the Visual Analogue Scale (VAS). Patients' interpretations of the 0 to 10 VAS vary, and chronic pain patients may describe their pain as "always at 8" or even "never below 12."

ASSESSMENT OF PATIENTS

Perioperative Pain Management

Every patient undergoing surgery should have a perioperative pain management plan, even if this is simple and straightforward. The most important components of multi-modal pain management include non-opioid systemic pain medications, sometimes called "adjunctive" pain medications; nerve blocks or regional anesthesia; and opioid analgesics. Pain management should use all three components where practical to reduce the reliance on and dosage of opioids. While this is a large topic, we address the basics here for convenience.

NON-OPIOID SYSTEMIC PAIN MEDICATIONS

Acetaminophen is safe and effective for postoperative pain and tends to reduce opioid requirements during the first postoperative day, although it may not reduce adverse effects of opioids.[9] Practice guidelines call for it to be used routinely for postoperative pain.[10] Nonsteroidal anti-inflammatory drugs (NSAIDs) have greater analgesic effect and reduce adverse effects from opioids, but the risk of adverse effects including renal impairment and bleeding may restrict their use.[11] A meta-analysis suggested that ketorolac did not increase the risk of surgical bleeding; however, other studies have suggested that the risk of bleeding at the surgical site and in the gastrointestinal tract is significant in elderly surgical patients.[12,13] There is also a concern that NSAIDs may increase the risk of colorectal anastomosis leakage, a recent meta-analysis was inconclusive but suggestive of this.[14] Celecoxib, a COX-2 inhibitor, may be safer in that it does not affect platelet function, but it carries a risk of ischemic heart disease.[15] Gabapentin has been shown to be helpful preoperatively and may also be helpful to continue postoperatively with an opioid-sparing effect.[16] The most common adverse effect is sedation.

Certain intravenous (IV) medications have also been shown to be moderately beneficial for postoperative pain. Ketamine is an N-methyl-D-aspartate receptor antagonist which can be used for anesthesia but also as an adjunct in lower doses, which do not tend to cause psychotomimetic adverse effects. These lower-dose infusions may help reduce pain and reverse opioid tolerance to exert an opioid-sparing effect.[17] Intravenous lidocaine after colon surgery reduces postoperative pain, reduces opioid requirements, and improves time until return of bowel function and time until discharge.[18,19]

REGIONAL AND PERIPHERAL NERVE BLOCKS

The application of local anesthetic to a nerve, nerve root, or nerve plexus can have a powerful analgesic effect by blocking the transmission of nociceptive signals to the central nervous system. This may allow the surgery to be done without general anesthetic and also may dramatically reduce pain and analgesic use postoperatively.[20] This may also significantly reduce hospital stays and postoperative complications such as nausea and vomiting. When performed as a single-shot block, the result is a dense block that is excellent for surgery but tends to wear off after 10 to 24 hours, which may mean the patient wakes up in pain. At least one study has shown less opioid use with continuous nerve catheter use for shoulder surgery.[21]

Continuous nerve blocks with a catheter may be prolonged for multiple days, but the catheters may interfere with mobilization and rehabilitation.[22] Epidurals have marked benefits in providing bilateral analgesia over several dermatomes and promote early return of bowel function over opioid analgesia alone.[23] Opioids may also be included in the epidural infusion, in which case the patient should not be given oral or IV opioids. Epidural anesthesia is associated with a risk of hypotension due to sympathetic blockade.[24] Peripheral nerve and epidural catheters are also considered a contraindication to anticoagulation other than subcutaneous heparin or daily enoxaparin.[25] While these guidelines are primarily intended to reduce the risk of epidural complications such as hematoma, more specific guidelines for other nerve blocks are not currently available.

OPIOID THERAPY FOR PAIN MANAGEMENT

Patients with previous surgical experience may have particular preferences which most of the time may be followed. For surgeries expected to be more painful, or where the opioids requirements are difficult to establish, the patient should be managed with IV opioids postoperatively for the first one or two days, then transitioned to oral medications. PCA is the easiest and safest way of accomplishing this in most cases, unless the patient is unable to use the button effectively due to cognitive or motor impairment.[26] Family members must be educated never to press the PCA button and not to wake the patient up to press it. Hydromorphone is the usual medication of choice for the PCA, although morphine and fentanyl may also be used. Once the patient is able to eat, he or she should be transferred to oral opioids, such as oxycodone or hydromorphone. Tramadol is a weak opioid that also has norepinephrine and serotonin reuptake inhibitory properties.[27] It may be useful in elderly patients who are very sensitive to sedation from other opioids. Long-acting opioids should not be used to treat acute postoperative pain in most cases. Meperidine is not used for acute pain due to risk of toxic metabolite accumulation and seizures.[28] This medication is still sometimes used in small doses for postoperative shivering.

PATIENTS ON CHRONIC OPIOID THERAPY

Patients who are on chronic opioid therapy should be identified prior to surgery and their doses verified if possible. Patients on a chronic long-acting opioid, such as extended-release oxycodone or morphine or fentanyl patches, should continue this treatment throughout the surgical period as much as possible. This will preserve the level of opioids that the patient has become tolerant to and allow the acute pain to be treated with short-acting medications. Otherwise, opioid requirements will predictably be very high due to the need to treat the patient's opioid withdrawal as well as his or her acute pain. Patients on methadone, whether it is given daily or multiple times a day, should likewise continue this during their hospitalization.

Patients receiving long-acting opioids together with short-acting opioids for pain or PCA analgesia should be closely observed to ensure that they are receiving adequate analgesia without overmedication. Ketamine may be particularly effective in these patients.

POTENTIAL COMPLICATIONS

Respiratory suppression is a potentially lethal complication of opioid analgesia with huge human and medical costs. It may occur at lower doses in the setting of lung disease, obstructive sleep apnea, or benzodiazepine use.[29] Often the first sign of this syndrome is excessive sedation, so medical and nursing staff caring for postoperative patients should be educated to further assess sedated patients, in particular checking their respiratory rate, oxygen saturation, and pupil size. Early intervention with naloxone and dose reduction may prevent respiratory failure and avoid the need for more dramatic interventions, such as intensive care unit transfer.

Sedation due to opioids can be difficult to distinguish from confusion and quiet delirium, especially in vulnerable populations and those who are not able to communicate. A recent study suggests that delirium is more common in patients with preoperative risk factors as well as those with severe postoperative pain and those with high opioid doses.[30] It may be helpful to reduce but not eliminate opioid analgesics while pursuing an evaluation for other causes of confusion such as infection or other medication and instituting behavioral and pharmacological treatments for delirium.

PATIENTS WITH ADDICTION

Patients rarely develop opioid use disorder due to short-term opioid treatment for acute pain. However, a Canadian study found that elderly patients receiving opioids after day surgeries were 44% more likely to be on opioids a year later than controls of the same age.[31] Opioid and other substance use disorders are common in the general population and may not be easy to recognize. Patients may present with multiple substance use disorders in various stages of intoxication and withdrawal and elective surgery may need to be delayed while this is addressed. The multimodal approach to analgesia outlined previously can be very helpful with these patients.[32] Patients injecting drugs are at higher risk for infectious complications and may not be suitable for regional anesthesia. Clonidine, an alpha-2 antagonist, can be very useful for patients with substance use disorders, especially in the setting of partially treated withdrawal.

Opioid use disorder patients may be enrolled in medication-assisted therapy, which may affect perioperative pain management. Methadone for opioid use disorder should be continued perioperatively, like any other long-acting opioid, and combined with a short-acting opioid given orally or via PCA.[33]

Postoperatively, the patient will need to follow up with the methadone maintenance clinic for their treatments and get tapered off the short-acting opioids at the surgical or pain clinic responsible for postoperative pain care.

Buprenorphine, prescribed together with naloxone as Suboxone, is a treatment for opioid use disorder that is increasingly popular and available. Since buprenorphine is a partial agonist of the mu-opioid receptor, it will interfere with other opioids and make pain management difficult. If surgeries are expected to be more than minimally painful, the patient should be taken off buprenorphine five days early and put on full agonist opioids instead.[33] Naltrexone may also be prescribed for opioid use disorder and will block the analgesic effects of opioids. Surgery should again be delayed until the naltrexone has worn off, which could be up to 30 days for the injectable depot form.

ELDERLY PATIENTS AND THOSE WITH IMPAIRED METABOLISM

The elderly and patients with central nervous disease and liver and renal dysfunction are particularly vulnerable for the complications mentioned previously. These patients often have decreased metabolism of medications and may have polypharmacy and reduced cognitive reserve. These factors mean that patients often benefit from cautious prescribing starting at lower doses and titrating as needed.

Patients with renal impairment may use fentanyl and methadone, which are not renally excreted, and hydromorphone and oxycodone with caution.[34,35] Morphine and codeine are not recommended due to active neurotoxic metabolites that can accumulate. NSAIDs are typically not recommended in renal impairment. Gabapentin dosage must be reduced depending on the estimated the glomerular filtration rate.

Liver impairment results in decreased clearance of many hepatically medications. Methadone and fentanyl are usually not strongly affected, while morphine, oxycodone, and hydromorphone have decreased clearance.[36] The dose of acetaminophen must be reduced to 2 grams/day in severe liver disease, and NSAIDs are not recommended. Gabapentin dosing is not affected.

PREGNANT AND NURSING PATIENTS

Pregnancy is associated with a host of physical and physiologic changes that go beyond the bounds of this review. Many medications have higher risks, or unknown risks, in pregnancy, so acetaminophen and opioids are mainstays of perioperative analgesia. NSAIDs are contraindicated in pregnancy since they may close the ductus arteriosus too soon.[37] Chronic opioids should be avoided to avoid fetal dependence and abstinence syndrome upon birth. Gabapentin is a class C drug and should be avoided in pregnancy.

In nursing mothers, the question is typically whether the patient may breast-feed her infant postoperatively. The physiology of lactation is complex, and the expression of medications into breast milk depends on the timing of the drug's administration versus the timing of breastfeeding and the degree of protein binding of the drug. Anesthetics and single doses of opioids perioperatively did not appear to result in significant levels of opioids within the breast milk. Ongoing opioid treatment appears to result in significant expression of opioids in milk, which may result in sedation of the infant. This includes use of opioids in epidural catheters, by mouth, or by PCA for postoperative pain. Ideally, opioids should be used at the lowest possible dose for the shortest time and the infant monitored for signs of lethargy. Neonates are more sensitive to opioids than older babies. Some mothers may choose to use a breast pump and discard some milk to minimize exposure while preserving their ability to breastfeed in the future.

Codeine should be avoided due to the small risk of very high blood levels in the event of a CYP2D6 polymorphism.[38] Opioids given by intrathecal pumps typically result in minimal blood levels and should not affect breastfeeding. There is a report of a patient with a 100 mcg/hr fentanyl patch with very low fentanyl levels in her milk.[39] NSAIDs are safe, especially when administered at time of breastfeeding so that they will have the maximum time to metabolize before the next feeding. Local anesthetics are considered safe in breastfeeding women.

CONCLUSION

Prevention of adverse events associated with perioperative pain management starts with the preoperative visit. It is essential while speaking with the patient to obtain an accurate pain history and also to set realistic goals for pain care. In most cases, use of multimodal pain treatment will improve pain control while reducing opioid consumption, which will in turn reduce the incidence of serious complications. Recognition of chronic pain, chronic opioid use, anxiety, and addiction will allow the provider to shape a care plan to address these issues. Recognizing other medical conditions and vulnerabilities may require reduction or avoidance of some elements of the pain care plan. There are many problems that can complicate a surgical treatment, but many of them may be mitigated through early detection. Where possible, surgical providers should seek to develop partners in perioperative care among allied specialties, particularly in anesthesia, pain medicine, and psychiatry. Nurses too have a great deal to offer in perioperative pain care beyond the provision of medication and reassurance. Providers working in an environment without ready access to pain consultants, psychiatrists, maternal-fetal medicine specialists, and so on will benefit all the more from a standardized approach to evaluation and management of these issues.

REFERENCES

1. Egbert LD, Battit GE, Welch CE, Bartlett MK. Reduction of postoperative pain by encouragement and instruction of patients: a study of doctor-patient rapport. *N Engl J Med.* 1964;270(16):825–827.
2. Carr DB, Goudas LC. Acute pain. *Lancet.* 1999;353(9169):2051–2058.
3. Williams JB, Alexander KP, Morin J-F, et al. Preoperative anxiety as a predictor of mortality and major morbidity in patients aged> 70 years undergoing cardiac surgery. *Am J Cardiol.* 2013;111(1):137–142.
4. Rasouli MR, Menendez ME, Sayadipour A, Purtill JJ, Parvizi J. Direct cost and complications associated with total joint arthroplasty in patients with preoperative anxiety and depression. *J Arthroplasty.* 2016;31(2):533–536.
5. Kiecolt-Glaser JK, Page GG, Marucha PT, MacCallum RC, Glaser R. Psychological influences on surgical recovery: perspectives from psychoneuroimmunology. *Am Psychologist.* 1998;53(11):1209.
6. Theunissen M, Peters ML, Bruce J, Gramke H-F, Marcus MA. Preoperative anxiety and catastrophizing: a systematic review and meta-analysis of the association with chronic postsurgical pain. *Clin J Pain.* 2012;28(9):819–841.
7. Riddle DL, Keefe FJ, Nay WT, McKee D, Attarian DE, Jensen MP. Pain coping skills training for patients with elevated pain catastrophizing who are scheduled for knee arthroplasty: a quasi-experimental study. *Arch Phys Med Rehab.* 2011;92(6):859–865.
8. Alanazi AA. Reducing anxiety in preoperative patients: a systematic review. *Br J Nurs.* 2014;23(7):387–393.
9. Remy C, Marret E, Bonnet F. Effects of acetaminophen on morphine side-effects and consumption after major surgery: meta-analysis of randomized controlled trials. *Br J Anaesth.* 2005;94(4):505–513.
10. American Society of Anesthesiologists Task Force on Acute Pain Management. Practice guidelines for acute pain management in the perioperative setting: an updated report by the American Society of Anesthesiologists Task Force on Acute Pain Management. *Anesthesiology.* 2012;116(2):248.

11. Elia N, Lysakowski C, Tramèr M. Does multimodal analgesia with acetaminophen, nonsteroidal antiinflammatory drugs, or selective cyclooxygenase-2 inhibitors and patient-controlled analgesia morphine offer advantages over morphine alone? Meta-analyses of randomized trials. *Anesthesiology.* 2005;103(6):1296.

12. Gobble RM, Hoang HL, Kachniarz B, Orgill DP. Ketorolac does not increase perioperative bleeding: a meta-analysis of randomized controlled trials. *Plast Reconstruct Surg.* 2014;133(3):741–755.

13. Hernandez-Diaz S, Rodriguez LAG. Association between nonsteroidal anti-inflammatory drugs and upper gastrointestinal tract bleeding/perforation: an overview of epidemiologic studies published in the 1990s. *Arch Intern Med.* 2000;160(14):2093.

14. Burton TP, Mittal A, Soop M. Nonsteroidal anti-inflammatory drugs and anastomotic dehiscence in bowel surgery: systematic review and meta-analysis of randomized, controlled trials. *Dis Colon Rectum.* 2013;56(1):126–134.

15. Gupta A, Jakobsson J. Acetaminophen, nonsteroidal anti-inflammatory drugs, and cyclooxygenase-2 selective inhibitors: an update. *Plast Reconst Surg.* 2014;134(4 Suppl 2):24S–31S.

16. Yan PZ, Butler PM, Kurowski D, Perloff MD. Beyond neuropathic pain: gabapentin use in cancer pain and perioperative pain. *Clin J Pain.* 2014;30(7):613–629.

17. Laskowski K, Stirling A, McKay WP, Lim HJ. A systematic review of intravenous ketamine for postoperative analgesia. *Can J Anesth.* 2011;58(10):911–923.

18. Koppert W, Weigand M, Neumann F, et al. Perioperative intravenous lidocaine has preventive effects on postoperative pain and morphine consumption after major abdominal surgery. *Anesthes Analg.* 2004;98(4):1050–1055.

19. Herroeder S, Pecher S, Schönherr ME, et al. Systemic lidocaine shortens length of hospital stay after colorectal surgery: a double-blinded, randomized, placebo-controlled trial. *Ann Surg.* 2007;246(2):192.

20. Liu SS, Strodtbeck WM, Richman JM, Wu CL. A comparison of regional versus general anesthesia for ambulatory anesthesia: a meta-analysis of randomized controlled trials. *Anesth Analg.* 2005;101(6):1634–1642.

21. Goebel S, Stehle J, Schwemmer U, Reppenhagen S, Rath B, Gohlke F. Interscalene brachial plexus block for open-shoulder surgery: a randomized, double-blind, placebo-controlled trial between single-shot anesthesia and patient-controlled catheter system. *Arch Orthopaed Trauma Surg.* 2010;130(4):533–540.

22. Capdevila X, Ponrouch M, Choquet O. Continuous peripheral nerve blocks in clinical practice. *Curr Opin Anesth.* 2008;21(5):619–623.

23. Jørgensen H, Wetterslev J, Møiniche S, Dahl JB. Epidural local anaesthetics versus opioid-based analgesic regimens for postoperative gastrointestinal paralysis, PONV and pain after abdominal surgery. *Cochrane Database Syst Rev.* 2001;1.

24. Wheatley R, Schug S, Watson D. Safety and efficacy of postoperative epidural analgesia. *Br J Anaesth.* 2001;87(1):47–61.

25. Horlocker TT, Wedel DJ, Rowlingson JC, Enneking FK. Executive summary: regional anesthesia in the patient receiving antithrombotic or thrombolytic therapy: American Society of Regional Anesthesia and Pain Medicine Evidence-Based Guidelines. *Reg Anesth Pain Med.* 2010;35(1):102–105.

26. Walder B, Schafer M, Henzi I, Tramer M. Efficacy and safety of patient-controlled opioid analgesia for acute postoperative pain. *Acta Anaesth Scand.* 2001;45(7):795–804.

27. Houmes R-JM, Voets MA, Verkaaik A, Erdmann W, Lachmann B. Efficacy and safety of tramadol versus morphine for moderate and severe postoperative pain with special regard to respiratory depression. *Anesth Analg.* 1992;74(4):510–514.

28. Simopoulos TT, Smith HS, Peeters-Asdourian C, Stevens DS. Use of meperidine in patient-controlled analgesia and the development of a normeperidine toxic reaction. *Arch Surg.* 2002;137(1):84–88.

29. Melamed R, Boland LL, Normington JP, et al. Postoperative respiratory failure necessitating transfer to the intensive care unit in orthopedic surgery patients: risk factors, costs, and outcomes. *Periop Med.* 2016;5(1):19.

30. Leung JM, Sands LP, Lim E, Tsai TL, Kinjo S. Does preoperative risk for delirium moderate the effects of postoperative pain and opiate use on postoperative delirium? *Am J Geriatr Psychiatry.* 2013;21(10):946–956.

31. Alam A, Gomes T, Zheng H, Mamdani MM, Juurlink DN, Bell CM. Long-term analgesic use after low-risk surgery: a retrospective cohort study. *Arch Intern Med.* 2012;172(5):425–430.

32. Stromer W, Michaeli K, Sandner-Kiesling A. Perioperative pain therapy in opioid abuse. *Eur J Anaesthesiol.* 2013;30(2):55–64.

33. Bryson EO. The perioperative management of patients maintained on medications used to manage opioid addiction. *Curr Opin Anesthesiol.* 2014;27(3):359–364.

34. Launay-Vacher V, Karie S, Fau J-B, Izzedine H, Deray G. Treatment of pain in patients with renal insufficiency: the World Health Organization three-step ladder adapted. *J Pain.* 2005;6(3):137–148.

35. O'connor NR, Corcoran AM. End-stage renal disease: symptom management and advance care planning. *Am Fam Physician.* 2012;85(7):705–710.

36. Chandok N, Watt KD. Pain management in the cirrhotic patient: the clinical challenge. Paper presented at Mayo Clinic Proceedings, 2010.

37. Lucas S. Medication use in the treatment of migraine during pregnancy and lactation. *Curr Pain Headache Rep.* 2009;13(5):392–398.

38. Koren G, Cairns J, Chitayat D, Gaedigk A, Leeder SJ. Pharmacogenetics of morphine poisoning in a breastfed neonate of a codeine-prescribed mother. *Lancet.* 2006;368(9536):704.

39. Cohen RS. Fentanyl transdermal analgesia during pregnancy and lactation. *J Hum Lact.* 2009;25(3):359–361.

19 Management of Neuropathic Postoperative Pain

Ean Saberski and Lloyd Saberski

Surgery invariably causes pain. This pain is routinely self-limited and temporally restricted to the perioperative period. The consensus opinion by the International Association for the Study of Pain (IASP) published in 2011 states that routine postoperative pain is expected to resolve within two months.[1] At this time point, the processes of acute pain transition to physiologically distinct processes of chronic pain.[2] Nociceptive signals are the root source for acute pain perception, while more complex neural pathways drive chronic pain. Persistent nociception is of course a potential etiology, but the most likely etiology of chronic postoperative pain is neuropathic pain.[3]

Overall, 20% to 50% of surgical cases are complicated by an element of chronic postoperative pain with 2% to 10% resulting in severe, debilitating pain.[4] The morbidity of chronic postoperative pain is significant, with persistent suffering and decreased quality of life for all affected patients.[5] A tremendous burden is also shared by elevated health care costs and social support systems in managing chronic postoperative pain.[6]

The effective management of postoperative neuropathic pain first requires an understanding of the physiological processes contributing to routine postoperative pain. Armed with this understanding, the observant surgeon recognizes the transition from acute pain to chronic pain and tailors treatment to address the underlying pathology.

PHYSIOLOGY OF ROUTINE POSTOPERATIVE PAIN

Surgical intervention routinely requires operative exposure, necessitating the division and dissection of anatomic structures. This tissue damage elicits a physiologically normal yet unpleasant protective pain response.[7] No matter if tissue damage is induced by surgery or trauma, pain perceived by a patient is the culmination of a common cascade of events.[8] These events are broadly categorized into four major processes: transduction, transmission, decoding, and modulation.[9]

Transduction

Through the process of transduction, noxious stimuli are converted into neural signals by primary afferent nociceptors found in the terminal branches of A-delta and C fibers. Nociceptive signal demonstrates a graded response correlating the rate of receptor firing to the intensity of noxious stimulus.[10] In the context of postoperative pain, deforming mechanical force and tissue damage serve as relevant stimuli for transduction. Damaged tissues release various substances that initiate multiple inflammatory pathways, subsequently increasing the transduction of painful signal. Prostaglandins and leukotrienes are members of the arachidonic acid pathway involved in reducing the nociceptor activation threshold, which further amplifies pain transduction.[11-13] Kinins such as bradykinin and kallidin also affect the milieu for pain transduction by releasing prostaglandins, promoting the release of free radicals, degranulating mast cells, and stimulating sympathetic tone on local blood vessels.[14] Histamine, neurokinins such as substance P, serotonin, interleukins, and cytokines also each contribute to the noxious stimulus found at the tissue level that initiates a localized nociceptive pain signal.[8,15,16]

Transmission

After a noxious stimulus is transduced at the nociceptor end organ, its signal is transmitted cephalad through A-delta and C fibers in the peripheral nervous system to the superficial Rexed laminae in the dorsal horn of the spinal cord. Presynaptic first order neurons release multiple neurotransmitters such as substance P and calcitonin gene-related peptide that contribute to a process of enhanced excitability mediated by calcium influx in postsynaptic neurons.[17-19] During this period of enhanced excitability, excitatory amino acids including aspartate and glutamate act on the α-amino-3-hydroxy-5-methyl-4-isoxazolepropionic acid (AMPA) and N-methyl-D-aspartate (NMDA) receptors with heightened effect.[20-23]

Decoding

Afferent pain signals continue from the dorsal horn of the spinal cord along second-order nociceptive neurons to the central nervous system. The afferent signal travels cephalad in the spinothalamic tract and is routed to the reticular formation and through the brainstem before terminating in the thalamus. From the thalamus, afferent information is projected to the somatosensory cortex and centers such as the reticularis gigantocellularis for sensory processing. Branches terminating in the reticular formation coordinate an emotional response to the nociceptive signal. It is also at this level that complex networks of neural connections regulate somatic and autonomic motor reflexes associated with pain.[24,25]

While afferent nociceptive signals ascend cephalad, efferent pathways modulate pain by means of inhibitory neuronal systems. Signals propagated in the motor cortex, hypothalamus, and periaqueductal gray matter relay inhibition at synapses throughout the nervous system. In the dorsal horn, Gamma-amino butyric acid (GABA) and glycine are released as inhibitory neurotransmitters that act on the NMDA receptor.[26] In normal physiology, peripheral inflammation leads to upregulation of GABA receptors and increased sensitivity to descending inhibition.[27] Supraspinal modulation occurs vastly throughout the central nervous system, chiefly employing norepinephrine, somatostatin, and endorphins to temper the perception of pain.[28,29] The inhibition achieved through modulation is conceptually achieved by closing "gates."[30] These gates act as checkpoints in the transmission of pain and are effectively closed by adequate inhibitory signals. Gate closure terminates the cephalad progression of nociceptive signals, thereby reducing the electrical signal available for decoding.

PHYSIOLOGY OF NEUROPATHIC POSTOPERATIVE PAIN

Chronic nociceptive signaling precipitates a cascade of biochemical changes in the peripheral and central nervous systems. These changes represent a wide spectrum of deviations from normal physiology and beget the aberrant physiology of neuropathic pain after approximately two months of continued noxious stimulus. Unlike acute pain, chronic neuropathic pain signals do not initiate with tissue damage. Instead, neuropathic pain signals are independent entities that occur as the result of changes in the processing of pain signals.

Neuropathic Changes During Transduction

Persistent tissue damage and inflammation will propagate persistent ascending nociceptive signaling. In neuropathic pain, however, there is not necessarily a connection between tissue damage and ascending signals. Neuromas are capable of ectopic electrogenesis, through which ascending signals are initiated without any tissue damage.[31] Ectopic signals can also be generated in response to neuritis and nerve compression.[32]

Neuropathic Changes During Transmission

During periods of prolonged signaling, the neurons of the dorsal horn are flooded with excitatory amino acids and substance P, causing enhanced depolarization and calcium influx.[33] These changes promote a hyperexcitable state, which leads to increased transmission through the dorsal horn. C-fos protein is also expressed at higher concentration in the dorsal horn in response to persistent pain signaling.[34]

Neuropathic Changes During Decoding

The central nervous system response to chronic nociceptive input is to undergo a process known as central sensitization. Through central sensitization, allodynia is facilitated by a perturbation in the sensory modalities.[35] Through various molecular pathways, the cortical response to ascending input is altered and associated with pain.[36]

Neuropathic Changes During Modulation

The role of modulation is to act as a descending inhibitory pathway, in effect damping the pain response. The typical response to peripheral painful stimulus is to upregulate spinal GABA receptors, in turn inhibiting the ascending nociceptive signal.[27] In cases of neuropathic pain, this upregulation is inadequate, and the ascending signal progresses unimpeded.[26]

THERAPEUTIC TARGETS IN PAIN MANAGEMENT

The processes of transduction, transmission, decoding, and modulation provide targeted opportunities to provide analgesia. Every analgesic agent provides a therapeutic benefit at a specific target, and a synergistic effect is created when multiple agents are used to affect multiple targets. Taking advantage of the synergism between different chemotherapies lowers the dose of each agent needed to achieve analgesia. With lower doses prescribed, the likelihood of unwanted side effect is reduced, in turn reducing postoperative morbidity.

Targeting Transduction

The first opportunity to intervene therapeutically in the development of pain is during the process of transduction. Nociceptive signals are spawned at the tissue level during transduction, and agents that affect transduction either raise the threshold for or reduce the frequency of nociceptive signaling. Local anesthetic agents block afferent nociceptive impulses and, when used in local field blocks, limit the transmission from mechanoreceptors detecting tissue deformation. Nonsteroidal anti-inflammatory drugs (NSAIDs) disrupt the expansion of the inflammatory milieu associated with tissue injury by inhibiting prostaglandin production.[37] NSAIDs also work to stabilize cellular membranes during tissue injury, which further leads to decreased prostaglandin release, a phenomenon also observed with the administration of glucocorticoids, tricyclic antidepressants, and antiarrhythmics.[38] Capsaicin is another agent known to reduce the impulse of nociceptive signaling at the tissue level.[39]

Targeting Transmission

Nociceptive transmission is the second target for postoperative analgesia. The goal in targeting transmission is to blunt afferent signal progression and thereby blunt the degree of glutamate and aspartate acting at the synapse. Transmission of nociceptive signals is most effectively tempered by means of regional anesthesia blockade. Neural axial blocks, plexus blocks, and somatic blocks each dampen the degree of pain signal that ultimately excites the second-order neurons in the dorsal horn.

Targeting Decoding

The process of decoding affords a third opportunity to pharmaceutically intervene in pain signaling. Agents that affect nociceptive decoding do so by altering the perception of pain. When decoding is altered, normal nociceptive signals arrive at their terminus without restriction but do not elicit a painful sensation. General anesthetics and opioids are both known to depress the activity of major nociceptive processing centers.[40-42] Targeting nociceptive decoding with opioids is the gold standard approach to perioperative analgesia because it is reliable and efficacious. The protracted use of opioids is ill advised, however, because of increased risk of dependence, tolerance, and untoward side effects.

Psychotropic modulation also influences nociceptive decoding by augmenting the emotional context for pain processing. Management of underlying anxiety and depression, either pharmaceutically or therapeutically, profoundly impacts pain decoding.[43]

Targeting Modulation

The final opportunity to therapeutically manage pain is during modulation. Pharmaceutical agents that target modulation achieve clinically significant pain reduction by amplifying inhibitory signals. Gabapentin and pregabalin both increase GABA concentration at the synapse, in turn reducing glutamate release and decreasing signal transmission, effectively closing the gate of nociceptive transmission. Other pharmaceutical agents modulate nociception through complex and incompletely understood mechanisms. Tricyclic antidepressants and serotonin/norepinephrine reuptake inhibitors both achieve a modulatory effect at synaptic gates through a pathway involving adrenoreceptors.[44] The modulatory effect of opioids is complex but well documented. Opioid receptors are distributed throughout the central and peripheral nervous system and augment the transmission of nociceptive signal.

MANAGING NEUROPATHIC POSTOPERATIVE PAIN

As with the management of routine postoperative pain, the management of chronic neuropathic postoperative pain is most effective when interventions and therapeutics are applied thoughtfully to specific targets in the nociceptive pathway.

Diagnosis of Neuropathic Postoperative Pain

The effective management of chronic postoperative pain hinges on timely and accurate diagnosis. At approximately two months status postsurgical intervention, the routine expectation is for near resolution of pain. Persistent pain at the two-month postoperative time point warrants concern for the development of chronic pain physiology.

Clinical investigation must always start with a detailed history examining the nature and quality of the pain. It is important to understand if the pain quality evolved during the postoperative course. A change in the pain quality can correlate with the development of chronic pain, which is classically described as "electrical" in quality. Subjective paresthesia can also correlate to neuropathic pain.

Targeted examination includes inspection and palpation of the surgical site. Ongoing edema and ecchymoses may suggest ongoing tissue damage and perhaps provide evidence for continued acute nociceptive signaling. The ability to reproduce the pain by palpation is also suggestive of an active transductive process. Increased pain sensitivity, also known as hyperalgesia, is often present in neuropathic pain. Allodynia is the perception of pain in response to a typically nonpainful stimulus and is also a common element of neuropathic pain. Examination should also qualify hyperesthesia or hypoesthesia in the affected area.

Management of Neuropathic Postoperative Pain

Effective management of neuropathic postoperative pain relies on the distillation of the components of the pain response. Based on the history and physical, the examiner must synthesize a concept of which nociceptive processes are aberrant and tailor the analgesic approach appropriately. For example, patients with active nociceptive transduction require analgesic agents that reduce transduction. Conversely, patients with no active transductive process do not need agents that target transduction.

KNOWN NEUROPATHIC POSTOPERATIVE PAIN DIAGNOSES

While any surgical intervention may be complicated by neuropathic pain, there are particular interventions with documented heightened postoperative risk profiles. The two best investigated and reported in the literature are postherniorrhaphy pain syndrome and persistent pain after breast cancer surgery.

Postherniorrhaphy Pain Syndrome

Chronic pain following inguinal hernia repair is a well-documented phenomenon, affecting 11% to 39% of patients.[45,46] The underlying etiology of this chronic pain is categorized into one of three groups: group 1 is neuropathic pain, group 2 is nonneuropathic pain, and group 3 is a tender spermatic cord.[47] Patients from group 1 typically sustain an injury to a neural structure at the time of surgery, ultimately leading to neuropathic pain. The patients in groups 2 and 3 do not develop neuropathic pain, and their exam is often more consistent with periostitis pubis or a recurrent hernia.

The ilioinguinal, iliohypogastric, and genitofemoral nerves are all at risk of injury in inguinal hernia surgery. Nerve damage by transection as well as by entrapment is possible. Nerve entrapment can occur when suture, staple, or prosthetic material impinge and compress a neural structure. Nerves under compression from a surgically placed material will provide chronic nociceptive signals that will ultimately spur neuropathic physiological changes and potentially lead to ectopic signaling.

The most effective management strategy to reduce the prevalence of postherniorrhaphy syndrome is to meticulously identify all neurological structures at the time of surgery and ensure they are preserved or deliberately managed. Management of postherniorrhaphy pain syndrome is dependent on the accurate diagnosis and categorization of the presentation. Patients from groups 2 and 3 are best if approached for symptom management and reoperation if clinically indicated. The patients with neuropathic pain in group 1 respond well to approaches that are well described for neuropathic pain management. Surgical release and decompression of the compressed nerves does effectively eliminate ongoing nociceptive signaling, but oftentimes the transition to ectopic nociception has occurred before secondary surgery.

Persistent Pain After Breast Cancer Surgery

Persistent pain after breast cancer was first recognized as an entity in the literature as postmastectomy pain syndrome in 1978.[48] It was further formally recognized by the IASP in 1986. In the intervening decades, breast cancer surgery has become less invasive, yet a subset of patients with chronic pain persists.[49] Up to 50% of patients report persistent pain following breast surgery, with approximately 10% of patients experiencing severe pain.[50,51]

Injury to the intercostal, medial, or lateral pectoral; long thoracic; thoracodorsal; and intercostal brachial nerves is often unavoidable during surgical extirpation of breast cancer. Injury to any of these nerves initiates the common cascade of events implicit in acute pain. Chronic pain develops in a subset of patients as their pain signaling transitions from acute to chronic physiology. A recent study suggested that central sensitization is the primary mechanism through which persistent pain after breast cancer surgery develops.[52] Risk factors for persistent pain after breast cancer surgery include axillary lymph node dissection, radiation therapy, and chemotherapy.[53]

The most prudent approach to reduce the incidence of persistent postmastectomy pain is to minimize perioperative pain. In minimizing perioperative pain, the degree of nociceptive signal is limited, which lessens the odds of developing painful neuropathy. Consistent with this logic, the most efficacious means by which risk is reduced is by avoiding axillary lymph node dissection when clinically appropriate.[54,55]

There is no clearly defined ideal management algorithm for patients who do present with persistent pain after breast cancer. However, the principals of managing neuropathic postoperative pain are translatable to breast cancer patients. Pharmacological therapy should be tailored to deliberately address aberrant physiology in nociceptive processes. Local anesthetic paravertebral or intercostal blockade are effective temporary measures for patients refractory to medical therapy.[56]

REFERENCES

1. Ballantyne JC. Pain medicine: repairing a fractured dream. *Anesthesiology.* 2011;114(2):243–246.
2. Katz J, Seltzer Z. Transition from acute to chronic postsurgical pain: risk factors and protective factors. *Expert Rev Neurother.* 2009;9(5):723–744.
3. Kehlet H, Jensen TS, Woolf CJ. Persistent postsurgical pain: risk factors and prevention. *Lancet.* 2006;367(9522):1618–1625.
4. Macrae WA. Chronic post-surgical pain: 10 years on. *Br J Anaesth.* 2008;101(1):77–86.
5. Blyth FM, March LM, Cousins MJ. Chronic pain-related disability and use of analgesia and health services in a Sydney community. *Med J Aust.* 2003;179(2):84–87.
6. Engoren M. Cost-effectiveness of different postoperative analgesic treatments. *Expert Opin Pharmacother.* 2003;4(9):1507–1519.
7. Woolf CJ. What is this thing called pain? *J Clin Invest.* 2010;120(11):3742–3744.

8. Julius D, Basbaum AI. Molecular mechanisms of nociception. *Nature.* 2001;413(6852):203–210.

9. Kelly DJ, Ahmad M, Brull SJ. Preemptive analgesia I: physiological pathways and pharmacological modalities. *Can J Anaesth.* 2001;48(10):1000–1010.

10. Mendell LM. Physiological properties of unmyelinated fiber projection to the spinal cord. *Exp Neurol.* 1966;16(3):316–332.

11. Birrell GJ, McQueen DS, Iggo A, Coleman RA, Grubb BD. PGI2-induced activation and sensitization of articular mechanonociceptors. *Neurosci Lett.* 1991;124(1):5–8.

12. Cohen RH, Perl ER. Contributions of arachidonic acid derivatives and substance P to the sensitization of cutaneous nociceptors. *J Neurophysiol.* 1990;64(2):457–464.

13. Levine JD, Fields HL, Basbaum AI. Peptides and the primary afferent nociceptor. *J Neurosci.* 1993;13(6):2273–2286.

14. Walker K, Perkins M, Dray A. Kinins and kinin receptors in the nervous system. *Neurochem Int.* 1995;26(1):1–16; discussion 17–26.

15. Lisowska B, Siewruk K, Lisowski A. Substance P and Acute Pain in Patients Undergoing Orthopedic Surgery. *PLoS One.* 2016;11(1):e0146400.

16. McMahon SB. *Wall and Melzack's Textbook of Pain,* 6th ed. Philadelphia, PA: Elsevier/Saunders; 2013.

17. Murase K, Randic M. Actions of substance P on rat spinal dorsal horn neurones. *J Physiol.* 1984;346:203–217.

18. Skofitsch G, Jacobowitz DM. Calcitonin gene-related peptide coexists with substance P in capsaicin sensitive neurons and sensory ganglia of the rat. *Peptides.* 1985;6(4):747–754.

19. Schaible HG, Neugebauer V, Geisslinger G, Beck U. The effects of S- and R-flurbiprofen on the inflammation-evoked intraspinal release of immunoreactive substance P—a study with antibody microprobes. *Brain Res.* 1998;798(1-2):287–293.

20. Dougherty PM, Willis WD. Enhancement of spinothalamic neuron responses to chemical and mechanical stimuli following combined micro-iontophoretic application of N-methyl-D-aspartic acid and substance P. *Pain.* 1991;47(1):85–93.

21. Kangrga I, Larew JS, Randic M. The effects of substance P and calcitonin gene-related peptide on the efflux of endogenous glutamate and aspartate from the rat spinal dorsal horn in vitro. *Neurosci Lett.* 1990;108(1-2):155–160.

22. Schneider SP, Perl ER. Selective excitation of neurons in the mammalian spinal dorsal horn by aspartate and glutamate in vitro: correlation with location and excitatory input. *Brain Res.* 1985;360(1-2):339–343.

23. Willcockson WS, Chung JM, Hori Y, Lee KH, Willis WD. Effects of iontophoretically released amino acids and amines on primate spinothalamic tract cells. *J Neurosci.* 1984;4(3):732–740.

24. Bowsher D. Role of the reticular formation in responses to noxious stimulation. *Pain.* 1976;2(4):361–378.

25. Price DD, Dubner R, Hu JW. Trigeminothalamic neurons in nucleus caudalis responsive to tactile, thermal, and nociceptive stimulation of monkey's face. *J Neurophysiol.* 1976;39(5):936–953.

26. Yaksh TL. Behavioral and autonomic correlates of the tactile evoked allodynia produced by spinal glycine inhibition: effects of modulatory receptor systems and excitatory amino acid antagonists. *Pain.* 1989;37(1):111–123.

27. Dickenson AH. Spinal cord pharmacology of pain. *Br J Anaesth.* 1995;75(2):193–200.

28. Besson JM, Chaouch A. Peripheral and spinal mechanisms of nociception. *Physiol Rev.* 1987;67(1):67–186.

29. Fields HL, Heinricher MM, Mason P. Neurotransmitters in nociceptive modulatory circuits. *Annu Rev Neurosci.* 1991;14:219–245.

30. Melzack R, Wall PD. Pain mechanisms: a new theory. *Science.* 1965;150(3699):971–979.

31. Mao J, Price DD, Coghill RC, Mayer DJ, Hayes RL. Spatial patterns of spinal cord [14C]-2-deoxyglucose metabolic activity in a rat model of painful peripheral mononeuropathy. *Pain.* 1992;50(1):89–100.

32. Bove GM, Ransil BJ, Lin HC, Leem JG. Inflammation induces ectopic mechanical sensitivity in axons of nociceptors innervating deep tissues. *J Neurophysiol.* 2003;90(3):1949–1955.

33. Dray A. Inflammatory mediators of pain. *Br J Anaesth.* 1995;75(2):125–131.

34. Tolle TR, Castro-Lopes JM, Coimbra A, Zieglgansberger W. Opiates modify induction of c-fos proto-oncogene in the spinal cord of the rat following noxious stimulation. *Neurosci Lett.* 1990;111(1-2):46–51.

35. Devor M. Centralization, central sensitization and neuropathic pain. Focus on "sciatic chronic constriction injury produces cell-type-specific changes in the electrophysiological properties of rat substantia gelatinosa neurons." *J Neurophysiol.* 2006;96(2):522–523.

36. Nitzan-Luques A, Devor M, Tal M. Genotype-selective phenotypic switch in primary afferent neurons contributes to neuropathic pain. *Pain.* 2011;152(10):2413–2426.

37. Dahl JB, Kehlet H. Non-steroidal anti-inflammatory drugs: rationale for use in severe postoperative pain. *Br J Anaesth.* 1991;66(6):703–712.

38. Kitahata LM. Pain pathways and transmission. *Yale J Biol Med.* 1993;66(5):437–442.

39. Vergne P, Bertin P, Bonnet C, Treves R. [Morphine and neuropathic pain]. *Therapie.* 1999;54(2):257–258.

40. Kikuchi H, Kitahata LM, Collins JG, Kawahara M, Nio K. Halothane-induced changes in neuronal activity of cells of the nucleus reticularis gigantocellularis of the cat. *Anesth Analg.* 1980;59(12):897–901.

41. Mosso JA, Kruger L. Spinal trigeminal neurons excited by noxious and thermal stimuli. *Brain Res.* 1972;38(1):206–210.

42. Ohtani M, Kikuchi H, Kitahata LM, et al. Effects of ketamine on nociceptive cells in the medial medullary reticular formation of the cat. *Anesthesiology.* 1979;51(5):414–417.

43. Wylde V, Trela-Larsen L, Whitehouse MR, Blom AW. Preoperative psychosocial risk factors for poor outcomes at 1 and 5 years after total knee replacement. *Acta Orthop.* 2017:1–7.

44. Bohren Y, Tessier LH, Megat S, et al. Antidepressants suppress neuropathic pain by a peripheral beta2-adrenoceptor mediated anti-TNFalpha mechanism. *Neurobiol Dis.* 2013;60:39–50.

45. Aasvang EK, Bay-Nielsen M, Kehlet H. Pain and functional impairment 6 years after inguinal herniorrhaphy. *Hernia.* 2006;10(4):316–321.

46. Massaron S, Bona S, Fumagalli U, Battafarano F, Elmore U, Rosati R. Analysis of postsurgical pain after inguinal hernia repair: a prospective study of 1,440 operations. *Hernia.* 2007;11(6):517–525.

47. Loos MJ, Roumen RM, Scheltinga MR. Classifying post-herniorrhaphy pain syndromes following elective inguinal hernia repair. *World J Surg.* 2007;31(9):1760–1765; discussion 1766–1767.

48. Wood KM. Intercostobrachial nerve entrapment syndrome. *South Med J.* 1978;71(6):662–663.

49. Vadivelu N, Schreck M, Lopez J, Kodumudi G, Narayan D. Pain after mastectomy and breast reconstruction. *Am Surg.* 2008;74(4):285–296.

50. Gartner R, Jensen MB, Nielsen J, Ewertz M, Kroman N, Kehlet H. Prevalence of and factors associated with persistent pain following breast cancer surgery. *JAMA.* 2009;302(18):1985–1992.

51. Macdonald L, Bruce J, Scott NW, Smith WC, Chambers WA. Long-term follow-up of breast cancer survivors with post-mastectomy pain syndrome. *Br J Cancer.* 2005;92(2):225–230.

52. van Helmond N, Steegers MA, Filippini-de Moor GP, Vissers KC, Wilder-Smith OH. Hyperalgesia and persistent pain after breast cancer surgery: a prospective randomized controlled trial with perioperative COX-2 inhibition. *PLoS One.* 2016;11(12):e0166601.

53. Wang L, Guyatt GH, Kennedy SA, et al. Predictors of persistent pain after breast cancer surgery: a systematic review and meta-analysis of observational studies. *CMAJ.* 2016;188(14):E352–E361.

54. Giuliano AE, Hunt KK, Ballman KV, et al. Axillary dissection vs no axillary dissection in women with invasive breast cancer and sentinel node metastasis: a randomized clinical trial. *JAMA.* 2011;305(6):569–575.

55. Abdullah TI, Iddon J, Barr L, Baildam AD, Bundred NJ. Prospective randomized controlled trial of preservation of the intercostobrachial nerve during axillary node clearance for breast cancer. *Br J Surg.* 1998;85(10):1443–1445.

56. Cheng GS, Ilfeld BM. An evidence-based review of the efficacy of perioperative analgesic techniques for breast cancer-related surgery. *Pain Med.* 2017;18(7):1344–1365.

20 Perioperative Pain Management in Hand and Upper Extremity Surgery

Marc E. Walker, David M. Tsai,
and J. Grant Thomson

INTRODUCTION

As the focus on health care cost and quality has sharpened over the past three decades, there has been a dramatic shift in the delivery of care. In response, the number of outpatient surgery centers has risen exponentially. Along with major advancements in medical technology and the wide availability of improved anesthetic agents, this growth of outpatient facilities (whether affiliated with hospitals or not) has led to a notable surge in demand for ambulatory surgery.

According to the Healthcare Cost and Utilization Project, between 1992 and 2012 the number of outpatient surgeries performed in community hospitals grew by more than 20%, accounting for 65% of all surgeries.[1-2] Hand and upper extremity surgery is no exception, and, in many respects, with the modern advancements in anesthesia care, surgery of the hand is one of the best-suited fields for such change.[3]

New developments in perioperative pain management have contributed largely to this shift, as options ranging from general anesthesia to regional nerve blocks to wide-awake local-only techniques have enabled hand surgeons to meet this growing demand.

PHYSIOLOGIC ASPECTS

Pain is a physiologic phenomenon rendered via a complex cascade from the periphery to the central nervous system. Primary somatosensory neurons relay noxious stimuli to the dorsal horn of the spinal cord, where then synapse with secondary neurons. From there, they decussate and conduct to higher levels, synapsing with tertiary neurons in the thalamus and different nuclei in the brainstem including the periaqueductal gray and nucleus raphe magnus. Tertiary neurons project to somatosensory cortices and limbic structures, which are involved with the sensory and emotional components of pain, respectively. Excitatory and inhibitory neurons modulate pain at all levels in both ascending and descending paths.[4-5]

Nociceptors are the free nerve endings found throughout the body such as skin, periosteum, and joint surfaces that detect potentially harmful mechanical, thermal, or chemical stimuli and transmit the signals to the spinal cord. When tissue insult occurs, bradykinins, histamine, serotonin, adenosine triphosphate, interleukins, interferon, tumor necrosis factor, and various substances are released. These proinflammatory and pronociceptive factors incite the initial cascade.[4-5]

Three groups of afferent fibers exist, differing in their role, diameter, and conduction velocity: Aβ, Aδ, and C. Aβ fibers are large myelinated fibers that conduct nonnociceptive input such as touch, vibration, and movement but also participate in pain modulation as described in the gate control theory, whereby activation of these fibers inhibit nociceptive input from the same region. Aδ fibers are large myelinated fibers that rapidly conduct the initial sharp localization and sensation of pain, sometimes referred to as first pain. C fibers are the slowest due to their small caliber and lack of myelin. They are responsible for the delayed, deep throbbing, burning pain, known as second pain.[4-5]

Constant recruitment of C fibers can lead to central sensitization, in which prolonged activation of N-methyl-D-aspartate receptors induce downstream changes in the permeability and recruitment threshold of secondary neurons. These neuronal plastic consequences ultimately lead to hyperalgesia and allodynia that may long persist after the initial injury. Understanding the impact of this sensitization and taking preemptive measures is crucial in preventing chronic pain.[4-5]

PHARMACOLOGY

Local Anesthetics

Local anesthetics are indispensable in hand and upper extremity procedures. They are particularly advantageous in an ambulatory setting, where their strategic use can help obviate the need for general anesthesia and its untoward risks.

Local anesthetic agents may be classified as either amides or esters and can be delivered in a local, topical, intravenous, or regional fashion. After administration, the agent passively diffuses across neuronal cell membranes and blocks the sodium channels, thereby inhibiting the generation of action potentials and thus pain. The onset of action for each agent relates to the agent's pKa, impacting the ratio of ionized to un-ionized forms with only the latter basic form capable of penetrating cell membranes. The closer the agent's pKa is to physiologic pH, the greater the proportion of molecules in the un-ionized forms. These anesthetic agents cross membranes more readily and have a faster onset of action. Other important pharmacokinetic factors are an agent's lipid solubility, protein-binding capacity, and vasodilatory effects, which are important in determining potency and duration of action.[6-7]

Esters tend to have a shorter plasma half-life as they rapidly undergo hydrolysis by circulating pseudocholinesterases. Historically, these were the first developed local anesthetics in the form of cocaine and procaine. Amides were later developed, and they quickly replaced the use of esters due to a faster onset and longer duration of action. Amides are metabolized primarily in the liver. Common amides include lidocaine, bupivacaine, mepivacaine, prilocaine, etidocaine, and ropivacaine.[6-7]

The esters, procaine and chloroprocaine, and the amides, lidocaine and prilocaine, are the most commonly available short-acting agents. They last about one to two hours and have a relatively quick onset of action. Lidocaine is by far the most commonly used of these agents, as it can be combined with epinephrine to increase duration of action and provide hemostatic effect. These anesthetics are most useful in the ambulatory or emergency room setting.

Amides such as bupivacaine and ropivacaine tend to have a longer onset to action (up to 15 minutes) but have the added benefit of a longer duration of anesthetic effects (240 to 480 minutes). These agents are valuable in providing postprocedural analgesia and reducing the consumption of opioids or need for oral medications.[6-7]

Recently, extended-release liposomal formulations of bupivacaine (Exparel®) have garnered increasing attention in the surgical literature. A single-shot injection is boasted to provide postoperative pain relief up to 96 hours. A randomized, multicenter, double-blinded phase 3 clinical study showed that compared with placebo, patients treated with Exparel® were pain free up to 48 hours after bunionectomy and required substantially less opioids in the initial 24 hours postoperatively.[8]

In the hand literature, a recent study of Exparel® use in wide-awake trigger finger release demonstrated that 50% of patients treated with both Marcaine® and Exparel® required no additional pain medications and maintained the lowest pain scores through postoperative day 3 compared with the use lidocaine or Marcaine® alone. Aside from local infiltration, Exparel® holds much promise as an agent for peripheral nerve blockade. Active studies are underway with phase 2 and 3 trials approved by the Food and Drug Administration to further investigate its value in this area.[8]

Topical Anesthetics

Topical anesthetic formulations can be a useful adjunct for pediatric populations or for patients with high anxiety and poor pain tolerance. Applied 30 to 60 minutes prior to a procedure, they can help mitigate the initial pain of injections. The most popular agent is a eutectic mixture of local anesthetics (EMLA), comprised of 25 mg lidocaine and 50 mg prilocaine per gram. Unfortunately, these agents do little to lessen the burning pain associated with the infiltration. Coupled with the "blow slow before you go" technique, making sure that the anesthetic agent leads the needle tip while it advances, Lalonde proposes that one could avoid the pain from the sharpened needle tip experienced during analgesia administration.[7-9] Despite taking all available steps to reduce the pain of injection, however, there are some patients who will always find this procedure painful, possibly due to a decreased pain threshold, anxiety, or both.

Use of Epinephrine in Hand Surgery

Local anesthetics with epinephrine are now routine in hand surgery. The old mantra prohibiting its use in the digits has generally been debunked, and its safety is well established in the literature. Historically, it was thought that epinephrine causes irreversible vasoconstriction and eventual digital necrosis. This was based on several case reports in the first half of the 20th century, where the use of procaine or cocaine with epinephrine caused digital infarction.[10-11] However, it was noted that there were also several other cases where just plain procaine or cocaine without epinephrine was used. The true culprit was later attributed to the acidity of procaine and its use in an era when anesthetic expiration dates were not yet established. Furthermore, rescue agents such as phentolamine did not become available until after 1957. Subsequent studies have since demonstrated the safety of injectable epinephrine in the modern era.

Thomson and Lalonde demonstrated in a randomized, double-blind comparison using 30 volunteers who underwent digital blocks that the addition of 1:100,000 epinephrine to 2% lidocaine solution extends the duration of action two-fold with no detrimental effect. Of note, in this particular study, only 1.8 mL of anesthetic solution was administered in the central volar surface of the fingers; this is less volume than is typically administered for preoperative digital blockage.[12] The largest report to date includes a prospective study of 3,110 cases by nine surgeons, in which none of the patients experienced tissue loss.[13]

The advantage of epinephrine is two-fold. It increases the duration of action of anesthetics by causing local vasoconstriction and increasing the concentration of anesthetic molecules available to act on nerve cells. Moreover, it has the tremendous added benefit of providing a bloodless field without the use of a tourniquet. It is frequently used at concentrations of 1:100,000 or 1:200,000 but can be effective even at 1:1,000,000. For maximum vasoconstriction, 26 minutes is the optimal wait time after injection of 1:100,000.[14]

Despite the overall safety and success of epinephrine, caution should still be exercised in patients with inherent vascular compromise or if its integrity is in question from trauma or acute disease processes. Phentolamine should always be considered as a rescue option to reverse effects of vasoconstriction.

GENERAL ANESTHESIA

General anesthesia and narcotic medications are, perhaps, the most important innovations in the growth of the field of surgery. The combination of inhalational and intravenous agents has demonstrated a long history of safety and efficacy and has allowed surgeons to offer the full spectrum of hand and upper extremity procedures.[8]

The use of general anesthesia, however, does not come without risks. In developing an appropriate anesthesia plan, several important side effects must be considered including but not limited to the potential for intraoperative hypotension, decreased cardiac output, central nervous system depression, respiratory depression, loss of airway and related protective reflexes, and need for tracheal intubation and mechanical ventilation, as well as residual anesthetic effects. As such, there will be patients for whom upper extremity surgery is indicated but for whom general anesthesia might preclude a necessary intervention. In these cases, other avenues of anesthesia must be explored.

One major concern and a common question for both the patient and his or her surgeon is which mode of anesthesia will allow for the best postoperative pain control. Several comparative reports have been published addressing this topic. While patient-reported pain control following general anesthesia was found to be equivalent outside of the immediate postoperative period (during days 1–14),[15] multiple reports have demonstrated that immediate postoperative recovery, time to discharge, and overall cost are more favorable with alternate modes of perioperative pain management including peripheral and intravenous nerve blocks.[16-18]

PERIPHERAL REGIONAL BLOCKADE

First described by William Stuart Halstead in 1885, peripheral regional blocks (PRBs) have been used for more than a century as both an adjunct to general anesthesia as well as the primary mode of surgical analgesia in hand and upper extremity surgery.[19]

In addition to more comprehensive perioperative pain management, the primary clinical benefit of PRBs is the avoidance of risks associated with general anesthesia. As such, peripheral blocks should be considered when developing an anesthesia plan for patients who may be more vulnerable.

The clinical indications for PRB use include (a) surgery limited to a region between the shoulder and fingers; (b) no intraoperative or immediate postoperative need for examination of function of the blocked extremity; (c) no contraindications such as coagulopathy, allergy, or hypersensitivity to local anesthetics, injection site skin infection, or severe needle phobia and/or anxiety; and (d) patient preference for PRB over other anesthesia options.

In general, PRBs are performed by an anesthesiologist under ultrasound guidance where the anesthetic agent is injected in the area of the brachial plexus. A wide variety of targets have been described to address each anatomic site of interest and have been found to deliver 12 to 24 hours of pain relief.[20-21]

The primary sites for peripheral nerve blocks in hand and upper extremity surgery include the interscalene, supraclavicular, infraclavicular, suprascapular, and axillary blocks.[20] The axillary and suprascapular blocks may be employed for procedures limited to the shoulder. For procedures involving the shoulder, distal clavicle, and proximal humerus, the interscalene block may be performed at the root-trunk level of the brachial plexus.[20-28] For procedures distal to the elbow, both the supraclavicular (anterior and posterior divisions) and infraclavicular (at the level of the cords) blocks may be administered for regional anesthetic effect.[29-30]

Peripheral nerve blocks do not come without risks, which may include pneumothorax, peripheral neuropathy, spinal cord injury, and a range of iatrogenic blockades (i.e., recurrent laryngeal, phrenic, and sympathetic chain), all of which can be minimized with the ultrasound-guided technique.[31] Ultrasound-guided techniques have not shown to be more effective, however, in the degree of analgesia or duration of effect.[29-30]

PRBs have been identified as an acceptable and cost-effective alternative to general anesthesia for intraoperative and postoperative pain control, minimizing narcotic use and related complications, leading to shorter hospital stays, and resulting in increased patient satisfaction.[16,20-28,30,32]

INTRAVENOUS REGIONAL ANESTHESIA

Intravenous regional anesthesia was developed in the early 20th century by Dr. August Bier. This method of perioperative pain management has a proven safety record and remains in common use today for upper extremity surgery. In patients for whom general anesthesia may not be an option, the Bier block technique can provide complete anesthesia without the additional risks of endotracheal intubation.

The technique requires that a tourniquet be placed above the elbow and inflated to achieve arterial occlusion. This allows for a bloodless field and maintains the intravenous anesthetic in the upper extremity for the duration of the procedure. After inflation of the tourniquet, intravenous injection of a rapid-onset local anesthetic (typically 0.5% lidocaine at 1.5–3 mg/kg) is performed and can be administered by either an anesthesiologist or the surgeon.[33-34]

While this technique can be effective intraoperatively, some patients will require additional sedation due to tourniquet discomfort, which comes with an additional set of risks including postoperative nausea and vomiting as well as prolonged time to discharge.[35]

Several local and systemic complications have been reported in the literature associated with intravenous regional anesthesia, particularly upon deflation of the tourniquet. These include compartment syndrome, seizures, cardiac arrest, and death from systemic pharmacologic toxicity.[33-39] However, a recent systemic review demonstrates that the incidence is low, and thus the Bier block technique remains a safe alternative to general anesthesia for upper extremity surgery.[37]

Several modifications have been made to the Bier block technique to further mitigate risks and complications. Historically, a minimum tourniquet time of 30 minutes has been employed to allow for adequate diffusion and reduce the bolus dose of anesthetic released into the bloodstream following deflation. More recent modifications to the technique including cyclical tourniquet release and forearm positioning of the tourniquet have allowed for decreased doses of anesthetic and, thus, decreased tourniquet time to just over 10 minutes.[38]

The Bier block solution has also been modified over the years to improve its efficacy both intra- and postoperatively. While plain lidocaine remains the mainstay of treatment, several agents have been used for or added to the injection solution, including short- and long-acting anesthetics (i.e., bupivacaine, mepivacaine, prilocaine), opiates (i.e., morphine, fentanyl, meperidine), nonsteroidal anti-inflammatory drugs (NSAIDs; ketorolac), alpha-2 adrenergic agonists, sodium bicarbonate, and muscle relaxants with varying degrees of improvement.[14,36,38-42] While still available, the Bier block has been largely replaced by the PRB techniques, as these have been found to achieve increased success on multiple parameters including rate of administration, speed of onset, duration of action, and safety as discussed earlier in this chapter.

WIDE-AWAKE HAND SURGERY

Background and Technique

With the advent of literature debunking the long-standing myth that injecting epinephrine directly into the human finger would result in tissue ischemic and necrosis,[10,43] the wide-awake local anesthesia no tourniquet (WALANT) technique was first described by Lalonde et al. in 2005.

The WALANT technique involves the injection of local anesthetic with epinephrine for analgesia and hemostasis without a tourniquet in the wide-awake patient. Lalonde advocates for the use of bicarbonate in the anesthetic solution as well as slow injection via small caliber needle (no larger than 27-gauge) to minimize patient discomfort during administration.[11-13]

Intraoperative Considerations and Outcomes

This WALANT technique has been shown to provide adequate anesthesia and a hemostatic field for a wide variety of upper extremity procedures ranging from carpal tunnel release to arthroplasties and tendon transfers,[44-47] all while minimizing patient risk by avoiding more invasive forms of perioperative anesthesia and analgesia as well as decreasing costs and increasing patient satisfaction.[48-51]

Perhaps one of the most advantageous aspects of the WALANT technique is that the patient may be engaged in the operating room at the time of surgery to assess the efficacy of the procedure while it is being performed, such as with tendon repair or trigger finger release.[8,45]

As national attention turns to minimizing narcotic use, wide-awake local anesthesia has been shown to reduce demand for postoperative opiates from 67% to 5% when compared to sedated patients.[52]

POSTOPERATIVE PAIN MANAGEMENT

Opiate Medications

Opioids have had a prevalent role in both inpatient and outpatient surgery. When administered they bind to specific opioid receptors, delta (δ), kappa (κ), and mu (μ), within the central nervous system and lead to analgesic effects similar to endogenous endorphins, enkephalins, and dynorphins. These substances are metabolized by the liver and cleared by the kidney and should be avoided in patients with hepatic or renal dysfunction.[8,53]

Opioids are frequently prescribed after elective procedures and can help mitigate acute moderate or severe postoperative pain; however, their side effect profile frequently calls into question whether other modalities should be first-line. The adverse events are many and include nausea, vomiting, constipation, sedation, respiratory depression, and substance dependence.[8,53]

Within the last two decades, the amount of opioids prescribed and the deaths from opioid overdoses have quadrupled. In the late 1990s, it was thought that pain had been largely undiagnosed and left inadequately untreated.[54-56] This lead to the adoption of pain as a fifth vital sign. Yet despite the surge in opioids there has been no overall change in the perception of pain reported by Americans. Instead, it has led to an opioid prescription epidemic.[54-56] Consequently, the medical community now looks to other means of pain management that are safer and more efficacious, such as PRB, to minimize postoperative pain as discussed earlier.

Non-Opiate Medications

Non-opiate medications can be used as an adjunct or an alternative to opioids. The goal is to complement and minimize the need for and consumption of opioid substances while still providing sufficient pain control.[8]

Acetaminophen is perhaps the most utilized analgesic worldwide. It is available in oral and intravenous formulations. It can be administered alone or co-prescribed with oxycodone, hydrocodone, or tramadol. It is safe, inexpensive, and has a relatively favorable side effect profile. It is usually preferred over NSAIDs, since it does not inhibit platelet function, irritate gastric lining, or carry the risk of renal insufficiency. Though effective, one must be wary that the maximum daily dose should not exceed 4 g, as greater doses can cause hepatotoxicity.[3,8]

NSAIDs are also effective and commonly used. In addition to analgesic effects, NSAIDs also have anti-inflammatory properties that help to minimize postsurgical swelling. They are prevalent in most ambulatory pain regimens and are generally well tolerated.[3,8]

NSAIDs act by inhibiting COX enzymes, which are involved in the synthesis of prostaglandins and also play an important role in platelet aggregation. Two isoforms exist, with COX-1 involved in maintenance of gastric mucosa and renal blood flow and COX-2 with inflammatory response. Consequently, careful consideration must be given before prescribing these analgesics to patients with known gastric ulcers, bleeding issues, or renal disease.[3,8]

Ketorolac is a NSAID that was first approved in 1997. Since then it has gained increasing popularity as an adjunct in the postoperative period. It minimizes opioid requirements as much as 25% to 50%.[8]

Other non-opiate medications with some success include gabapentin and dexamethasone. Both have beneficial effects on postoperative analgesia and an ability to decrease opiate need. Gabapentin has also been shown to decrease the risk of chronic pain. Dexamethasone can reduce postoperative nausea and vomiting.[8,57]

Multimodal Approaches

Overall, a multimodal approach to pain management is best, one that combines different methods of pain modulation in a way that lessens the side effects of each. Pain control should be an active consideration throughout the entire process from preoperative, intraoperative, to postoperative in all fields of surgery. However, in hand and upper extremity surgery, the combination of oral medications with the perioperative administration of extended local and/or peripheral regional nerve blocks when appropriate can provide a longer duration of optimal analgesia and ultimately minimize opioid consumption.

REFERENCES

1. Wier LM, Steiner CA, Owens PL. Surgeries in hospital-owned outpatient facilities, 2012. Statistical Brief #188. Rockville, MD: Agency for Healthcare Research and Quality; February 2015.
2. American Hospital Association. Utilization and volume. In: *Trends Affecting Hospitals and Health Systems*. Washington, DC: American Hospital Association. http://www.aha.org/research/reports/tw/chartbook/index.shtml. Accessed March 7, 2017.
3. Chung F, Ritchie E, Su J. Postoperative pain in ambulatory surgery. *Anesth Analg*. 1997;85(4):808–816.
4. Marchand S. The physiology of pain mechanisms: from the periphery to the brain. *Rheum Dis Clin North Am*. 2008 May;34(2):285–309. doi:10.1016/j.rdc.2008.04.003

5. Millan MJ. The induction of pain: an integrative review. *Prog Neurobiol.* 1999 Jan;57(1):1–164.

6. Katz RD, LaPorte DM. Use of short-acting local anesthetics in hand surgery patients. *J Hand Surg Am.* 2009 Dec;34(10):1902–1905. doi:10.1016/j.jhsa.2009.07.001

7. Becker DE, Reed KL. Essentials of local anesthetic pharmacology. *Anesth Progress.* 2006;53(3):98–109.

8. Ketonis C, Ilyas AM, Liss F. Pain management strategies in hand surgery. *Orthop Clin North Am.* 2015 Jul;46(3):399–408.

9. Farhangkhoee H, Lalonde J, Lalonde DH. Teaching medical students and residents how to inject local anesthesia almost painlessly. *Can J Plast Surg.* 2012;20(3): 169–172.

10. Denkler K. A comprehensive review of epinephrine in the finger: to do or not. *Plast Reconstr Surg* 2001;108(1):114–124.

11. Thomson CJ, Lalonde DH, Denkler KA. A critical look at the evidence for and against elective epinephrine use in the finger. *Plast Reconstr Surg.* 2007;119(1):260.

12. Thomson CJ, Lalonde DH. Randomized double-blind comparison of duration of anesthesia among three commonly used agents in digital nerve block. *Plast Reconstr Surg.* 2006;188(2):429–432.

13. Lalonde DH, Bell M, Benoit P, Sparkes G, Denkler K, Chang P. A multicenter prospective study of 3110 consecutive cases of elective epinephrine use in the fingers and hand: the Dalhousie Project clinical phase. *J Hand Surg Am.* 2005;30:1061.

14. Reuben SS, Steinberg RB, Klatt JL, Klatt ML. Intravenous regional anesthesia using lidocaine and clonidine. *Anesthesiology.* 1999;91(3):654–658.

15. D'Alessio JG, Rosenblum M, Shea KP, Freitas DG. A retrospective comparison of interscalene block and general anesthesia for ambulatory surgery shoulder arthroscopy. *Reg Anesth.* 1995;20(1):62–68.

16. Brown AR, Weiss R, Greenberg C, Flatow EL, Bigliani LU. Interscalene block for shoulder arthroscopy: a comparison with general anesthesia. *Arthroscopy.* 1993;9(3):295–300.

17. Chan VWS, Peng PWH, Kaszas Z. A comparative study of general anesthesia, intravenous regional anesthesia, and axillary block for outpatient hand surgery: clinical outcome and cost analysis. *Anesth Analg.* 2001;93(5):1181–1184.

18. McCartney CJ, Brull R, Chan VWS, et al. Early but no long-term benefit of regional compared to general anesthesia for ambulatory hand surgery. *Anesthesiology.* 2004;101(2):461–467.

19. Halsted WS. Practical comments on the use and abuse of cocaine; suggested by its invariably successful employment in more than a thousand minor surgical operations. *New York Med J.* 1885 Sept;42:294–295.

20. Gohl MR, Moeller RK, Olson RL, Vacchiano CA. The addition of interscalene block to general anesthesia for patients undergoing open shoulder procedures. *AANA J.* 2011;69(2):105–109.

21. Kinnard P, Truchon R, St-Pierre A, Montreuil J. Interscalene block for pain relief after shoulder surgery: a prospective randomized study. *Clin Orthop Relat Res.* 1994;(304):22–24.

22. Ciccone WJ, Busey TD, Weinstein DM, Walden DL, Elias JJ. Assessment of pain relief provided by interscalene regional block and infusion pump after arthroscopic shoulder surgery. *Arthroscopy.* 2008 Jan;24(1):14–19.

23. Ilfield BM et al. Ambulatory continuous interscalene nerve blocks decrease time to discharge readiness after total shoulder arthroplasty: a randomized, triple-masked, placebo-controlled study. *Anesthesiology.* 2006 Nov;105(5):999–1007.

24. Ilfield BM, Vandenborne K, Duncan PW, et al. Joint range of motion after total shoulder arthroplasty with and without a continuous interscalene nerve block: a retrospective, case-controlled study. *Reg Anesth Pain Med.* 2005 Sept-Oct;30(5):429–433.

25. Lee HY, Kim SH, So KY, Kim DJ. Effects of interscalene brachial plexus block to intraoperative hemodynamics and postoperative pain for arthroscopic shoulder surgery. *Korean J Anesthesiol.* 2012 Jan;62(1):30–34.

26. Mariano ER, Afra R, Loland VJ, et al. Continuous interscalene brachial plexus block via an ultrasound-guided approach: a randomized, triple-masked, placebo-controlled study. *Anesth Analg.* 2009 May;108(5):1688–1694.

27. Singelyn FJ, Lhotel L, Fabre B. Pain relief after arthroscopic shoulder surgery: a comparison of intraarticular analgesia, suprascapular nerve block, and interscalene brachial plexus block. *Anesth Analg.* 2004 Aug;99(2):589–592.

28. Wu CL, Rouse LM, Chen JM, Miller RJ. Comparison of postoperative pain in patients receiving interscalene block or general anesthesia for shoulder surgery. *Orthopedics.* 2002 Jan;25(1):45–48.

29. Vazin M, Jensen K, Kristensen DL, et al. Low-volume brachial plexus block providing surgical anesthesia for distal arm surgery comparing supraclavicular, infraclavicular, and axillary approach: a randomized observer blind trial. *Biomed Res Int.* 2016;2016:7094121.

30. Chin KJ, Alakkad H, Adhikary SD, Singh M. Infraclavicular brachial plexus block for regional anaesthesia of the lower arm. *Cochrane Database Syst Rev.* 2013 Aug 28;8:CD005487.

31. Russon K, Pickworth T, Harrop-Griffiths W. Upper extremity limb blocks. *Anaesthesia.* 2010;65(Suppl 1):48–56.

32. Srikumaran U, Stein BE, Tan EW, Freehill MT, Wilckens JH. Upper-extremity peripheral nerve blocks in the perioperative pain management of orthopaedic patients: AAOS exhibit selection. *J Bone Joint Surg Am.* 2013;95(24):e197(1–13).

33. Brill S, Middleton W, Brill G, Fisher A. Bier's block: 100 years old and still going strong! *Acta Anaesthesiol Scand.* 2004;48(1):117–122.

34. Colburn E. The Bier block for intravenous regional anesthesia: technic and literature review. *Anesth Analg.* 1970;49(6):935–940.

35. Chiao FB, Chen J, Lesser JB, Resta-Flarer F, Bennett H. Single-cuff forearm tourniquet in intravenous regional anaesthesia results in less pain and fewer sedation requirements than upper arm tourniquet. *Br J Anaesth.* 2013;111(2):271–275.

36. Joshi GP. Recent developments in regional anesthesia for ambulatory surgery. *Curr Opin Anaesthesiol.* 1999;12(6):643–647.

37. Guay J. Adverse events associated with intravenous regional anesthesia (Bier block): a systematic review of complications. *J Clin Anesth.* 2009;21(8):585–594.

38. Arslanian B, Mehrzad R, Kramer T, Kim DC. Forearm Bier block: a new regional anesthetic technique for upper extremity surgery. *Ann Plast Surg.* 2014;73(2):156–157.

39. Pickering SA and JB Hunter. Bier's block using prilocaine: safe, cheap and well-tolerated. *Surgeon.* 2003;1(5):283–285.

40. Singh R, Bhagwat A, Bhadoria P, Kohli A. Forearm IVRA, using 0.5% lidocaine in a dose of 1.5 mg/kg with ketorolac Forearm IVRA, using 0.5% lidocaine in a dose of 1.5 mg/kg with ketorolac 0.15 mg/kg for hand and wrist surgeries. *Minerva Anestesiol.* 2010;76(2):109–114.

41. Gupta A, Björnsson A, Sjöberg F, Bengtsson M. Lack of peripheral analgesic effect of low-dose morphine during intravenous regional anesthesia. *Reg Anesth.* 1993;18(4):250–253.

42. Armstrong P, Power I, Wildsmith JA. Addition of fentanyl to prilocaine for intravenous regional anaesthesia. *Anaesthesia*. 1991;46(4):278–280.

43. Krunic AL, Wang LC, Soltani K, Weitzul S, Taylor RS. Digital anesthesia with epinephrine: an old myth revisited. *J Am Acad Dermatol*. 2004;51(5):755–759.

44. Farhangkhoee H, Lalonde J, Lalonde DH. Wide awake trapeziectomy: video detailing local anesthetic injection and surgery. *Hand*. 2011;6(4):466–467.

45. Bezuhly M, Sparkes GL, Higgins A, Neumeister MW, Lalonde DH. Immediate thumb extension following extensor indicis proprius-to-extensor pollicus longus tendon transfer using the wide-awake approach. *Plast Reconstr Surg*. 2007;119(5):1507–1512.

46. Lalonde DH. How the wide-awake approach is changing hand surgery and hand therapy: inaugural AAHS sponsored lecture at the ASHT meeting, San Diego 2012. *J Hand Ther*. 2013;26(2):175–178.

47. Lalonde DH, Wong A. Dosage of local anesthesia in wide-awake hand surgery. *J Hand Surg Am*. 2013;38(10):2025–2028.

48. Bismil M, Bismil Q, Harding D, Harris P, Lamyman E, Sansby L. Transition to total one-stop wide-awake hand surgery service-audit: a retrospective review. *JRSM Short Rep*. 2012;3(4):23.

49. Lalonde DH. Reconstruction of the hand with wide awake surgery. *Clin Plast Surg*. 2011;38(4):761–769.

50. Nelson R. The wide-awake approach to Dupuytren's disease: fasciectomy under local anesthetic with epinephrine. *Hand*. 2010;5(2):117–124.

51. Davison PG, Cobb T, Lalonde DH. The patient's perspective on carpal tunnel surgery related to the type of anesthesia: a prospective cohort study. *Hand*. 2013;8(1):47–53.

52. Marcus JR, Tyrone JW, Few JW, Fine NA, Mustoe TA. Optimization of conscious sedation in plastic surgery. *Plast Reconstr Surg*. 1999;104(5):1338–1345.

53. Brunton LM, Laporte DM. Use of opioids in hand surgery. *J Hand Surg Am*. 2009 Oct;34(8):1551–1554. doi:10.1016/j.jhsa.2009.04.022

54. Centers for Disease Control and Prevention. Wide-ranging online data for epidemiologic research (WONDER). Atlanta, GA: Centers for Disease Control and Prevention, National Center for Health Statistics; 2016. http://wonder.cdc.gov

55. Chang HY, Daubresse M, Kruszewski SP, Alexander GC. Prevalence and treatment of pain in emergency departments in the United States, 2000–2010. *Amer J Emerg Med*. 2014; 32(5): 421–431.

56. Daubresse M, Chang H, Yu Y, et al. Ambulatory diagnosis and treatment of nonmalignant pain in the United States, 2000–2010. *Medical Care*. 2013;51(10):870–878.

57. Beaussier M, Sciard D, Sautet A. New modalities of pain treatment after outpatient orthopaedic surgery. *Orthop Traumatol Surg Res*. 2016 Feb;102(1 Suppl):S121–S124. doi:10.1016/j.otsr.2015.05.011

21 Migraine Headaches: Surgery and Pain Management

William G. Austen Jr. and John Hulsen

INTRODUCTION

The diagnosis and management of migraine headache is challenging and often frustrates the patient as well as the clinician. Migraine is incompletely understood, and its nomenclature is frequently confused or misused by lay people and medical professionals alike. Unfortunately, this miscommunication can lead to inaccurate diagnosis and improper therapeutic measures. The result of this is adverse medical side effects and, most importantly, continued pain, disability, and a lower patient quality of life.

The International Classification of Headache Disorders 3rd Edition (beta version) (ICHD-3 beta) recognizes two major subtypes of migraine: migraine with and without aura.[1] A review of the diagnostic subtleties of each migraine subset is beyond the scope of this chapter. However, accepted basic diagnostic criteria for migraine with and without aura have been published.[1] For the most comprehensive and up-to-date criteria, see the most recent version of the ICHD. As this text is specifically directed toward surgeons, the authors recommend that patients receive proper diagnosis and care from a trained neurologist with expertise in headache medicine.

EPIDEMIOLOGY

The Global Burden of Disease Study 2015 ranked migraine as the third leading cause of years lived with disability for ages 25 to 29 and the seventh leading cause for all age groups worldwide.[2] The American Migraine Prevalence and Prevention cross-sectional study estimates that in the United States approximately 4 out of every 10 women and 2 in 10 men will suffer from migraine headaches in their lifetime.[3] The prevalence of migraine has been consistent over 10 years and affects a reported 17.2%

of women and 6% of men.[4,5] The age of onset is typically before the third decade, with half of the cases occurring before age 25 and 75% prior to age 35.[3]

THE PATHOGENESIS OF MIGRAINE AND THE PERIPHERAL TRIGGER THEORY

Presently, there is an incomplete understanding of the complex pathophysiologic mechanisms leading to the activation of migraine headache pain.[6] Both central and peripheral etiologies are implicated, the latter being more controversial and the subject of recent intense investigation and debate.[7-14]

Conceptually, migraine is a primary disorder of the brain.[6,15] It is a neurovascular dysfunction attributable to a genetically linked deficiency of cortical regulatory mechanisms leading to a predisposition for cortical excitability.[16-18] It is believed that this predisposition for neural excitation lowers a migraineurs threshold for the initiation of cortical spreading depression (CSD).[6] Generally, induced CSD is believed to be responsible for migraine aura and increased neuropeptide release with subsequent vasodilation/increased meningeal blood flow, and it is a mediator of neurogenic inflammation. This sterile meningeal inflammation, along with CSD, may sensitize and sustain the activation of perivascular meningeal nociceptors and trigeminal neurovascular pathways, resulting in the diverse symptoms and debilitating pain of migraine headache.[19]

The peripheral trigger site theory of migraine headaches contends that irritation of trigeminal nerve branches in the head and neck, which are anatomically vulnerable to insult from muscle, fascia, bone, contact points, or vessels, generates a centrally conducted stimulus.[8,20,21] These peripherally generated/centrally conducted stimuli, when superimposed onto a genetically predisposed patient possessing a structurally susceptible brain (baseline diminished threshold for cortical depolarization), are believed to be one of many triggers in the activation of migraine pathology.[17]

Interestingly, recent physiologic research has added basic science support to the peripheral trigger theory. A direct anatomic and functional link between intracranial and extracranial structures has been described.[22,23] Afferent fibers from the trigeminal innervation of the cranial dura mater form functional collateral axons that exit the skull to innervate extracranial tissues.[22-24] Peripheral extracranial stimuli is conducted via these collateral axons centrally to the cranial dura and is antidromically transmitted along the intracranial branches.[22] Proinflammatory vasoactive neuropeptide (substance P, calcitonin gene-related peptide [CGRP]) release occurs, causing vasodilitation and results in increased meningeal blood flow as well as nociception at the meninges.[17,22,25]

The precise neurobiologic circumstances that lead to genesis of a migraine attack are incompletely understood and the subject of ongoing investigation and debate.[6] A variety of mechanisms are likely at play given the heterogenous clinical spectrum of this disorder.[6] The current body of clinical evidence for peripheral trigger deactivation in migraine is now finding indirect support at the basic science level.[15,17,22,23] Surgically targeting these sites in well-selected patients has reliably produced successful outcomes in multiple centers and has engendered enthusiasm from surgeons, basic scientists, some neurologists, and, most importantly, treated patients with improved quality of life.[26,27]

DIAGNOSTIC TESTS AND IMAGING

Migraine is a clinical diagnosis reserved for patients who provide sufficient history and physical examination to fulfill the current ICHD diagnostic criteria as previously outlined.[1] A thorough history is essential to properly characterize the headache and to identify concerning and potentially dangerous features that would prompt neuroimaging.[28]

Once a clinical diagnosis is established, multiple tools are available to assist the surgeon in uncovering potential craniofacial trigger sites for migraine headaches.[29] Trigger sites are areas of pain where the migraine begins and are anatomically associated with segments of muscle, fascia, bone, or blood vessels (in isolation or combination) that cause compression or irritation of major or minor peripheral nerve branches.[29,30] Meticulous history and physical examination along with a strong foundation in three-dimensional head and neck anatomy is essential to identify the offending tissue structural component(s) hypothesized to contribute to nerve irritation at a trigger site. Experienced surgeons may reliably localize peripheral targets using only an in-depth appreciation for site-specific patterns of pain and constellation of symptoms.[29,31-33] Fortunately, an observant novice headache surgeon can predictably identify peripheral trigger sites by using well-described diagnostic protocols while experience and clinical acumen is honed.

Of note, careful historical attention must be given to the circumstances and results of prior diagnostic tests performed by another practitioner. The circumstances and results of patient-reported diagnostic testing performed outside of one's practice must be critically evaluated. The results should be clear and logical.

Computerized Tomography Scan

A careful nasal speculum exam should be supplemented with computerized tomography (CT) imaging should patient history and constellation of symptoms suggest a rhinogenic trigger (Site III, septonasal). A non-contrast, thin section, three-view CT scan of the head and neck is indicated.[29] This CT data is crucial to elucidate potential triggers from intranasal or sinus pathology including septal deviation, septal spur, contact points, septal/middle concha bullosa, sinus disease, and paradoxically turned turbinates that may be amenable to surgical correction.[29,30,34,35]

Peripheral Nerve Block

Diagnostic nerve blocks can yield a bevy of information regarding suspected trigger sites when utilized appropriately and correctly interpreted. First, the patient must have active pain at the trigger site at the time of examination. Additionally, the pain must be of a sufficient intensity for the patient to make an honest comparison of symptoms pre- and postinjection (typically ≥ 5/10 on a numerical scale, with 0 being no pain and 10 being the worst pain). Some authors believe the sensitivity of the diagnostic block is decreased if the patient has had prolonged pain in the proposed block site. The underlying rational is the anesthetic is less likely to influence a chronically "inflamed" or irritated trigeminal nerve tree.[29]

The block is performed by first asking the patient to point with one finger directly to the area of maximum pain or precisely to the location where he or she believes the pain originated.[29] This area is marked with an indelible marker for reference if needed. An injection of 1 to 5 mL of local anesthetic (the volume depends on the trigger site) exactly into the identified area (the depth/plane depends on the trigger site). A positive response will be complete or nearly complete pain relief. This occurs almost immediately or possibly in 5 to 10 minutes postinjection depending on the anesthetic used. A poor responder shows minimal to no improvement of pain/migraine attack or merely numbness of the anesthetized area with continued pain. Again, the results should be interpreted carefully based on the chronicity of the pain at the trigger site as well in light of the patient's verbal and nonverbal cues. Professional judgment must be exercised to assure patients respond objectively and do not simply reply (either intentionally or unintentionally) with the response they wish for or what they expect a clinician to see. If there is any doubt, the block can be repeated on a separate date.

Botox® (Onabotulinumtoxin A) Injection

Neurotoxin injection into a muscle group suspected of undue compression or irritation of potential trigger site has a paralytic effect that best replicates the surgical resection of the muscle(s) in question.[36,37] In early experiences within the field of migraine surgery, a positive response to Botox® was part of the standard protocol for the selection of patients for surgery.[36–39] While experienced surgeons may find diagnostic Botox® unnecessary when selecting patients for surgery, a favorable preoperative response to Botox® has shown to be a significant prognosticator of surgical success.[40]

As with diagnostic blocks, before and immediately following injection it is vitally important not to "prime" the patient to relay an affirmative or negative response to the injection. Botox® blocks neuromuscular transmission by cleaving a presynaptic protein, thereby preventing docking and release of acetylcholine from vesicles within muscle nerve endings. Maximum effect of the neurotoxin should not be seen until several days following injection. Be wary of the patient who insists the injection relieved pain nearly immediately (as in a block). Additionally, one should consider alternate sources of offending tissue besides muscle at a trigger site (fascial band, bony foramen, and vessel) should Botox® be ineffective. Each of these sources of nerve irritation would be amenable to diagnostic block +/- epinephrine.

Doppler

The use of a simple hand-held ultrasonic doppler is often helpful when localizing a suspected vascular trigger or if the location of patient-reported point of maximal pain is atypical. Preoperatively, the patient is asked to point to the site of maximal pain with a single finger. Should the patient not have an active headache at the time of examination, he or she is still encouraged to recall and point directly to the usual site of maximal pain. The site is marked and the area probed with the doppler. An arterial signal is often identified, and photographs of the patient-localized mark and positive signal may be taken for intraoperative reference. A diagnostic/therapeutic nerve block may also be directed here in the setting of active pain.[41]

Clinical experience and cadaveric dissection has demonstrated potential deleterious nerve-artery relationships in susceptible migraineurs. Single cross-over (nerve over artery or artery over nerve) and helical intertwining of the neurovascular structures have been reported. The most common interactions occur at site IV (greater occipital nerve), Site V (temporal, auriculotemporal), and site VI (lesser occipital nerve). In these areas, the occipital artery has been shown to intersect the greater occipital nerve (or branches thereof) in 54% of cases, while the superficial temporal artery intersects the auriculotemporal nerve (or branches thereof) in 34% of cases, and occipital artery branches intersect the lesser occipital nerve (or branches thereof) 55% of the time.[29,42–44] A recent study reviewed a series of patients who underwent auricluotemporal deactivation with a preoperative positive doppler signal over the point of maximal pain. A branch of the superficial temporal artery was found at the time of surgery in 100% of patients with a preoperatively identified doppler signal.[41]

Additionally, so-called minor trigger sites that do not follow a typical main peripheral nerve branch may be present. These unusual sites, often located near the hairline or scalp vertex, may represent terminal nerve branches and are often associated with an identifiable arterial doppler signal at the point of maximal pain. These nerve-artery relationships can be important sources of nerve irritation and a potential source of unrecognized or untreated trigger sites.[29,41]

MANAGEMENT

Lifestyle Modification

There are at least 60 described factors or "external" triggers (distinguished from anatomic migraine trigger sites) of an acute migraine attack in susceptible individuals.[45,46] Over 75% of migraineurs report generally having migraine triggers.[46] This figure increases to nearly 95% when these patients are presented with a specific list of potential triggers.[46] Commonly reported factors known to incite a migraine include stress, fasting, certain foods, weather changes, altered sleep patterns, hormones in women, and certain odors including perfumes, to name a few.[45–47]

Encouraging patients to keep a headache diary and record the chronological relationship of their own unique factors to their migraine is advocated.[46] While triggers such as changes in weather patterns are difficult to control, strategies for stress management, dietary restrictions, and sleep hygiene empower migraineurs with a degree of personal control over their headaches.[46] It is important to recognize that lifestyle modifications that successfully control unique triggers should be maintained even after adequate medical or surgical therapy.

Medical Treatment

Introduction

Numerous drug therapies have been used for the prevention of migraine. Appropriate medical treatment should be individualized to the patient as commonly used therapy spans a variety of drug classes—each with specific indications and side-effect profiles. A tailored medication regimen should consider patient age, gender, and comorbid conditions. Should a particular medication prove ineffective, another within the same class, or a different class altogether, may be attempted as predicting the most effective medication regimen for an individual is often challenging.[48,49]

Unfortunately, drug therapy has many drawbacks that may prevent compliance/optimum medical treatment including medication intolerance and adverse side-effect profiles, and many are not recommended during pregnancy.[50] Up to almost 50% of migraine patients report lack of drug efficacy and over 50% have cited intolerable side effects as reasons for discontinuation of prophylactic therapy.[51] Of those who are fortunate enough to tolerate their regimen, just two-thirds can expect a 50% reduction in the frequency of headaches.[52]

Pharmacologic Therapy

Pharmacotherapy is generally divided into two main categories: abortive treatment for acute migraine pain attack and preventative treatment to reduce the frequency, severity, and duration of migraine. A number of supplemental and herbal therapies have also been proposed for the prevention of migraine with varying degrees of success and limited clinical evidence. Of note, unless specified, the medication classes and specific drug therapies described here are for the treatment of episodic migraine. However, despite comparatively limited clinical research, chronic migraineurs generally follow iterations of prophylactic pharmacotherapy trial and error similar to those who suffer from episodic migraine. A notable exception to this paradigm is the Food and Drug Administration (FDA)–approved use of Botox® for the treatment of chronic migraine headaches.

Abortive Treatment

Analgesics

Nonsteroidal Anti-Inflammatory Medications and Acetaminophen General analgesics in the form of oral nonsteroidal anti-inflammatory medications and acetaminophen, alone or in combination, are commonly utilized for in the treatment of mild to moderate migraine.[53] Multiple drugs within this class have been shown to provide pain relief.[54–56] Adverse effects in healthy patients are rare, and occasional ingestion of standard doses of acetaminophen is considered safe in pregnant women.[53]

Opioids and Barbiturates Acute and chronic migraine pain is frequently treated with powerful nonspecific narcotic analgesics in spite of numerous guidelines and recommendations to the contrary.[49,57,58] Opioid or barbiturate use has been reported in approximately 20% of patients presenting to headache clinics despite generally inferior efficacy compared to migraine-specific medications and the potential for overuse, tolerance, and dependence.[49,58] A patient's first prescriber of opioids is often the emergency department (ED) clinician.[57,58] Ironically, patients with migraine who were treated with opioids as a first-line therapy in the ED setting were twice as likely to return to the same ED within one week with headache pain.[57] Although some opioids are probably effective in the treatment of migraine, if properly monitored under the correct conditions, they are not recommended for regular use.[49] In addition, preoperative narcotic use is associated with worse outcomes following trigger site deactivation surgery.[59]

Triptans The triptans are mainstays of therapy in the treatment of migraine headaches.[49] This class of medication includes numerous short- and long-acting serotonin 5-HT$_{1B/1D}$ receptor agonists.[53] They have been proven effective for acute migraine pain and have similar efficacy between drugs within this class.[60,61] Triptans are considered migraine-specific therapy as they are believed to target a component of the underlying pathophysiologic disturbance in migraine. Agonists of the 5-HT$_{1B/1D}$ serotonin receptor in the periaqueductal gray area have been shown to modulate dural nociception.[62] Additionally, some triptans may inhibit action potentials generated in the trigeminal nucleus caudalis as well as inhibit the release of neuropeptides, including CGRP, seen in trigeminal ganglion stimulation.[62] Conveniently, certain triptans have variable formulations including oral, subcutaneous injection, or nasal spray, each with unique bioavailability profiles that can be tailored to the desired rate of onset.[53]

Failure to respond to one triptan does not predict response to additional drugs within this class, and proper selection may require trial and error.[61] Certain triptans should be used with caution, or may be contraindicated, in patients with known renal or hepatic impairment, cardiac or vascular disease, and diabetes.[53] They should not be taken with other triptans or ergots and should be carefully timed in relation to use of monoamine oxidase inhibitor medications.[53] The use of triptans during pregnancy has not been shown to increase the risk of birth defects.[53]

Ergots Historically, migraine headache pain was often treated with the ergot alkaloids. These drugs have a multimechanistic action which includes alpha-adrenergic blockade and 5-HT$_{1B/1D}$ serotonin receptor agonism.[63] Ergotamine is often prepared in combination with caffeine and is an alternative to triptan therapy.[53] Dihydroergotamine has multiple formulations that can be delivered via various routes including subcutaneous, intramuscular, intravenous, or intranasal administration.[53] Vasoconstrictive side effects and propensity to induce nausea and/or vomiting limit the appeal of ergots.[53] They are contraindicated for use in pregnancy as well as with concurrent comorbid hypertension or peripheral vascular disease.[53]

Antiemetics At least limited data has demonstrated the effectiveness of various antiemetics in the treatment of migraine pain or as adjunctive therapy including metoclopramide, chlorpromazine, and haloperidol.[64–66]

Preventative Treatment
Beta Blockers Beta blockers are often prescribed for migraine prophylaxis. At the time of this writing, only propranolol and timolol are indicated by the FDA for the prevention of migraines.[67] However, other beta blockers have been studied and found to be effective.[67] The therapeutic benefit of beta blockers in the prevention of migraines often takes weeks to be fully realized.[68] Following proper titration, the medication should be maintained for at least three months to assess efficacy.[60,68]

The side effects of beta blocker therapy are not trivial and often these medications can exacerbate many comorbid conditions. They should not be used in patients with decompensated heart failure and are relatively contraindicated in patients with underlying asthma.[53] Beta blockers have been associated with growth retardation and congenital anomalies in pregnancy.[53] They also have limited use in those with underlying depression, diabetes, erectile dysfunction, fatigue, bradycardia, hypotension, or structural heart disease.[53]

Anticonvulsants The classic antiepileptic medications for the prevention of migraine headaches are valproate and topiramate. Both drugs are indicated by the FDA for migraine prophylaxis. Large trials of topiramate have shown that approximately half of properly dosed migraineurs can expect at least a 50% reduction in headache frequency.[69] Adverse effects with anticonvulsants appear to be dose dependent—with higher doses showing improved migraine outcomes at the expense of increased side effects. Typical adverse effects of topiramate include paresthesia, impairment of memory and concentration, nausea, anorexia, and weight loss.[53] Conversely, valproate is known to cause weight gain in addition to drowsiness and alopecia.[53] The use of topiramate or valproate in pregnancy has been associated with numerous fetal malformations including (but not limited to) oral clefts and open neural tube defects.[70] Neither drug should be used for headache prevention in women of childbearing age.[70]

Antidepressants The American Academy of Neurology endorses the tricyclic antidepressant (TCA) amitriptyline and serotonin-norepinephrine reuptake inhibitor (SNRI) venlafaxine as "probably effective" in migraine prophylaxis.[60] Numerous TCAs are used for the prevention of migraine; however, only amitriptyline has demonstrated efficacy in large clinical trials.[71] Data regarding commonly prescribed SNRIs efficacy in headache prevention is less convincing while their side effect profile can include nausea, tachycardia, hypertension, and urinary retention.[53] SNRI use during pregnancy has also been associated with an increased risk of perinatal complications.[72,73] TCAs are commonly sedating and can cause confusion, dry mouth, constipation, urinary retention, as well as seizures in infants if taken during pregnancy.[53]

Botox® (Onabotulinumtoxin A) Injection Botox® recently received FDA approval for the preventative treatment of chronic migraine in adults based on two large randomized double-blind trials, PREEMPT 1 and PREEMPT 2.[74,75] These studies showed a modest, however significant, reduction in headache days per month as well as headache duration. The recommended dosage and protocol for this indication is an intramuscular injection of 155 units divided between 31 sites in the head and neck every 12 weeks.[74,75] Botox is not currently FDA approved for the treatment of episodic migraine.[76] Initiation of headache, neck pain or weakness, and eyelid ptosis are commonly reported adverse effects.[74,75] Unfortunately, the stringent FDA-approved protocol allows little flexibility to use less total toxin in focused injections of anatomically described trigger sites in favor of a fixed site and fixed unit dosing of expensive neurotoxin.

Other Medication Therapy Additional classes of drugs with limited or conflicting efficacy data have been used in the prevention of migraine with variable success. A small effect has been shown with calcium channel blockers, particularly verapamil,[77,78] as well as angiotensisn-converting enzyme inhibitors[79] and angiotensin receptor blockers.[80,81]

Other Procedural/Interventions

Additional interventional approaches to migraine pain are utilized to varying degrees including peripheral nerve stimulation and radiofrequency ablation of nerves.[14] A recent systematic review of peripheral nerve interventions for chronic headaches revealed a pooled success rates of 68% for nerve stimulation and 55% for radiofrequency therapy.[82] Implantable nerve stimulators had nearly one in three rate of complications requiring reoperation.[82]

Surgical Treatment

Anatomical Basis of Peripheral Trigger Sites

In the relatively short history of migraine surgery, numerous authors have advanced or refined the basic understanding of the regional anatomic foundations of potential peripheral trigger sites in the head and neck through clinical experience and cadaveric dissection. Sites are often grouped by anatomic region and given a numerical designation for ease of discussion as recently outlined by Forootan et al.[30] Familiarity with regional head and neck anatomy is essential, and the reader is encouraged to review the key cited anatomic and surgical references for each trigger site. Equipped with this knowledge, surgeons today are better able to diagnose, plan, and safely approach and execute the surgical deactivation of the offending triggers with improved patient outcomes.

Surgical Technique

Introduction

The various surgical techniques employed to treat offending triggers at each site are described below. With the exception of perhaps site IV (greater occipital nerve [GON]/third occipital nerve [TON]) and site III (septonasal), each of these procedures can be performed in a properly equipped and lighted office-based procedure room under local anesthesia with or without sedation. Combining the deactivation of multiple "major" trigger sites may increase patient discomfort, and a brief day surgery under general anesthesia is often favored by patients and surgeons alike.

Site I: Supraorbital Nerve/Supratrochlear Nerve[83–87]

An endoscopic or transpalpebral approach may be used to access this site. The latter is useful if a conventional upper eyelid blepharoplasty is to be concurrently performed and requires no special equipment. The patient is marked in the upright position. Ophthalmic ointment lubricated corneal shields are placed. Preoperative markings are confirmed, reinforced, and injected with epinephrine containing local anesthetic. Additional anesthetic is infiltrated within the glabellar muscle group for pain control and hemostasis. Adequate time is allowed for the hemostatic effect of epinephrine.[88,89]

The upper eyelid skin is incised and dissection is carried through the orbicularis occuli muscle to the orbital septum. Cephalic retraction of the upper incision allows dissection with low power electrocautery towards the orbital rim. A supraperiosteal dissection is undertaken with an elevator from lateral to medial to facilitate identification of branches of the supraorbital and supratrochlear nerve exiting the orbit along the orbital rim. The nerves are carefully freed from muscle, fascia, bone, and vascular sources of compression/irritation. A direct osteotomy is performed if the nerve exits the orbit through a bony foramen. If a supraorbital notch is present, any fascial band or bony spicule constricting the nerve is sharply released. A total versus subtotal resection of the corrugator supercilii muscles and any additional offending depressor supercilii or lateral procerus muscle is performed via avulsion or with electrocautery. Complete nerve release and hemostasis is confirmed. A pedicled flap of adipose tissue from the medial fat pad is elevated and used to envelop and securely protect both nerves. The upper eyelid incision or blepharoplasty is closed in a standard fashion.

Site II: Temporal, Zygomaticotemporal Nerve[83,90,91]
The zygomaticotemporal branch may be accessed through an endoscopic[90] or transpalpebral[83] approach (with or without a lateral extension of the incision) while simultaneously deactivating the supraorbital nerve/supratrochlear nerve (SON/STN) as described earlier. Alternately, the ZTN can be approached directly through an incision posterior to the temporal hairline in the hair bearing scalp as described by Peled[92]. The lateral portion of the transpalpebral incision affords easy access to this nerve and is the authors preferred technique. Dissection proceeds along the inferior lateral orbital rim. A small lighted retractor aids in visualization in this area. A periosteal elevator is used to lift the superficial temporal fascia off the deep temporal fascia. Accessing the proper plane is essential to ensure the protection of the frontal branch of the facial nerve. The sentinel vein is identified and protected. The ZTN is identified inferior to the sentinel vein and avulsed with a hemostat. Hemostasis is achieved and the transpalpebral incision is closed in the standard fashion.

Site III: Septonasal (Rhinogenic)[34,35]
Surgery of the septonasal trigger site is individualized according to the identified pathology. Contact points from a deviated septum are addressed with standard septoplasty. Turbinate pathology can be addressed by closed outfracture or size reduction through mucosal cauterization, microdebrider resection, or submucous resection. Complete resection of the turbinate is discouraged so as not to disrupt airflow warmth and humidification through the nose.

Site IV: Greater Occipital Nerve/Third Occipital Nerve[93–97]
The posterior midline of the neck is marked from the occipital protuberance to the caudal hairline with the patient awake in the sitting position. General anesthesia is induced, and the patient is placed on the operating table in the prone position. A mayfied headrest may be helpful in positioning. Undue pressure over the eyes must be avoided. The posterior scalp hair is either combed and taped out of the field or a small track is shaved with surgical clippers. Local anesthetic with epinephrine is injected along the incision line and into the deeper tissue planes. Adequate time is allowed for hemostatic effect.[88,89] The scalp is incised and dissection is deepened to the median raphae. The TON, sometimes referred to as the dorsal branch of the occipital nerve, is often identified within the surgical field in a more caudal location than the expected position of the GON. If encountered, the TON may be avulsed or resected under traction and allowed to retract into soft tissue without consequence.

Continuing just lateral to the median raphae, the trapezius fascia and obliquely oriented fibers of the trapezius muscle are identified. This fascia/muscle is incised exposing the deeper, vertically oriented fibers of the semispinalis capitis muscle. The emergence of the GON is identified as it pierces the semispinalis capitis muscle approximately 3 cm below the occipital protuberance and 1.5 cm lateral to the midline. The nerve may be ensnared with a vessel loop for atraumatic handling. It is then completely freed from all musculofascial and vascular compression from proximal to distal. A small medial section of the semispinalis capitis muscle that abuts the GON is resected. The deepest point of compression is released between the obliquus capitis inferior and semispinalis. The nerve is then traced distally and freed from the surrounding trapezius fascia and muscle (the so-called trapezial tunnel) as it courses lateral and superficial towards the nuchal line. The occipital artery may be seen to be crossing or intertwined with the nerve at this level. Any artery-nerve crossover or intimate association that could cause nerve irritation is addressed and the artery ligated. Hemostasis is achieved. The GON is then shielded with a three-sided fat flap from the scalp secured to the median raphae. A surgical drain is placed and the incision is closed in layers with absorbable suture.

Site V: Temporal, Auriculotemporal Nerve[43,92,98,99]

The auriculotemporal nerve is found lateral to the superficial temporal artery in the preauricular area of the temple. This site is accessed through at temporal hairline incision and the superficial temporal artery (STA) is found within the superficial temporal fascia (temporoparietal fascia). Any direct contact of the auriculotemporal nerve (ATN) with the STA is addressed by dissecting the nerve free from the artery and ligating the vessel both distally and proximally.

Site VI: Lesser Occipital Nerve[44,95,100]

A separate lateral posterior scalp access incision is often used to reach the lesser occipital nerve. An approximately 4 cm obliquely oriented incision is made along or parallel to the posterior border of the sternocledomastoid (SCM). The lesser occipital nerve (LON) emerges from behind the SCM, travels in a cephalic direction and branches into medial and lateral segments before reaching the nuchal line. This nerve is often identified and avulsed or resected under traction to allow retraction of the stump into muscle to prevent neuroma. Alternately, the LON can be released from fascial compression/irritation points along its cephalic course to the nuchal line. If deactivation the GON and LON is planned, both can be accessed through a single midline posterior incision, as described previously for site IV, which is the author's preference. A counter incision near the SCM border can be utilized, though this is rarely necessary.

Minor Trigger Sites[30,41,101]

After careful examination, often with the assistance of the hand-held doppler, the point(s) of maximum tenderness are identified, often along the scalp vertex or hairline. The position of these sites often does not follow the main course or location of a major peripheral nerve or vessel but rather a minor branch. Again, for this site, the doppler has been a valuable tool for the localization of these minor triggers of small residual offending arterial branches that cross or intertwine minor nerve branches. The localized location(s) are incised and superficial dissected to the target vessel which is controlled and ablated along its proximal and distal course. Hemostasis is achieved and the incisions are closed with absorbable suture.

OUTCOMES

A review of the published outcomes and evidence in migraine surgery was recently summarized by Janis et al.[21] The "gold standard" of surgical investigation was performed by Guyuron et al.[102] in their 2009 placebo-controlled/sham surgery trial. At one-year follow-up, 83.7% of surgically treated patients showed improvement (57.1% had complete elimination of migraine pain). By contrast, 57.7% of sham surgery patients reported improvement with only one patient reporting complete elimination. A long-term follow-up report of five-year follow-up data for patients who underwent surgical deactivation of peripheral triggers demonstrated lasting improvement in frequency, duration, and intensity of migraine headache pain in 88% of patients with 29% reporting complete elimination of pain. The surgical success of this center has been robustly reproduced.[38,39,103] Additionally, since first reported by Guyuron et al.[104] in 2000, there have been numerous clinical and technical refinements to improve success.[31,105-108]

CONCLUSIONS

Migraine headache is a debilitating disease with a heterogeneous clinical presentation and complex mechanisms underlying the genesis and perception of pain. Both clinical and basic science progress has been made regarding the processes contributing to the activation of a migraine attack. Both central and peripheral etiologies are suspected, and now there is evidence that these processes are linked. While medical management is often sufficient for migraine, life-long therapy can be unpredictable and costly, produce adverse effects, or be contraindicated. Surgical deactivation of peripheral migraine triggers, in properly selected patients, has consistently produced successful outcomes in multiple centers and represents an exciting new frontier in the treatment of refractory migraine.

REFERENCES

1. Olesen J. The International Classification of Headache Disorders, 3rd Edition. *Cephalagia.* 2013;33(9):629–808. doi:10.1177/0333102413485658
2. Vos T, Allen C, Arora M, et al. Global, regional, and national incidence, prevalence, and years lived with disability for 310 diseases and injuries, 1990–2015: a systematic analysis for the Global Burden of Disease Study 2015. *Lancet.* 2016;388(10053):1545–1602. doi:10.1016/S0140-6736(16)31678-6
3. Stewart WF, Wood C, Reed ML, Roy J, Lipton RB. Cumulative lifetime migraine incidence in women and men. *Cephalalgia.* 2008;28(11):1170–1178. doi:10.1111/j.1468-2982.2008.01666.x
4. Lipton RB, Scher AI, Kolodner K, Liberman J, Steiner TJ, Stewart WF. Migraine in the United States: epidemiology and patterns of health care use. *Neurology.* 2002;58(6):885–894. http://www.ncbi.nlm.nih.gov/pubmed/11914403
5. Stewart WF, Lipton RB, Celentano DD, Reed ML. Prevalence of migraine headache in the United States. Relation to age, income, race, and other sociodemographic factors. *JAMA.* 1992;267(1):64–69. doi:10.1001/jama.267.1.64

6. Pietrobon D, Moskowitz MA. Pathophysiology of migraine. *Annu Rev Physiol.* 2013;75:365–391. doi:10.1146/annurev-physiol-030212-183717

7. Olesen J, Burstein R, Ashina M, Tfelt-Hansen P. Origin of pain in migraine: evidence for peripheral sensitisation. *Lancet Neurol.* 2009;8(7):679–690. doi:10.1016/S1474-4422(09)70090-0

8. Calandre EP, Hidalgo J, García-Leiva JM, Rico-Villademoros F. Trigger point evaluation in migraine patients: an indication of peripheral sensitization linked to migraine predisposition? *Eur J Neurol.* 2006;13(3):244–249. doi:10.1111/j.1468-1331.2006.01181.x

9. McGeeney BE. Migraine trigger site surgery is all placebo. *Headache.* 2015;55(10):1461–1463. doi:10.1111/head.12715

10. McGeeney BE. Migraine trigger site surgery is all placebo: a response. *Headache J Head Face Pain.* 2016;56(4):779–781. doi:10.1111/head.12812

11. Guyuron B. Is migraine surgery ready for prime time? The surgical team's view. *Headache.* 2015 Nov-Dec;55(10):1464–1473.

12. Diener HC, Bingel U. Surgical treatment for migraine: time to fight against the knife. *Cephalalgia.* 2015;35(6):465–468. doi:10.1177/0333102414545895

13. Ambrosini A, D'Alessio C, Magis D, Schoenen J. Targeting pericranial nerve branches to treat migraine: current approaches and perspectives. *Cephalalgia.* 2015;35(14):1308–1322. doi:10.1177/0333102415573511

14. Ambrosini A, Schoenen J. Invasive pericranial nerve interventions. *Cephalalgia.* 2016;36(12):1156–1169. doi:10.1177/0333102416639515

15. Guyuron B, Yohannes E, Miller R, Chim H, Reed D, Chance MR. Electron Microscopic and proteomic comparison of terminal branches of the trigeminal nerve in patients with and without migraine headaches. *Plast Reconstr Surg.* 2014;134(5):796e–805e. doi:10.1097/PRS.0000000000000696

16. Vecchia D, Pietrobon D. Migraine: A disorder of brain excitatory-inhibitory balance? *Trends Neurosci.* 2012;35(8):507–520. doi:10.1016/j.tins.2012.04.007

17. Bove GM. Lending a hand to migraine. *Pain.* 2013;154(9):1493–1494. doi:10.1016/j.pain.2013.05.025

18. Eikermann-Haerter K, Ayata C. Cortical spreading depression and migraine. *Curr Neurol Neurosci Rep.* 2010;10(3):167–173. doi:10.1007/s11910-010-0099-1

19. Waeber C, Moskowitz MA. Migraine as an inflammatory disorder. *Neurology.* 2005;64(10 Suppl 2):S9–S15. http://www.ncbi.nlm.nih.gov/pubmed/15911785

20. Perry CJ, Blake P, Buettner C, et al. Upregulation of inflammatory gene transcripts in periosteum of chronic migraineurs: implications for extracranial origin of headache. *Ann Neurol.* 2016;79(6):1000–1013. doi:10.1002/ana.24665

21. Janis JE, Barker JC, Javadi C, Ducic I, Hagan R, Guyuron B. A review of current evidence in the surgical treatment of migraine headaches. *Plast Reconstr Surg.* 2014;134(4 Suppl 2):131S–141S. doi:10.1097/PRS.0000000000000661

22. Schueler M, Messlinger K, Dux M, Neuhuber WL, De Col R. Extracranial projections of meningeal afferents and their impact on meningeal nociception and headache. *Pain.* 2013;154(9):1622–1631. doi:10.1016/j.pain.2013.04.040

23. Schueler M, Neuhuber WL, De Col R, Messlinger K. Innervation of rat and human dura mater and pericranial tissues in the parieto-temporal region by meningeal afferents. *Headache.* 2014;54(6):996–1009. doi:10.1111/head.12371

24. Kosaras B, Jakubowski M, Kainz V, Burstein R. Sensory innervation of the calvarial bones of the mouse. *J Comp Neurol.* 2009;515(3):331–348. doi:10.1002/cne.22049

25. Welch KM. Contemporary concepts of migraine pathogenesis. *Neurology.* 2003;61(8 Suppl 4):S2–S8. doi:10.1212/WNL.61.8_suppl_4.S2

26. Kung T, Guyuron B, Cederna PS. Migraine surgery: a plastic surgery solution for refractory migraine headache. *Plast Reconstr Surg.* 2011;127(1):181–189. doi:10.1097/PRS.0b013e3181f95a01

27. Kung T, Pannucci CJ, Chamberlain JL, Cederna PS. Migraine surgery practice patterns and attitudes. *Plast Reconstr Surg.* 2012;129(3):623–628. doi:10.1097/PRS.0b013e3182412a24

28. Katz M. The cost-effective evaluation of uncomplicated headache. *Med Clin North Am.* 2016;100(5):1009–1017. doi:10.1016/j.mcna.2016.04.009

29. Guyuron B, Nahabet E, Khansa I, Reed D, Janis JE. The current means for detection of migraine headache trigger sites. *Plast Reconstr Surg.* 2015;136(4):860–867. doi:10.1097/PRS.0000000000001572

30. Seyed Forootan NS, Lee M, Guyuron B. Migraine headache trigger site prevalence analysis of 2590 sites in 1010 patients. *J Plast Reconstr Aesthet Surg.* 2016;70(2):152–158. doi:10.1016/j.bjps.2016.11.004

31. Liu MT, Armijo BS, Guyuron B. A comparison of outcome of surgical treatment of migraine headaches using a constellation of symptoms versus botulinum toxin type A to identify the trigger sites. *Plast Reconstr Surg.* 2012;129(2):413–419. doi:10.1097/PRS.0b013e31823aecb7

32. Kurlander DE, Ascha M, Sattar A, Guyuron B. In-depth review of symptoms, triggers, and surgical deactivation of frontal migraine headaches (Site I). *Plast Reconstr Surg.* 2016;138(3):681–688. doi:10.1097/PRS.0000000000002479

33. Kurlander DE, Punjabi A, Liu MT, Sattar A, Guyuron B. In-depth review of symptoms, triggers, and treatment of temporal migraine headaches (Site II). *Plast Reconstr Surg.* 2014;133(4):897–903. doi:10.1097/PRS.0000000000000045

34. Behin F, Behin B, Bigal ME, Lipton RB. Surgical treatment of patients with refractory migraine headaches and intranasal contact points. *Cephalalgia.* 2005;25(6):439–443. doi:10.1111/j.1468-2982.2004.00877.x

35. Lee M, Erickson C, Guyuron B. Intranasal pathology in the migraine surgery population. *Plast Reconstr Surg.* 2017;139(1):184–189. doi:10.1097/PRS.0000000000002888.

36. Guyuron B, Kriegler JS, Davis J, Amini SB. Comprehensive surgical treatment of migraine headaches. *Plast Reconstr Surg.* 2005;115:1–9. doi:10.1097/01.PRS.0000145631.20901.84

37. Guyuron B, Tucker T, Davis J. Surgical treatment of migraine headaches. *Plast Reconstr Surg.* 2002;109(7):2183–2189. doi:10.1097/00006534-200206000-00001

38. Janis JE, Dhanik A, Howard JH. Validation of the peripheral trigger point theory of migraine headaches: single-surgeon experience using botulinum toxin and surgical decompression. *Plast Reconstr Surg.* 2011;128(1):123–131. doi:10.1097/PRS.0b013e3182173d64

39. Poggi JT, Grizzell BE, Helmer SD. Confirmation of surgical decompression to relieve migraine headaches. *Plast Reconstr Surg.* 2008;122(1):115–224. doi:10.1097/PRS.0b013e31817742da

40. Lee M, Monson M, Liu MT, Reed D, Guyuron B. Positive botulinum toxin type a response is a prognosticator for migraine surgery success. *Plast Reconstr Surg.* 2013;131(4):751–757. doi:10.1097/PRS.0b013e3182818b7f

41. Guyuron B, Riazi H, Long T, Wirtz E. Use of a Doppler signal to confirm migraine headache trigger sites. *Plast Reconstr Surg.* 2015;135(4):1109–1112. doi:10.1097/prs.0000000000001102

42. Janis JE, Hatef D, Ducic I, et al. The anatomy of the greater occipital nerve: part II. Compression point topography. *Plast Reconstr Surg.* 2010;126(5):1563–1572. doi:10.1097/PRS.0b013e3181ef7f0c

43. Janis JE, Hatef D, Ducic I, et al. Anatomy of the auriculotemporal nerve: variations in its relationship to the superficial temporal artery and implications for the treatment of migraine headaches. *Plast Reconstr Surg*. 2010;125(5):1422–1428. doi:10.1097/PRS.0b013e3181d4fb05

44. Lee M, Brown M, Chepla K, et al. An anatomical study of the lesser occipital nerve and its potential compression points: implications for surgical treatment of migraine headaches. *Plast Reconstr Surg*. 2013;132(6):1551–1556. doi:10.1097/PRS.0b013e3182a80721

45. Rose FC. Trigger factors and natural history of migraine. *Funct Neurol*. 1(4):379–384. http://www.ncbi.nlm.nih.gov/pubmed/3301558

46. Kelman L. The triggers or precipitants of the acute migraine attack. *Cephalalgia*. 2007;27(5):394–402. doi:10.1111/j.1468-2982.2007.01303.x

47. Finocchi C, Sivori G. Food as trigger and aggravating factor of migraine. *Neurol Sci*. 2012;33(Suppl 1):9–12. doi:10.1007/s10072-012-1046-5

48. Becker WJ. Acute migraine treatment in adults. *Headache*. 2015;55(6):778–793. doi:10.1111/head.12550

49. Marmura MJ, Silberstein SD, Schwedt TJ. The acute treatment of migraine in adults: the American Headache Society evidence assessment of migraine pharmacotherapies. *Headache*. 2015;55(1):3–20. doi:10.1111/head.12499

50. Whyte CA, Tepper SJ. Adverse effects of medications commonly used in the treatment of migraine. *Expert Rev Neurother*. 2009;9(9):1379–1391. doi:10.1586/ern.09.47

51. Blumenfeld AM, Bloudek LM, Becker WJ, et al. Patterns of use and reasons for discontinuation of prophylactic medications for episodic migraine and chronic migraine: Results from the second international burden of migraine study (IBMS-II). *Headache*. 2013;53(4):644–655. doi:10.1111/head.12055

52. Goadsby PJ, Lipton RB, Ferrari MD. Migraine--current understanding and treatment. *N Engl J Med*. 2002;346(4):257–270. doi:10.1056/NEJMra010917

53. Letter TM. Drugs for migraine. *Med Lett Drugs Ther*. 2017;59(1514):27–32. http://www.ncbi.nlm.nih.gov/pubmed/28170366

54. Prior MJ, Codispoti JR, Fu M. A randomized, placebo-controlled trial of acetaminophen for treatment of migraine headache. *Headache*. 2010;50(5):819–833. doi:10.1111/j.1526-4610.2010.01638.x

55. Suthisisang CC, Poolsup N, Suksomboon N, Lertpipopmetha V, Tepwitukgid B. Meta-analysis of the efficacy and safety of naproxen sodium in the acute treatment of migraine. *Headache*. 2010;50(5):808–818. doi:10.1111/j.1526-4610.2010.01635.x

56. Suthisisang C, Poolsup N, Kittikulsuth W, Pudchakan P, Wiwatpanich P. Efficacy of low-dose ibuprofen in acute migraine treatment: systematic review and meta-analysis. *Ann Pharmacother*. 2007;41(11):1782–1791. doi:10.1345/aph.1K121

57. Colman I, Rothney A, Wright SC, Zilkalns B, Rowe BH. Use of narcotic analgesics in the emergency department treatment of migraine headache. *Neurology*. 2004;62(10):1695–1700. doi:10.1212/01.WNL.0000127304.91605.BA

58. Minen MT, Lindberg K, Wells RE, et al. Survey of opioid and barbiturate prescriptions in patients attending a tertiary care headache center. *Headache*. 2015;55(9):1183–1191. doi:10.1111/head.12645

59. Adenuga P, Brown M, Reed D, Guyuron B. Impact of preoperative narcotic use on outcomes in migraine surgery. *Plast Reconstr Surg*. 2014;134(1):113–119. doi:10.1097/PRS.0000000000000281

60. Silberstein SD, Holland S, Freitag F, et al. Evidence-based guideline update: pharmacologic treatment for episodic migraine prevention in adults: report of the Quality Standards Subcommittee of the American Academy of Neurology and

the American Headache Society. *Neurology*. 2012;78(17):1337–1345. doi:10.1212/WNL.0b013e3182535d20

61. Dahlöf CGH. Infrequent or non-response to oral sumatriptan does not predict response to other triptans—review of four trials. *Cephalalgia*. 2006;26(2):98–106. doi:10.1111/j.1468-2982.2005.01010.x

62. Tfelt-Hansen P, De Vries P, Saxena PR. Triptans in migraine: a comparative review of pharmacology, pharmacokinetics and efficacy. *Drugs*. 2000;60(6):1259–1287. doi:10.2165/00003495-200060060-00003

63. Raskin NH. Repetitive intravenous dihydroergotamine as therapy for intractable migraine. *Neurology*. 1986;36(7):995–997. http://www.ncbi.nlm.nih.gov/pubmed/3520384

64. Kelley NE, Tepper DE. Rescue therapy for acute migraine, part 2: neuroleptics, antihistamines, and others. *Headache*. 2012;52(2):292–306. doi:10.1111/j.1526-4610.2011.02070.x

65. John M. Eisenberg Center for Clinical Decisions and Communications Science. Acute Migraine Treatment in Emergency Settings; 2007. http://www.ncbi.nlm.nih.gov/pubmed/24156113

66. Honkaniemi J, Liimatainen S, Rainesalo S, Sulavuori S. Haloperidol in the acute treatment of migraine: a randomized, double-blind, placebo-controlled study. *Headache*. 2006;46(5):781–787. doi:10.1111/j.1526-4610.2006.00438.x

67. Loder E, Burch R, Rizzoli P. The 2012 AHS/AAN guidelines for prevention of episodic migraine: a summary and comparison with other recent clinical practice guidelines. *Headache J Head Face Pain*. 2012;52(6):930–945. doi:10.1111/j.1526-4610.2012.02185.x

68. Rosen JA. Observations on the efficacy of propranolol for the prophylaxis of migraine. *Ann Neurol*. 1983;13(1):92–93. doi:10.1002/ana.410130119

69. Mulleners WM, McCrory DC, Linde M. Antiepileptics in migraine prophylaxis: an updated Cochrane review. *Cephalalgia*. 2015;35(1):51–62. doi:10.1177/0333102414534325

70. Weston J, Bromley R, Jackson CF, et al. Monotherapy treatment of epilepsy in pregnancy: congenital malformation outcomes in the child. *Cochrane Database Syst Rev*. 2016;11:CD010224. doi:10.1002/14651858.CD010224.pub2

71. Dodick DW, Freitag F, Banks J, et al. Topiramate versus amitriptyline in migraine prevention: a 26-week, multicenter, randomized, double-blind, double-dummy, parallel-group noninferiority trial in adult migraineurs. *Clin Ther*. 2009;31(3):542–559. doi:10.1016/j.clinthera.2009.03.020

72. Bellantuono C, Vargas M, Mandarelli G, Nardi B, Martini MG. The safety of serotonin-noradrenaline reuptake inhibitors (SNRIs) in pregnancy and breastfeeding: a comprehensive review. *Hum Psychopharmacol*. 2015;30(3):143–151. doi:10.1002/hup.2473

73. Banzi R, Cusi C, Randazzo C, Sterzi R, Tedesco D, Moja L. Selective serotonin reuptake inhibitors (SSRIs) and serotonin-norepinephrine reuptake inhibitors (SNRIs) for the prevention of tension-type headache in adults. *Cochrane Database Syst Rev*. 2015;(5):CD011681. doi:10.1002/14651858.CD011681

74. Aurora SK, Dodick DW, Turkel CC, et al. Onabotulinumtoxin: a for treatment of chronic migraine: results from the double-blind, randomized, placebo-controlled phase of the PREEMPT 1 trial. *Cephalalgia*. 2010;30(7):793–803. doi:10.1177/0333102410364676

75. Diener HC, Dodick DW, Aurora SK, et al. Onabotulinumtoxin: a for treatment of chronic migraine: results from the double-blind, randomized, placebo-controlled phase of the PREEMPT 2 trial. *Cephalalgia*. 2010;30(7):804–814. doi:10.1177/0333102410364677

76. Letter TM. Botulinum toxin for chronic migraine. *Med Lett Drugs Ther*. 2011;53(1356):7–8. http://www.ncbi.nlm.nih.gov/pubmed/21252842

77. Solomon GD, Steel JG, Spaccavento LJ. Verapamil prophylaxis of migraine: a double-blind, placebo-controlled study. *JAMA*. 1983;250(18):2500–2502. http://www.ncbi.nlm.nih.gov/pubmed/6355533

78. Markley HG, Cheronis JC, Piepho RW. Verapamil in prophylactic therapy of migraine. *Neurology*. 1984;34(7):973–976. http://www.ncbi.nlm.nih.gov/pubmed/6539877

79. Schrader H, Stovner LJ, Helde G, Sand T, Bovim G. Prophylactic treatment of migraine with angiotensin converting enzyme inhibitor (lisinopril): randomised, placebo controlled, crossover study. *BMJ*. 2001;322:1–5.

80. Tronvik E, Stovner LJ, Helde G, Sand T, Bovim G. Prophylactic treatment of migraine with an angiotensin II receptor blocker: a randomized controlled trial. *JAMA*. 2003;289(1):65–69. http://www.ncbi.nlm.nih.gov/pubmed/12503978

81. Gales BJ, Bailey EK, Reed AN, Gales MA. Angiotensin-converting enzyme inhibitors and angiotensin receptor blockers for the prevention of migraines. *Ann Pharmacother*. 2010;44(2):360–366. doi:10.1345/aph.1M312

82. Ducic I, Felder JM, Fantus S. A systematic review of peripheral nerve interventional treatments for chronic headaches. *Ann Plast Surg*. 2014;72(4):439–445. doi:10.1097/SAP.0000000000000063

83. Gfrerer L, Maman DY, Tessler O, Austen WG. Non-endoscopic deactivation of nerve triggers in migraine headache patients: surgical technique and outcomes. *Plast Reconstr Surg*. 2014:771–778. doi:10.1097/PRS.0000000000000507

84. Janis JE, Hatef DA, Hagan R, et al. Anatomy of the supratrochlear nerve. *Plast Reconstr Surg*. 2013;131(4):743–750. doi:10.1097/PRS.0b013e3182818b0c

85. Fallucco M, Janis JE, Hagan RR. The anatomical morphology of the supraorbital notch: clinical relevance to the surgical treatment of migraine headaches. *Plast Reconstr Surg*. 2012;130(6):1227–1233. doi:10.1097/PRS.0b013e31826d9c8d

86. McKinney PW. Anatomy of the corrugator supercilii muscle: part I. Corrugator topography. *Yearb Plast Aesthetic Surg*. 2009;2009:76. doi:10.1016/S1535-1513(08)79060-X

87. Janis JE, Ghavami A, Lemmon J, Leedy JE, Guyuron B. The anatomy of the corrugator supercilii muscle: part II. Supraorbital nerve branching patterns. *Plast Reconstr Surg*. 2008;121(1):233–240. doi:10.1097/01.prs.0000299260.04932.38

88. Mckee DE, Lalonde DH, Thoma A, Dickson L. Achieving the optimal epinephrine effect in wide awake hand surgery using local anesthesia without a tourniquet. *Hand*. 2015;10(4):613–615. doi:10.1007/s11552-015-9759-6

89. McKee DE, Lalonde DH, Thoma A, Glennie DL, Hayward JE. Optimal time delay between epinephrine injection and incision to minimize bleeding. *Plast Reconstr Surg*. 2013;131(4):811–814. doi:10.1097/PRS.0b013e3182818ced

90. Totonchi A, Pashmini N, Guyuron B. The zygomaticotemporal branch of the trigeminal nerve: an anatomical study. *Plast Reconstr Surg*. 2005;115(1):273–277. doi:10.1016/S1535-1513(08)70457-0

91. Janis JE, Hatef D, Thakar H, et al. The zygomaticotemporal branch of the trigeminal nerve: part II. Anatomical variations. *Plast Reconstr Surg*. 2010;126(2):435–442. doi:10.1097/PRS.0b013e3181e094d7

92. Peled ZM. A novel surgical approach to chronic temporal headaches. *Plast Reconstr Surg*. 2016;137(5):1597–1600. doi:10.1097/PRS.0000000000002051

93. Janis JE, Hatef D, Reece EM, McCluskey PD, Schaub T, Guyuron B. Neurovascular compression of the greater occipital nerve: implications for migraine headaches. *Plast Reconstr Surg*. 2010;126(6):1996–2001. doi:10.1097/PRS.0b013e3181ef8c6b

94. Mosser SW, Guyuron B, Janis JE, Rohrich RJ. The anatomy of the greater occipital nerve: implications for the etiology of migraine headaches. *Plast Reconstr Surg.* 2004;113(2):693–700. doi:10.1097/01.PRS.0000101502.22727.5D

95. Dash KS, Janis JE, Guyuron B. The lesser and third occipital nerves and migraine headaches. *Plast Reconstr Surg.* 2005;115(6):1752–1758. doi:10.1097/01.PRS.0000161679.26890.EE

96. Junewicz A, Katira K, Guyuron B. Intraoperative anatomical variations during greater occipital nerve decompression. *J Plast Reconstr Aesthetic Surg.* 2013;66(10):1340–1345. doi:10.1016/j.bjps.2013.06.016

97. Ducic I, Moriarty M, Al-Attar A. Anatomical variations of the occipital nerves: implications for the treatment of chronic headaches. *Plast Reconstr Surg.* 2009;123(3):859–863; discussion 864. doi:10.1097/PRS.0b013e318199f080

98. Sanniec K, Borsting E. Decompression–avulsion of the auriculotemporal nerve for treatment of migraines and chronic headaches. *Plast Reconstr Surg.* 2016;4(4):e678. doi:10.1097/GOX.0000000000000663

99. Chim H, Okada HC, Brown MS, et al. The auriculotemporal nerve in etiology of migraine headaches: compression points and anatomical variations. *Plast Reconstr Surg.* 2012;130(2):336–341. doi:10.1097/PRS.0b013e3182589dd5

100. Peled ZM, Pietramaggiori G, Scherer S. Anatomic and compression topography of the lesser occipital nerve. *Plast Reconstr Surg—Glob Open.* 2016;4(3):e639. doi:10.1097/GOX.0000000000000654

101. Punjabi A, Brown M, Guyuron B. Emergence of secondary trigger sites after primary migraine surgery. *Plast Reconstr Surg.* 2016;137(4):712e–716e. doi:10.1097/PRS.0000000000002011

102. Guyuron B, Reed D, Kriegler JS, Davis J, Pashmini N, Amini S. A placebo-controlled surgical trial of the treatment of migraine headaches. *Plast Reconstr Surg.* 2009;124(2):461–468. doi:10.1097/PRS.0b013e3181adcf6a

103. Dirnberger F, Becker K. Surgical treatment of migraine headaches by corrugator muscle resection. *Plast Reconstr Surg.* 2004;114(3):652–657. doi:10.1097/01.PRS.0000131906.27281.17

104. Guyuron B, Varghai A, Michelow BJ, Thomas T, Davis J. Corrugator supercilii muscle resection and migraine headaches. *Plast Reconstr Surg.* 2000;106(2):435–437. doi:10.1097/00006534-200008000-00030

105. Larson K, Lee M, Davis J, Guyuron B. Factors contributing to migraine headache surgery failure and success. *Plast Reconstr Surg.* 2011;128(5):1069–1075. doi:10.1097/PRS.0b013e31822b61a1

106. Lee M, Lineberry K, Reed D, Guyuron B. The role of the third occipital nerve in surgical treatment of occipital migraine headaches. *J Plast Reconstr Aesthetic Surg.* 2013;66(10):1335–1339. doi:10.1016/j.bjps.2013.05.023

107. Chmielewski L, Liu MT, Guyuron B. The role of occipital artery resection in the surgical treatment of occipital migraine headaches. *Plast Reconstr Surg.* 2013;131(3):351e–356e. doi:10.1097/PRS.0b013e31827c6f71

108. Hagan RR, Fallucco MA, Janis JE. Supraorbital rim syndrome. *Plast Reconstr Surg—Glob Open.* 2016;4(7):e795. doi:10.1097/GOX.0000000000000802

22 New Vistas in Perioperative Pain Management

Timothy Furnish and Engy Said

INTRODUCTION

Opioids remain the gold standard for treatment of acute postoperative pain despite the significant adverse effects related to tolerance, respiratory depression, sedation, gastrointestinal dysmotility, and dependence. The search for alternative analgesic agents has had very limited successes for either acute or chronic pain. Development of truly novel analgesic compounds has been met with significant failures, and much of the recent innovation in the area of perioperative analgesia has been the expansion and systemization of multimodal analgesic regimens and reformulation of older compounds into new delivery mechanisms with a handful of potentially exciting new compounds on the horizon.

A significant area of promise has been the perioperative use of gabapentinoids and the increasing use of multimodal analgesic regimens.[1-4] An emerging field of research and discussion in both in the fields of anesthesiology and surgery has been the concept of enhanced recovery after surgery (ERAS) programs. The idea of ERAS is to use protocols and care pathways, including multimodal analgesic regimens, to improve outcomes and reduce costs. The growth in use of expert-led acute pain services can aid in meeting the goals of an ERAS program.

The outlook for new perioperative analgesic options involves multiple pathways. New analgesic drugs coming to market or recently introduced have primarily been reformulations of existing drugs to be delivered via novel routes or in sustained-release or abuse-deterrent forms. A handful of drugs not commonly used for postoperative systemic analgesia have been studied for this purpose. Truly novel compounds are in development that may provide an improvement over currently available opioids with a promise of opioid-quality analgesia with fewer opioid-related adverse effects.

ENHANCED RECOVERY AFTER SURGERY

ERAS is a perioperative care pathway with standardized protocols designed to reduce surgical stress, improve patient outcomes, and reduce costs. Dr. Henrik Kehlet, a colorectal surgeon from Copenhagen University Hospital in Denmark, first described the concept of ERAS in 1990. He proposed a system of multimodal interventions that could lead to a reduction of surgical stress and thus accelerate recovery and reduce postoperative morbidity and overall costs.[5] This approach has proven to be successful in achieving those goals in colorectal surgery.[6-9] It has since expanded to include many other procedures, including orthopedics, gynecology, and urology.

The ERAS pathway can be divided into three broad components (Figure 22.1):

1. *Preoperative phase*: This phase starts in the preoperative care clinic and has a focus on the preparation of patients and their families in managing expectations. Detailed information about surgical and anesthetic procedures, especially postoperative pain management, is provided in order to reduce day-of-surgery anxiety. Evidence-based instructions on limiting fasting prior to surgery that allows free intake of clear fluids up to two hours before anesthesia are emphasized. Likewise, routine bowel preparation is avoided as both factors together have been linked to decreased patient thirst and overall improved well-being.[10] Similarly, patients with a high risk of morbidity such as smokers and those abusing alcohol are guided to rehabilitation resources as deemed appropriate. The patient is also provided with details regarding antimicrobial and thromboembolism prophylaxes, as well as skin preparation.

2. *Intraoperative phase*: Once the patient arrives in the preoperative area on the day of surgery, he or she is counseled regarding a preemptive multimodal analgesia plan, which includes a combination of non-opioid analgesics and regional anesthesia nerve blocks. After major abdominal surgeries, return of bowel function is an important milestone in postoperative recovery. Optimization of intraoperative fluid management and the minimization of

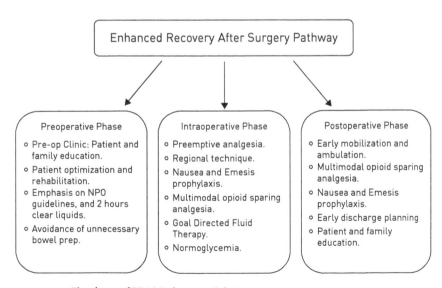

FIGURE 22.1. The phases of ERAS Pathways and their components.

intravenous (IV) opioids are two important intraoperative factors that may facilitate the return of bowel function.[11]

3. *Postoperative phase*: During the recovery phase, the focus is on continued minimization of opioid consumption, early ambulation, early oral nutrition, and safe discharge planning.

Enhanced Recovery: The Role of Multimodal Pain Management and an Acute Pain Service

One of the most significant limiting factors for early recovery after major abdominal surgery is the return of bowel function.[12] Postoperative ileus can be secondary to many causes including gastrointestinal autonomic nervous system dysfunction, inflammatory response, hormone disruption, as well as anesthetic and opioid administration.[13] Minimizing both the stress response as well as opioid consumption not only has the benefit of patient comfort but also the reduction of ileus. One commonly implemented strategy in an ERAS pathway is multimodal analgesia, which often includes the use of regional anesthesia techniques.

Opioids continue to be the mainstay of postoperative pain control but require careful monitoring and management of side effects, which include nausea, vomiting, somnolence, respiratory depression, and ileus. For this reason, many hospitals have introduced a multidisciplinary APS, which has been associated with decreases in pain intensity levels, improved patient satisfaction, and fewer adverse events.[14] The cornerstone of postoperative pain control with an APS is an evidence-based, multimodal approach to pain management that optimizes patient education while providing consistency and continuity of care. The multimodal technique highlights the effectiveness of individual agents in optimal dosages in order to maximize efficacy while minimizing opioids and their associated side effects. APS focuses on implementing multimodal therapy in the form of preemptive analgesia as well as preventive analgesia. This includes preoperative administration of non-opioid analgesics, including acetaminophen, nonsteroidal anti-inflammatory drugs (NSAIDs), anticonvulsants, and antiemetics. In contrast, preventive analgesia involves regional or neuraxial technique to help block central sensitization by blocking neural transmission of noxious stimuli.[15]

Thoracic epidural analgesia (TEA) plays an important role for patients undergoing open abdominal procedures. It is well recognized as a superior analgesic choice to IV opioids in patients undergoing major open abdominal surgery.[16] Likewise, several systematic reviews have documented that TEA reduces postoperative ileus duration after major abdominal surgery by an average of 36 hours.[11,17] The mechanism by which TEA may shorten the duration of ileus may include a decrease in sympathetic tone, stress response, and inflammatory processes. Despite these benefits, TEA has not been shown to decrease hospital length of stay.[11]

Transversus abdominis plane (TAP) block is gaining momentum as part of a multimodal approach to enhanced recovery in patients undergoing minimally invasive abdominal surgery and for those who are not TEA candidates. TAP blocks have the advantage of being a relatively safe and simple procedure, and studies have shown reduced postoperative morphine consumption as well as decreased nausea and vomiting.[18]

Enhanced Recovery: Goal-Directed Fluid Therapy and Length of Stay

Two other major goals of ERAS that go hand in hand with improving analgesia and reducing opioid requirements are the reduction of excess fluid administration and total hospital length of stay (LOS). Avoiding unnecessary fluid administration is a vital part of a ERAS pathway, as only 20% of IV crystalloids remain in circulation after one hour of administration.[19] Excess fluid contributes to bowel wall edema and prolonged ileus.[16] In a study by Brandstrup et al., the frequency of postoperative complications increased with increased fluid administration.[20] A primary goal of ERAS pathways is to reduce hospital LOS and associated health care costs. Investigators from the Department of Anesthesiology at Duke University have demonstrated that implementation of an ERAS protocol in patients undergoing colorectal surgery leads to decreased hospital LOS.[21] This reduction in LOS is comparable to other studies from diverse centers around the world.[9,22,23]

Enhanced Recovery: Conclusion

While some institutions have successfully started implementing ERAS pathways, there is still substantial need for further research to identify crucial interventions as well as dispensable ones. Likewise, a dedicated team such as APS can help fine-tune recommendations as well as guide research endeavors to enhance patients' recovery experience. The implementation of ERAS into a health care practice can be challenging, as it requires the commitment of multiple different teams in perioperative medicine. Barriers to its adoption include lack of time and personnel to spearhead the protocol, limited hospital resources, provider attitudes, and organizational and management logistics. However, when patients receive effective postoperative analgesia and optimal fluid therapy with the guidance of an ERAS pathway, postoperative morbidity can be reduced, recovery enhanced, hospital stay shortened, and patient satisfaction improved.

NEW FORMULATIONS OF OLD DRUGS

Much of what passes as innovation in the area of analgesics for either acute or chronic pain has involved the repurposing or reformulation of older drugs. A significant portion of this work has involved the creation of sustained-release formulations, transdermal delivery mechanisms, or transmucosal delivery of various opioids. The target market of most of these agents has been either cancer pain or chronic noncancer pain. A smaller segment of this trend has been analgesics reformulated for acute pain. The US introduction of an IV formulation of acetaminophen was a major player in this segment, but several other products have been approved or are being considered for such approval.

Intravenous NSAIDS

The category of IV NSAIDs with Food and Drug Administration (FDA) approval has grown in recent years. Ketorolac was approved in 1989 and remained the only IV

NSAID available in the United States for 20 years until an IV formulation of ibuprofen (Caldolor™) was introduced. More recently (December 2014) an IV formulation of diclofenac (Dyloject™) was introduced. NSAIDs have been highlighted in multiple guidelines for multimodal analgesia, but their use continues to be limited by concerns over perioperative bleeding and renal toxicity. One disadvantage to ketorolac is the limitation on duration of use to five days. The newer IV agents do not have this limit on duration of therapy. In a double-blind, placebo-controlled comparison in third molar extraction surgery, IV diclofenac had faster onset analgesia than ketorolac with similar duration of action but without superior analgesia.[24] There are no head-to-head studies comparing IV ibuprofen with ketorolac. Unlike the IV formulations of ketorolac and diclofenac, the IV formulation of ibuprofen cannot be administered as a low-volume bolus, only via infusion.[25,26]

Intravenous Tramadol

Tramadol is a synthetic, centrally acting analgesic with two different mechanisms of action. It acts as a weak agonist at the mu-opioid receptor as well as an inhibitor of norepinephrine and serotonin reuptake. It was FDA approved in an oral formulation in 1995 and has been used for both acute and chronic pain. It is available outside of the United States in an IV formulation which has been used in numerous studies of acute postsurgical pain.[27] In randomized, double-blind, comparative studies in cardiac surgery tramadol had equivalent efficacy to IV morphine or alfentanil for moderate to severe postoperative pain. Studies have also found tramadol equivalent to morphine when used in patient controlled analgesia (PCA) after multiple surgery types (laparoscopy, orthopedic, abdominal).[27]

Tramadol lowers the seizure threshold and carries a risk of seizures, especially in patients with a history of seizure disorder. Additionally, there is a risk of serotonin syndrome, especially when used in combination with other serotonergic drugs.[28] At doses equianalgesic to morphine, tramadol is less likely to depress respiratory rate or increase end-tidal carbon dioxide levels.[27] IV tramadol 50 mg to 150 mg is equianalgesic to morphine 5 mg to 15 mg in the treatment of moderate postoperative pain with a peak analgesic effect at one to two hours and a duration of five to six hours. The most common adverse events with IV tramadol are nausea and vomiting with similar rates compared with other IV opioids.[27,28] FDA approval for an IV formulation of tramadol is being pursued by Avenue Therapeutics.[29]

Oxycodone/Acetaminophen Sustained Release

Oral oxycodone and acetaminophen have been used separately and in combination products such as Percocet for acute postsurgical pain. A recently approved product combines both drugs into a single pill with both an immediate release component and a sustained-release component intended for twice-daily dosing.[30] The drug, Xartemis™, is FDA approved for the treatment of acute pain and was studied in a bunionectomy model. There are a number of studies using controlled-release oxycodone and immediate-release acetaminophen as part of a multimodal analgesic regimen. The potential benefit of a fixed-dose combination product would be a reduction in pill burden. However, the usual acetaminophen doses recommended for postoperative pain are generally higher than the 325 mg per dose provided in Xartemis™.[31]

Sublingual Sufentanil PCA

Sufentanil is a lipophilic, synthetic opioid, which is approximately 10 times as potent as fentanyl. It has mostly been used as an intraoperative short-acting opioid or for intrathecal injection. Due to its lipophilic nature, it is well absorbed across mucosal membranes and is being developed as a transmucosal PCA system for postoperative pain (Zalvizo; AcelRx Pharmaceuticals, Redwood City, CA).[32] The system does not require an IV catheter, and equilibration of sufentanil with the central nervous system is much faster than with morphine without active metabolites. In a noninferiority study, compared with morphine PCA 1 mg the sufentanil transmucosal PCA with a 15 mcg dose had superior analgesic efficacy with similar adverse effects between the two groups.[32] Additionally, the sufentanil group had faster onset of analgesic efficacy. The system is designed to minimize complexity with only one dose and lockout interval, thus reducing the risk of overdose due to programming errors. However, this limits its usefulness for opioid-tolerant patients who may need a higher dose PCA.

Transcutaneous Fentanyl PCA

The potent and lipophilic opioid fentanyl has been used for years as an intraoperative analgesic as well as in epidural and spinal analgesia. It can be used in standard IV PCAs in place of morphine or hydromorphone. A needle-free, transdermal PCA system that delivers fentanyl was approved by the FDA in April 2015. This inotophoretic transdermal system (IONSYS, The Medicines Company, Parsippany, NJ) uses a low-dose electric current to deliver a 40 mcg dose of fentanyl transdermally. The system requires no IV catheter. The device has an adhesive backing and is placed on the upper thorax or arm. Each dose is delivered over 10 minutes and it can deliver up to six doses each hour. The device is preprogrammed with no ability to change the dose or lockout parameters and is intended for hospital use only.[33]

In a multicenter study of the transdermal fentanyl PCA system versus IV PCA morphine, the transdermal fentanyl system was found to provide equivalent analgesic efficacy. The incidence of adverse events between groups was comparable. Patients rated the fentanyl transdermal system easier to use than the IV PCA morphine.[34] The lack of programming options to adjust dose or lockout may reduce the risk of overdose due to programming error but provides no flexibility for managing opioid-tolerant patients. One additional advantage may be improved mobility with ambulation and physical therapy since no external pump and tubing are required.

Liposomal Bupivacaine

The long-acting local anesthetic bupivacaine is commonly used in nerve blocks, epidural and spinal anesthetics, and for surgical incision infiltration. The clinical duration of bupivacaine in infiltration is four to six hours. An extended-duration formulation of bupivacaine (Exparel®, Pacira Pharmaceuticals) was FDA approved for surgical incision infiltration in 2011. In addition liposomal bupivacaine is approved to perfrom nerve blocks for shoulder surgery. In this product, bupivacaine is encapsulated in multilaminar liposomes to provide a sustained-release formulation. It was studied in a hemorrhoidectomy model where it provided significantly better analgesia than placebo for up to 72 hours.[35] In a phase 3 study with a bunionectomy model, liposomal bupivacaine provided significantly improved analgesia for up to 36 hours.[36] Both studies and others have found a morphine-sparing effect.[35-37] Some other studies have found no statistical effect on pain scores but still showed a significant reduction in morphine-equivalent consumption.[37] The rate of systemic absorption of bupivacaine, as with infiltration with any local anesthetic, will vary depending on the total dose of drug administered and the vascularity of the administration site. In a study total knee arthroscopy involving doses of up to 532 mg of liposomal bupivacaine, no significant cardiac events or electrocardiography changes were noted.[38]

NEW USES OF OLDER DRUGS

The extensive use of gabapentinoids as adjuvants for perioperative pain management is one example of the repurposing of an older agent for acute pain. The local anesthetic lidocaine has been investigated in recent years for use as an IV analgesic for postoperative pain. Medical marijuana has been legalized on the state level in nearly half of the United States and has received significant attention for the treatment of chronic and cancer pain. There is a limited amount of data regarding its use for postoperative pain.

Intravenous Lidocaine

Lidocaine has been used for years for infiltration local analgesia or nerve blocks. There have been a number of studies in the past few years evaluating the analgesic benefit of IV infusions of lidocaine performed during surgery. In meta-analyses and systematic reviews of intraoperative lidocaine infusions, the effect of IV lidocaine was shown to be superior to placebo for reducing pain and opioid consumption in the immediate postoperative period. The effect duration was somewhat limited and generally disappeared after 24 hours. The majority of positive IV lidocaine studies have involved either open or laparoscopic abdominal surgery. Those studies of nonabdominal surgery have generally failed to show a significant effect of lidocaine infusions.[39-41] In abdominal surgeries return of bowel function and hospital LOS was significantly shorter in the lidocaine group.[41] Unfortunately no studies have yet compared IV lidocaine infusions to thoracic epidurals. As a result, the use of IV lidocaine will likely remain a backup solution for patients undergoing major abdominal surgery who cannot receive an epidural.

Cannabinoids

Cannabinoids in various forms have been evaluated for the treatment of chronic pain, spasticity, neuropathic pain, and cancer pain. There have been only a handful of studies looking at cannabinoids for the treatment of acute pain. In a multicenter dose escalation study a cannabis-based extract showed significant reduction in pain at rest and reduction in rescue analgesia at higher doses. The extract included both delta-9-tetrahydrocannabinol (THC) and cannabidiol in a ratio of 1:0.5. The doses administered were 5, 10, and 15 mg of THC. Adverse effects were higher in at the 15 mg dose.[42] There are no cannabis-based extracts commercially available as a pharmaceutical in the United States. There are two synthetic cannabinoid pharmaceuticals with FDA approval for AIDS related wasting and chemotherapy induced nausea, dronabinol and nabilone. In a study of two different doses of nabilone (a THC analog) compared to placebo for postoperative pain there was no difference in opioid use. The higher dose nabilone group had significantly higher pain scores than either the low-dose or placebo group.[43] In a study of 5 mg of pure THC versus placebo for postoperative pain after abdominal hysterectomy, no analgesic benefit was found.[44] Given the limited number of studies and mixed efficacy, there needs to be more research before cannabinoids can be recommended as an acute pain analgesic option.

NEW DRUGS

Olicerinide μ-G-Protein Pathway Selective Modulator

Opioids such as morphine mediate both their analgesic and adverse effects via the μ-opioid receptors. There has been a desire for years to develop analgesics that have all the antinociceptive benefits of opioids without the respiratory depression, sedation, tolerance, and dependence issues associated with opioid agonists. Opioid receptors are categorized as g-protein coupled receptors (GPCRs). There are four known opioid receptor types, μ-opioid (MOR), δ-opioid, κ-opioid, and nociceptin opioid peptide receptors. Opioid ligands bind to μ-opioid receptors and nonselectively activate signaling pathways resulting in antinociception but also opioid-related adverse effects.[45,46]

In addition to the g-protein coupled activation, opioids also result in β-arrestin recruitment via the MOR. Studies of β-arrestin knockout mice have shown a reduction in tolerance, respiratory depression, and constipation with enhancement of analgesia.[47] The ability of a molecule to activate the GPCR without recruiting β-arrestin has been referred to as "biased agonism," "functional selectivity," or G-protein pathway selective (μ-GPS) modulation.[45,46] One such molecule in development is TRV-130, also known as olicerinide (Trevena Inc.). The effect of β-arrestin recruitment at the MOR not only results in respiratory depression and decreased gastrointestinal motility but also inhibits the GPCR activity, thus resulting in reduction of antinociception (see Figure 22.2). In a healthy volunteer study, TRV-130 resulted in higher peak analgesic efficacy, faster onset, and similar duration of action with less reduction in respiratory drive and nausea.[48] In a double-blind, placebo and active comparator, phase 2 clinical trial of patients undergoing bunionectomy, the analgesic efficacy of TRV-130 was comparable to morphine. This same trial found both TRV-130 and morphine had significantly more nausea than placebo.[49] In a phase 2b study comparing TRV-130 to morphine and placebo in PCA administration, TRV-130 had a similar analgesic effect to morphine but with significantly less nausea and respiratory depression.[50] Should olicerinide ultimately prove as effective as morphine with fewer opioid-related adverse effects, this μ-GPS opioid analgesic would be a major advance in perioperative pain management.

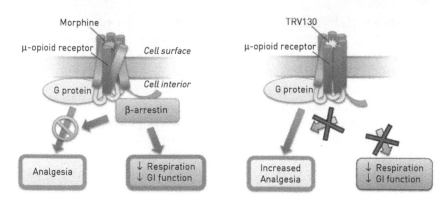

FIGURE 22.2. The G-protein selective pathway of mu-opioid agonists such as TRV130 lacks beta-arrestin activation and results in greater analgesia with decreased respiratory depression and reduced gastrointestinal dysmotility.

NKTR-181

The compound NKTR-181 (Nektar Therapeutics) is another promising opioid analgesic under development, which could play a role in acute pain management. A small but significant portion of opioid-naïve patients who undergo surgery will become long-term opioid users.[51,52] The addiction to prescription opioids has become a major public health problem in the United States.[53] This full agonist opioid compound has a polyethylene glycol polymer attached that modulates the rate of entry across the blood brain barrier (BBB). One measure of BBB penetration is the onset of miosis after administration of an opioid. Compared to oxycodone, which exhibits the onset of miosis 11 minutes after administration, NKTR-181 exhibited a delay in miosis onset of 2.8 hours. In abuse liability studies it has been indistinguishable from placebo in producing feelings of euphoria.[54] The slowed penetration of the BBB is thought to reduce euphoria and drug liking. The drug is being developed with the chronic pain market in mind. However, should it prove effective, with significantly lower abuse potential, it may have a role in postoperative pain for patients requiring opioids upon discharge home from the hospital.

CONCLUSION

While truly new analgesic drugs remain scarce, the development of novel opioid compounds with improved side effect profiles, whether μ-G-protein selective modulators or agents with slower BBB permeability, is a bright spot in the acute pain landscape with significant promise for improvement over standard opioid analgesics. Several more traditional analgesics with improvements in delivery mechanism or formulation are a welcome addition to the perioperative pain management armamentarium. Even more promising may be the systematic employment of multimodal analgesic regimens via ERAS protocols and pathways. These programs aim to maximize the use of non-opioid analgesics from the preoperative through the intraoperative phase and then transition postoperative pain management from early postoperative care to discharge. The cost-effective use of a thoughtful polypharmacy along with interventional and nonpharmacologic methods may be the future of perioperative pain care.

REFERENCES

1. American Society of Anesthesiologists Task Force on Acute Pain Management. Practice guidelines for acute pain management in the perioperative setting: an updated report by the American Society of Anesthesiologists Task Force on Acute Pain Management. *Anesthesiology.* 2012;116(2):248–273.

2. Chou R, Gordon DB, de Leon-Casasola OA, et al. Management of postoperative pain: a clinical practice guideline from the American Pain Society, the American Society of Regional Anesthesia and Pain Medicine, and the American Society of Anesthesiologists' Committee on Regional Anesthesia, Executive Committee, and Administrative Council. *J Pain.* 2016;17(2):131–157.

3. Mishriky BM, Waldron NH, Habib AS. Impact of pregabalin on acute and persistent postoperative pain: a systematic review and meta-analysis. *Br J Anaesth.* 2014;114(1):10–31.

4. Schmidt PC, Ruchelli G, Mackey SC, Carroll IR. Perioperative gabapentinoids: choice of agent, dose, timing, and effects on chronic postsurgical pain. *Anesthesiology.* 2013;119(5):1215–1221.

5. Kehlet H. Multimodal approach to control postoperative pathophysiology and rehabilitation. *Br J Anaesth.* 1997;78(5):606–617.

6. Basse L, Hjort Jakobsen D, Billesbølle P, Werner M, Kehlet H. A clinical pathway to accelerate recovery after colonic resection. *Ann Surg.* 2000;232(1):51–57.

7. Basse L, Raskov HH, Hjort Jakobsen D, et al. Accelerated postoperative recovery programme after colonic resection improves physical performance, pulmonary function and body composition. *Br J Surg.* 2002;89(4):446–453.

8. Wind J, et al. Perioperative strategy in colonic surgery: LAparoscopy and/or FAst track multimodal management versus standard care (LAFA trial). *BMC Surg.* 2006;6:16.

9. Khoo CK, Vickery CJ, Forsyth N, Vinall NS, Eyre-Brook IA. A prospective randomized controlled trial of multimodal perioperative management protocol in patients undergoing elective colorectal resection for cancer. *Ann Surg.* 2007;245(6):867–872.

10. Ljungqvist O, Søreide E. Preoperative fasting. *Br J Surg.* 2003;90(4):400–406.

11. Marret E, Remy C, Bonnet F, Postoperative Pain Forum Group. Meta-analysis of epidural analgesia versus parenteral opioid analgesia after colorectal surgery. *Br J Surg.* 2007;94(6):665–673.

12. Taguchi A, Sharma N, Saleem RM, et al. Selective postoperative inhibition of gastrointestinal opioid receptors. *N Engl J Med.* 2001;345(13):935–940.

13. Carroll J, Alavi K. Pathogenesis and management of postoperative ileus. *Clin Colon Rectal Surg.* 2009;22(1):47–50.

14. Werner MU, Søholm L, Rotbøll-Nielsen P, Kehlet H. Does an acute pain service improve postoperative outcome? *Anesth Analg.* 2002;95(5):1361–1372.

15. Kuusniemi K, Pöyhiä R. Present-day challenges and future solutions in postoperative pain management: results from PainForum 2014. *J Pain Res.* 2016;9:25–36.

16. Werawatganon T, Charuluxanun S. Patient controlled intravenous opioid analgesia versus continuous epidural analgesia for pain after intra-abdominal surgery. *Cochrane Database Syst Rev.* 2005;1:CD004088.

17. Jørgensen H, Wetterslev J, Møiniche S, Dahl JB. Epidural local anaesthetics versus opioid-based analgesic regimens on postoperative gastrointestinal paralysis, PONV and pain after abdominal surgery. *Cochrane Database Syst Rev.* 2000;4:CD001893.

18. Johns N, O'Neill S, Ventham NT, Barron F, Brady RR, Daniel T. Clinical effectiveness of transversus abdominis plane (TAP) block in abdominal surgery: a systematic review and meta-analysis. *Colorectal Dis Off J Assoc Coloproctol G B Irel.* 2012;14(10):e635–642.

19. Awad S, Dharmavaram S, Wearn CS, Dube MG, Lobo DN. Effects of an intraoperative infusion of 4% succinylated gelatine (Gelofusine®) and 6% hydroxyethyl starch (Voluven®) on blood volume. *Br J Anaesth.* 2012;109(2):168–176.

20. Brandstrup B, Tønnesen H, Beier-Holgersen R, et al. Effects of intravenous fluid restriction on postoperative complications: comparison of two perioperative fluid regimens: a randomized assessor-blinded multicenter trial. *Ann Surg.* 2003;238(5):641–648.

21. Miller TE, Thacker JK, White WD, et al. Reduced length of hospital stay in colorectal surgery after implementation of an enhanced recovery protocol. *Anesth Analg.* 2014;118(5):1052–1061.

22. Muller S, Zalunardo MP, Hubner M, Clavien PA, Demartines N, Zurich Fast Track Study Group. A fast-track program reduces complications and length of hospital stay after open colonic surgery. *Gastroenterology.* 2009;136(3):842–847.

23. Serclova Z, Dytrych P, Marvan J, et al. Fast-track in open intestinal surgery: prospective randomized study. *Clin Nutr.* 2009;28(6):618–624.

24. Christensen K, Daniels S, Bandy D, et al. A double-blind placebo-controlled comparison of a novel formulation of intravenous diclofenac and ketorolac for postoperative third molar extraction pain. *Anesth Prog.* 2011;58(2):73–81.

25. Bookstaver PB, Miller AD, Rudisill CN, Norris LB. Intravenous ibuprofen: the first injectable product for the treatment of pain and fever. *J Pain Res.* 2010;3:67–79.

26. Caldolor—intravenous ibuprofen package insert. Cumberland Pharmaceuticals, Apr 2016.

27. Scott LJ, Perry CM. Tramadol: a review of its use in perioperative pain. *Drugs.* 2000;60(1):139–176.

28. Beakley BD, Kaye AM, Kaye AD. Tramadol, pharmacology, side effects, and serotonin syndrome: a review. *Pain Physician.* 2015;18(4):395–400.

29. F. B. Inc. Coronado Biosciences in-licenses IV tramadol, a Phase III ready asset, from Revogenex Ireland Ltd. GlobeNewswire News Room, Feb 18, 2015. http://globenewswire.com/news-release/2015/02/18/707466/10120747/en/Coronado-Biosciences-In-Licenses-IV-Tramadol-a-Phase-III-Ready-Asset-From-Revogenex-Ireland-Ltd.html

30. Bekhit MH. Profile of extended-release oxycodone/acetaminophen for acute pain. *J Pain Res.* 2015;8:719–728.

31. McQuay HJ, Moore RA. Dose–response in direct comparisons of different doses of aspirin, ibuprofen and paracetamol (acetaminophen) in analgesic studies. *Br J Clin Pharmacol.* 2007;63(3):271–278.

32. Melson TI, Boyer DL, Minkowitz HS, et al. Sufentanil sublingual tablet system vs. intravenous patient-controlled analgesia with morphine for postoperative pain control: a randomized, active-comparator trial. *Pain Pract.* 2014;14(8):679–688.

33. Phipps JB, Joshi N, Regal KA, Li J, Sinatra RS. Pharmacokinetic characteristics of fentanyl iontophoretic transdermal system over a range of applied current. *Expert Opin Drug Metab Toxicol.* 2015;11(4):481–489.

34. Power I. Fentanyl HCl iontophoretic transdermal system (ITS): clinical application of iontophoretic technology in the management of acute postoperative pain. *Br J Anaesth.* 2007;98(1):4–11.

35. Gorfine SR, Onel E, Patou G, Krivokapic ZV. Bupivacaine extended-release liposome injection for prolonged postsurgical analgesia in patients undergoing

hemorrhoidectomy: a multicenter, randomized, double-blind, placebo-controlled trial. *Dis Colon Rectum*. 2011;54(12):1552–1559.

36. Golf M, Daniels SE, Onel E. A phase 3, randomized, placebo-controlled trial of DepoFoam® bupivacaine (extended-release bupivacaine local analgesic) in bunionectomy. *Adv Ther*. 2011;28(9):776–788.

37. Tong YCI, Kaye AD, Urman RD. Liposomal bupivacaine and clinical outcomes. *Best Pract Res Clin Anaesthesiol*. 2014;28(1):15–27.

38. Bramlett K, Onel E, Viscusi ER, Jones K. A randomized, double-blind, dose-ranging study comparing wound infiltration of DepoFoam bupivacaine, an extended-release liposomal bupivacaine, to bupivacaine HCl for postsurgical analgesia in total knee arthroplasty. *Knee*. 2012;19(5):530–536.

39. Vigneault L, Turgeon AF, Coˆté D, et al. Perioperative intravenous lidocaine infusion for postoperative pain control: a meta-analysis of randomized controlled trials. *Can J Anaesth*. 2011;58(1):22–37.

40. Weibel S, Jokinen J, Pace NL, et al. Efficacy and safety of intravenous lidocaine for postoperative analgesia and recovery after surgery: a systematic review with trial sequential analysis. *Br J Anaesth*. 2016;116(6):770–783.

41. McCarthy GC, Megalla SA, Habib AS. Impact of intravenous lidocaine infusion on postoperative analgesia and recovery from surgery: a systematic review of randomized controlled trials. *Drugs*. 2010;70(9):1149–1163.

42. Holdcroft A, Maze M, Dore C, Tebbs S, Thompson S. A multicenter dose-escalation study of the analgesic and adverse effects of an oral cannabis extract (Cannador) for postoperative pain management. *Anesthesiology*. 2006;104:1040–1046.

43. Beaulieu P. Effects of nabilone, a synthetic cannabinoid, on postoperative pain. *Can J Anaesth*. 2006;53(8):769–775.

44. Buggy DJ, Toogood L, Maric S, Sharpe P, Lambert DG, Rowbotham DJ. Lack of analgesic efficacy of oral delta-9-tetrahydrocannabinol in postoperative pain. *Pain*. 2003;106(1–2):169–172.

45. Burford NT, Traynor JR, Alt A. Positive allosteric modulators of the μ-opioid receptor: a novel approach for future pain medications. *Br J Pharmacol*. 2015;172(2):277–286.

46. Schneider S, Provasi D, Filizola M. How oliceridine (TRV-130) binds and stabilizes a μ-opioid receptor conformational state that selectively triggers g protein signaling pathways. *Biochemistry*. 2016;55(46):6456–6466.

47. Raehal KM, Walker JKL, Bohn LM. Morphine side effects in beta-arrestin 2 knockout mice. *J Pharmacol Exp Ther*. 2005;314(3):1195–1201.

48. Soergel DG, Subach RA, Burnham N, et al. Biased agonism of the μ-opioid receptor by TRV130 increases analgesia and reduces on-target adverse effects versus morphine: a randomized, double-blind, placebo-controlled, crossover study in healthy volunteers. *Pain*. 2014;155(9):1829–1835.

49. Viscusi ER, Webster L, Kuss M, et al. A randomized, phase 2 study investigating TRV130, a biased ligand of the μ-opioid receptor, for the intravenous treatment of acute pain. *Pain*. 2016 Jan;157(1): 264–272.

50. Minkowitz H, Skobieranda F, Soergel D, Burt D, Singla N. Oliceridine (TRV130), a novel μ receptor G protein pathway selective (μ-GPS) modulator, has enhanced titratability compared to morphine: analysis of PCA use in phase 2b. Presented at the 41st Annual ASRA Regional Anesthesiology and Acute Pain Medicine Meeting, New Orleans, LA, Apr 2016.

51. Alam A, Gomes T, Zheng H, Mamdani MM, Juurlink DN, Bell CM. Long-term analgesic use after low-risk surgery: a retrospective cohort study. *Arch Intern Med*. 2012;172(5):425–430.

52. Clarke H, Soneji N, Ko DT, Yun L, Wijeysundera DN. Rates and risk factors for prolonged opioid use after major surgery: population based cohort study. *BMJ.* 2014;348:1251.

53. Brady KT, McCauley JL, Back SE. Prescription opioid misuse, abuse, and treatment in the United States: an update. *Am J Psychiatry.* 2015;173(1):18–26.

54. Webster L, Smith S, Silowsky J, et al. Abuse potential assessment of novel opioid analgesic NKTR-181: Implications for labeling and scheduling. Presented at the College on Problems of Drug Dependence annual meeting, San Diego, CA, 2013.

Index

Page numbers followed by *f* and *t* refer to figures and tables, respectively.